Melanoma: From Molecular Pathology to Therapeutic Approaches

Melanoma: From Molecular Pathology to Therapeutic Approaches

Guest Editor

Michael Eccles

MDPI

Basel • Beijing • Wuhan • Barcelona • Belgrade • Novi Sad • Cluj • Manchester

Guest Editor
Michael Eccles
Department of Pathology
University of Otago
Dunedin
New Zealand

Editorial Office
MDPI AG
Grosspeteranlage 5
4052 Basel, Switzerland

This is a reprint of the Special Issue, published open access by the journal *International Journal of Molecular Sciences* (ISSN 1422-0067), freely accessible at: https://www.mdpi.com/journal/ijms/special_issues/XFL2P8303E.

For citation purposes, cite each article independently as indicated on the article page online and as indicated below:

Lastname, A.A.; Lastname, B.B. Article Title. *Journal Name* **Year**, *Volume Number*, Page Range.

ISBN 978-3-7258-6021-0 (Hbk)
ISBN 978-3-7258-6022-7 (PDF)
https://doi.org/10.3390/books978-3-7258-6022-7

Contents

About the Editor

Michael Eccles

Michael Eccles is Professor and Chair in Cancer Pathology in the Department of Pathology and Molecular Medicine, Dunedin School of Medicine, University of Otago. His interests include cancer, development, and disease. His current research interests include pathogenesis and progression of melanoma, kidney cancer, and polycystic kidney disease. Currently he heads the Developmental Genetics Laboratory, which focuses on genomic and epigenomic mechanisms in melanoma, including phenotype switching, and resistance to immune checkpoint inhibitor therapy. His group was one of the first to identify phenotype switching in melanoma. His lab also has an interest in genomic and epigenomic mechanisms in other cancer types, including kidney cancer, as well as in human autosomal dominant polycystic kidney disease. His group was the first to identify mutations in the human PAX2 gene.

Preface

Melanoma remains one of the most therapeutically challenging malignancies, characterized by complex molecular heterogeneity, intrinsic resistance to treatment, and dynamic interactions with the host immune system and tumour microenvironment. Despite significant advances in immunotherapy and targeted therapies, resistance and disease progression continue to present major clinical hurdles. A deeper understanding of the molecular pathology underlying these processes is therefore essential to the development of more effective and durable therapeutic strategies.

This Reprint brings together a curated collection of eight papers that collectively address both novel insights and comprehensive reviews concerning the molecular and therapeutic landscape of cutaneous and uveal melanoma. The included studies and reviews explore a broad spectrum of themes central to melanoma biology and treatment, encompassing topics such as therapeutic resistance, immune pathways and the tumour microenvironment, genomic, transcriptomic, and epigenetic determinants of therapeutic response, and emerging therapeutic strategies to overcome resistance and improve patient survival.

The reprint will be applicable to researchers, clinicians, and translational scientists, dedicated to improving the management of melanoma, who have an interest in current research integrating molecular investigation and innovative therapeutic development in melanoma.

Michael Eccles
Guest Editor

International Journal of *Molecular Sciences*

MDPI

Editorial

Special Issue "Melanoma: From Molecular Pathology to Therapeutic Approaches"

Michael R. Eccles [1,2]

[1] Department of Pathology, Dunedin School of Medicine, University of Otago, Dunedin 9016, New Zealand; michael.eccles@otago.ac.nz

[2] Maurice Wilkins Centre for Molecular Biodiscovery, Level 2, 3A Symonds Street, Auckland 1010, New Zealand

This Special Issue focuses on recent advances and innovations that have the potential to improve our understanding of the molecular pathology and therapeutic approaches associated with treating melanoma.

Globally, melanoma has a high incidence, accounting for the vast majority of skin cancer-related deaths [1]. Other forms of melanoma, such as uveal melanoma, also occur albeit more rarely, but they still contribute significantly to melanoma mortality [2]. Advanced melanoma is an aggressive cancer which is difficult to treat. Over the past two decades, there have been major advances in melanoma treatment, which include melanoma-targeted therapy as well as immune checkpoint inhibitor (ICI) immunotherapy, which have revolutionized melanoma treatment [3]. These advances have been driven by technical innovations and improved knowledge of molecular pathological biomarkers.

Despite recent therapeutic advances, a significant number of melanoma patients still do not benefit from these treatments [4,5]. In this issue, we have collated eight contributions, which can be accessed here: https://www.mdpi.com/journal/ijms/special_issues/XFL2P8303E (URL accessed on 7 November 2025). Their contributions to our knowledge of melanoma molecular pathology and therapeutic approaches are summarized in Figure 1. These papers address novel therapeutic approaches, as well as associated molecular pathologies, and they provide new angles for improving treatment outcomes for melanoma patients.

In the first contribution, Zanrè et al. investigated two antiretroviral drugs, doravirine and cabotegravir, and show that these drugs can influence apoptosis and cell proliferation in RAF-inhibitor-resistant melanoma cells, offering potential therapeutic strategies for overcoming drug resistance [Contribution 1].

Tura et al. focused on quercetin and showed that it impairs proliferation, viability, and metabolic activities while increasing oxidative stress in melanoma. The authors evaluated the effects of quercetin on the growth, survival, and glucose metabolism of the uveal melanoma cell line 92.1 [Contribution 2].

In the third contribution, Kuo et al. analyzed the transfer of mitochondria to melanoma cells from endothelial cells, which were found to increase M2-type macrophage polarization in a xenograft animal model, particularly through Nrf2/HO-1-mediated pathways. They found that the introduction of exogenous mitochondria from endothelial cells into melanoma cells promoted tumor growth [Contribution 3].

The fourth contribution by Liu et al. investigates Kinase Suppressor of RAS 1 (KSR1), which is a scaffolding protein for the RAS-RAF-MEK-ERK pathway. In this contribution, the authors examined the role of KSR1 in a BRAFV600E-transformed melanoma cell line, where they used CRISPR/Cas9 to knock out *KSR1*. Their results suggest that KSR1 directs ERK to phosphorylate substrates, which have a critical role in ensuring cell survival, and their results indicate that *KSR1* loss induces the activation of p38 Mitogen-Activated Protein Kinase (MAPK) and subsequent cell cycle aberrations and senescence [Contribution 4].

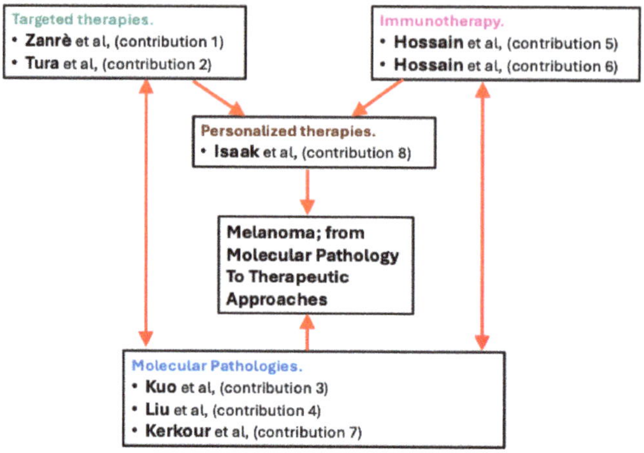

Figure 1. This figure summarizes the topics and papers in this Special Issue. The topics cover molecular pathologies, targeted therapies, and immunotherapy, which each have impacts on personalized therapies for melanoma. We have collected eight papers (Contribution 1 to Contribution 8) focused on different aspects of these topics, and which overall contribute to a better understanding of melanoma, from molecular pathology to therapeutic approaches.

The fifth contribution by Hossain et al. is a review article that asks what research should focus on to improve clinical outcomes in immune checkpoint inhibitor therapy for metastatic melanoma. The review summarizes current immune checkpoint inhibitors for melanoma and the factors involved in resistance to treatment, and also discusses emerging evidence that the host microbiome can impact ICI treatment outcomes by modulating tumor biology and anti-tumor immune function [Contribution 5].

In the sixth contribution, Hossain et al. review genomic and epigenomic biomarkers of immune checkpoint immunotherapy response in melanoma. In this contribution, the authors review established and emerging biomarkers of ICI response, and they then provide a focus on epigenomic and genomic alterations with the potential to guide single-agent ICI immunotherapy or ICI immunotherapy in combination with other ICI immunotherapies or agents [Contribution 6].

In the seventh contribution Kerkour et al. carry out a systematic review and meta-analysis of publications in the literature which have reported genetic alterations in the primary cutaneous melanoma and the matched metastasis, and determined the extent of genetic concordance between them [Contribution 7].

Finally, the eighth contribution by Isaak et al. in this Special Issue brings together new ideas to develop personalized strategies for precisely battling malignant melanoma. The authors review the current landscape, explore personalized oncology techniques, and provide an up-to-date summary of the tools available to circumvent common barriers faced when battling melanoma [Contribution 8].

We sincerely thank all the authors who submitted their work and contributed to this collection, as well as the staff of the *International Journal of Molecular Sciences* for their invaluable support in making this editorial project a success.

Conflicts of Interest: The authors declare no conflict of interest.

List of Contributions:

1. Zanrè, V.; Bellinato, F.; Cardile, A.; Passarini, C.; Di Bella, S.; Menegazzi, M. BRAF-Mutated Melanoma Cell Lines Develop Distinct Molecular Signatures After Prolonged Exposure to AZ628 or Dabrafenib: Potential Benefits of the Antiretroviral Treatments Cabotegravir or Doravirine on BRAF-Inhibitor-Resistant Cells. *Int. J. Mol. Sci.* **2024**, *25*, 11939. https://doi.org/10.3390/ijms252211939.
2. Tura, A.; Herfs, V.; Maaßen, T.; Zuo, H.; Vardanyan, S.; Prasuhn, M.; Ranjbar, M.; Kakkassery, V.; Grisanti, S. Quercetin Impairs the Growth of Uveal Melanoma Cells by Interfering with Glucose Uptake and Metabolism. *Int. J. Mol. Sci.* **2024**, *25*, 4292. https://doi.org/10.3390/ijms25084292.
3. Kuo, F.-C.; Tsai, H.-Y.; Cheng, B.-L.; Tsai, K.-J.; Chen, P.-C.; Huang, Y.-B.; Liu, C.-J.; Wu, D.-C.; Wu, M.-C.; Huang, B.; et al. Endothelial Mitochondria Transfer to Melanoma Induces M2-Type Macrophage Polarization and Promotes Tumor Growth by the Nrf2/HO-1-Mediated Pathway. *Int. J. Mol. Sci.* **2024**, *25*, 1857. https://doi.org/10.3390/ijms25031857.
4. Liu, Z.; Krstic, A.; Neve, A.; Casalou, C.; Rauch, N.; Wynne, K.; Cassidy, H.; McCann, A.; Kavanagh, E.; McCann, B.; et al. Kinase Suppressor of RAS 1 (KSR1) Maintains the Transformed Phenotype of BRAFV600E Mutant Human Melanoma Cells. *Int. J. Mol. Sci.* **2023**, *24*, 11821. https://doi.org/10.3390/ijms241411821.
5. Hossain, S.M.; Ly, K.; Sung, Y.J.; Braithwaite, A.; Li, K. Immune Checkpoint Inhibitor Therapy for Metastatic Melanoma: What Should We Focus on to Improve the Clinical Outcomes? *Int. J. Mol. Sci.* **2024**, *25*, 10120. https://doi.org/10.3390/ijms251810120.
6. Hossain, S.M.; Carpenter, C.; Eccles, M.R. Genomic and Epigenomic Biomarkers of Immune Checkpoint Immunotherapy Response in Melanoma: Current and Future Perspectives. *Int. J. Mol. Sci.* **2024**, *25*, 7252. https://doi.org/10.3390/ijms25137252.
7. Kerkour, T.; Zhou, C.; Hollestein, L.; Mooyaart, A. Genetic Concordance in Primary Cutaneous Melanoma and Matched Metastasis: A Systematic Review and Meta-Analysis. *Int. J. Mol. Sci.* **2023**, *24*, 16281. https://doi.org/10.3390/ijms242216281.
8. Isaak, A.J.; Clements, G.R.; Buenaventura, R.G.M.; Merlino, G.; Yu, Y. Development of Personalized Strategies for Precisely Battling Malignant Melanoma. *Int. J. Mol. Sci.* **2024**, *25*, 5023. https://doi.org/10.3390/ijms25095023.

References

1. Arnold, M.; Singh, D.; Laversanne, M.; Vignat, J.; Vaccarella, S.; Meheus, F.; Cust, A.E.; de Vries, E.; Whiteman, D.C.; Bray, F. Global Burden of Cutaneous Melanoma in 2020 and Projections to 2040. *JAMA Dermatol.* **2022**, *158*, 495–503. [CrossRef] [PubMed]
2. Kaštelan, S.; Pavičić, A.D.; Pašalić, D.; Nikuševa-Martić, T.; Čanović, S.; Kovačević, P.; Konjevoda, S. Biological characteristics and clinical management of uveal and conjunctival melanoma. *Oncol Res.* **2024**, *32*, 1265–1285. [CrossRef]
3. Qin, Z.; Zheng, M. Advances in targeted therapy and immunotherapy for melanoma. *Exp. Ther. Med.* **2023**, *26*, 416. [CrossRef] [PubMed]
4. Holder, A.M.; Dedeilia, A.; Sierra-Davidson, K.; Cohen, S.; Liu, D.; Parikh, A.; Boland, G.M. Defining clinically useful biomarkers of immune checkpoint inhibitors in solid tumours. *Nat. Rev. Cancer* **2024**, *24*, 498–512. [CrossRef] [PubMed]
5. Mourah, S.; Louveau, B.; Dumaz, N. Mechanisms of resistance and predictive biomarkers of response to targeted therapies and immunotherapies in metastatic melanoma. *Curr. Opin. Oncol.* **2020**, *32*, 91–97. [CrossRef] [PubMed]

International Journal of
Molecular Sciences

MDPI

Article

BRAF-Mutated Melanoma Cell Lines Develop Distinct Molecular Signatures After Prolonged Exposure to AZ628 or Dabrafenib: Potential Benefits of the Antiretroviral Treatments Cabotegravir or Doravirine on BRAF-Inhibitor-Resistant Cells

Valentina Zanrè [1], Francesco Bellinato [2], Alessia Cardile [1], Carlotta Passarini [1], Stefano Di Bella [3] and Marta Menegazzi [1,*]

1 Section of Biochemistry, Department of Neuroscience, Biomedicine and Movement Sciences, University of Verona, Strada Le Grazie 8, 37134 Verona, Italy; valentina.zanre@univr.it (V.Z.)
2 Section of Dermatology and Venereology, Department of Medicine, University of Verona, Piazzale Stefani 1, 37126 Verona, Italy; francesco.bellinato@univr.it
3 Clinical Department of Medical, Surgical and Health Sciences, University of Trieste, Piazzale Europa 1, 34127 Trieste, Italy; sdibella@units.it
* Correspondence: marta.menegazzi@univr.it

Abstract: Melanoma is an aggressive cancer characterized by rapid growth, early metastasis, and poor prognosis, with resistance to current therapies being a significant issue. BRAF mutations drive uncontrolled cell division by activating the MAPK pathway. In this study, A375 and FO-1, BRAF-mutated melanoma cell lines, were treated for 4–5 months with RAF inhibitor dabrafenib or AZ628, leading to drug resistance over time. The resistant cells showed altered molecular signatures, with differences in cell cycle regulation and the propensity of cell death. Dabrafenib-resistant cells maintained high proliferative activity, while AZ628-resistant cells, especially A375 cells, exhibited slow-cycling, and a senescent-like phenotype with high susceptibility to ferroptosis, a form of cell death driven by iron. Antiretroviral drugs doravirine and cabotegravir, known for their effects on human endogenous retroviruses, were tested for their impact on these resistant melanoma cells. Both drugs reduced cell viability and colony formation in resistant cell lines. Doravirine was particularly effective in reactivating apoptosis and reducing cell growth in highly proliferative resistant cells by increasing tumor-suppressor proteins $p16^{Ink4a}$ and $p27^{Kip1}$. These findings suggest that antiretroviral drugs can influence apoptosis and cell proliferation in RAF-inhibitor-resistant melanoma cells, offering potential therapeutic strategies for overcoming drug resistance.

Keywords: AXL; c-Met; BRAF; CRAF; SLC7A11; FTH1; GPX4; transferrin; retinoblastoma protein; cyclins

1. Introduction

Melanoma accounts for just 1% of all skin cancers, but it is highly aggressive and the leading cause of skin cancer-related deaths. Over the past 50 years, melanoma incidence in Europe has increased by 3–8% annually [1,2]. Approximately 50% of melanomas harbor harmful mutations in the BRAF kinase, which regulates the downstream mitogen-activated protein kinase (MAPK) signaling pathway [3]. RAF (V-raf murine sarcoma viral oncogene) proteins, downstream effectors of RAS (Rat sarcoma virus), are serine/threonine kinases that phosphorylate MEKs (MAP2Ks), which in turn activate ERKs (extracellular signal-regulated kinases). Under physiological conditions, the signaling pathway is transiently active. The MAPK activation is initiated extracellularly by the binding of growth factors to tyrosine kinase receptors, leading to the activation of RAF/MEK/ERK proteins [4], which generate signals that promote cell growth. In contrast, BRAF mutations result in a constitutively active MAPK signaling pathway that increases kinase activity up to 500-fold, ultimately driving cellular transformation [5,6]. The RAF kinase family consists of ARAF, BRAF, and CRAF, with BRAF being the primary activating kinase and the most frequently mutated [7].

Targeted therapy with BRAF inhibitors (BRAFi) has significantly improved response rates and extended median progression-free survival by several months compared to non-targeted chemotherapy. Second-generation BRAFi, designed as ATP-competitive small molecules, include vemurafenib and dabrafenib [8], which were approved by the Food and Drug Administration over a decade ago for treating patients with advanced BRAF-mutated metastatic melanoma. These BRAFi are predicted to be ineffective against dimeric RAF [9] because the inhibitor stabilizes the αC-helix in the inactive (OUT) position, a configuration that is not sterically permissible for both protomers in a RAF dimer. Consequently, when an αC-OUT inhibitor binds to the first protomer, it forces the αC-helix of the second protomer into the active (IN) position [10]. A third generation of targeted drugs has been developed to address the limitations of earlier therapies. AZ628, a member of this generation, is a selective and potent small molecule designed to target BRAF-mutated malignancies [11–13]. AZ628 stabilizes the αC-helix of the first protomer in the active (IN) position, allowing a second drug molecule to bind the second protomer, leading to the formation of imperfect dimers via a non-competitive allosteric inhibition mechanism [10]. As a result, αC-IN RAF inhibitors like AZ628 can hinder both BRAF and CRAF dimers, classifying them as 'pan-RAF inhibitors,' which may be particularly effective in RAF-mutant tumor cells where CRAF becomes the primary activator of ERK signaling [9,10]. However, increased CRAF protein levels can drive resistance to AZ628 [14]. To date, there are no ongoing trials studying the efficacy and safety of AZ628 in humans.

Despite initial benefits, the effectiveness of RAFi treatment is generally temporary, as patients eventually develop resistance, leading to disease progression [14,15]. Understanding the mechanisms of RAFi resistance is crucial for improving treatment outcomes in BRAF-mutated melanomas. Previous studies have explored acquired resistance to dabrafenib in melanoma cells and patients [16–18], and to AZ628 in cells [14]. Therefore, we studied and characterized the molecular features of two BRAF-mutated human cell lines, A375 and FO-1, following long-term treatment with increasing concentrations of dabrafenib or AZ628, and compared them to their respective parental cell populations. Our findings revealed significantly different molecular responses to each drug treatment.

Combination therapies targeting multiple pathways, such as DNA-damaging agents and BRAF inhibitors, have demonstrated enhanced tumor cell death both in vitro and in vivo, while also preventing melanoma re-growth after treatment discontinuation [19]. However, given the significant side effects of chemotherapy, there is an increasing preference to use more tolerable compounds, and combination treatments may lead to heightened side effects.

Recently, we investigated the potential benefits of administering antiretroviral drugs on the growth and invasive capabilities of various human melanoma cell lines, including A375 and FO-1 cells [20]. In this previous study, we demonstrated that lamivudine, doravirine, and cabotegravir affected the transcriptional activity of human endogenous retroviruses (HERV-K), leading to reduced cell growth, decreased clonogenic activity, and the induction of apoptosis or ferroptosis [20]. Although antiretroviral drugs have not yet been approved for melanoma treatment, several reverse transcriptase inhibitors have been shown to influence cell growth and differentiation in different cancers [21]. Remarkably, it is widely recognized that many antiretroviral drugs are safe for long-term use, as patients with HIV/AIDS typically require lifelong antiretroviral therapy, often with minimal side effects. Based on our previous findings, we selected the two most effective antiretroviral drugs to test their efficacy on A375 and FO-1 cells after they had developed resistance to dabrafenib or AZ628. Doravirine, a recently approved non-nucleoside reverse transcriptase inhibitor, and cabotegravir, a potent integrase strand transfer inhibitor, both retained anti-melanoma activity in melanoma cells resistant to targeted therapy. Their molecular effects on cell growth, and cell death pathways have been investigated.

2. Results

2.1. Cells' Sensitivity Following Prolonged Treatment with RAF Inhibitors

To mimic in vivo melanoma-acquired drug resistance, A375 and FO-1 cells were treated with increasing concentrations of dabrafenib or AZ628 (range: 10 nM–5 μM). After 4–5 months of treatment, the cells were tested for their sensitivity to dabrafenib or AZ628 and used for further experiments. In all cases, two days before starting new experiments, treatment with RAF inhibitors was stopped by changing the cell culture medium.

2.2. Cell Viability Assay

Our initial aim was to investigate whether A375 and FO-1 cells remained sensitive after prolonged treatment with increasing concentrations of the RAF inhibitors dabrafenib or AZ628. All experiments were conducted 72 h after drug administration.

To assess the viability of A375 and FO-1 cells, we performed a DAPI (4′,6-diamidino-2-phenylindole dihydrochloride) fluorescence assay. This method provides higher accuracy by selectively staining nucleated cells, making it suitable for cell line samples with varying viability, including those with high debris levels [22].

As expected, both A375 and FO-1 parental cells (A375P and FO-1P) are highly sensitive to the cytotoxic effects of dabrafenib or AZ628. Treatment with dabrafenib reduced cell viability to 41.6% in A375 and 33.5% in FO-1 at 10 nM (S.D. ± 8.3 and 5.6, respectively). At 50 nM, the viability rate decreased further to 22.1% in A375 and 26.7% in FO-1 (S.D. ± 1.7 and 1.8). Similarly, AZ628 reduced cell viability to 48.8% in A375P and 46.7% in FO-1P at 10 nM (S.D. ± 5.1 and 3.7) and to 32.3% and 25.7%, respectively, at 50 nM (S.D. ± 4.8 and 2.3) compared to untreated controls (set at 100%) (Figure 1).

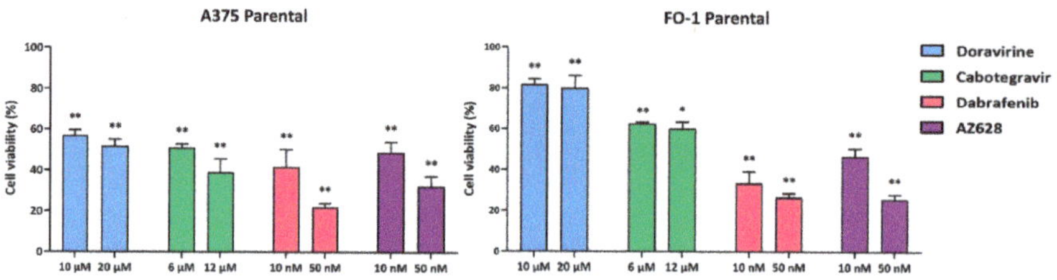

Figure 1. Parental A375 and FO-1 cell viability after antiretroviral or RAF inhibitor treatments. Cell viability was assessed using the DAPI fluorometric assay after 72 h of treatment with doravirine, cabotegravir, dabrafenib, or AZ628 in A375 and FO-1 cell lines. Data were acquired by calculating the mean ± S.D. of values from four independent experiments, each conducted in eight technical replicates, and then compared with the untreated control. Statistical significance was indicated as * $p < 0.05$; ** $p < 0.01$.

Conversely, administration of either dabrafenib or AZ628 at the same concentrations (10 and 50 nM) did not reduce cell viability in the cell lines treated for 4–5 months with increasing concentrations of each RAF inhibitor (Figure 2). Our results suggest that both cell lines have developed drug resistance. The resistant cell populations are designated as A375R and FO-1R for both inhibitors, with specific sub-designations as A375DR and FO-1DR (dabrafenib-resistant) or A375AR and FO-1AR (AZ628-resistant), in comparison to the parental A375P and FO-1P cells. Viability for A375DR was 103.5% at 10 nM and 98.6% at 50 nM (S.D. ± 0.8 and 1.1, respectively), while for FO-1DR, it was 94.6% at 10 nM and 99.7% at 50 nM (S.D. ± 2.3 and 3.7). Similarly, viability was 94.8% at 10 nM in A375AR and 94.5% at 50 nM (S.D. ± 2.3 and 6.4); in FO-1AR, it reached 99.6% at 10 nM and 78.7% at 50 nM (S.D. ± 4.1 and 19.1).

Next, we aim to test the effects of two different antiretroviral drugs on cell viability, specifically in the drug-resistant cell populations. Consistent with previous findings at lower concentrations [20], we confirmed that doravirine (10, 20 μM) and cabotegravir (6, 12 μM) significantly reduce cell viability in both parental cell lines. Notably, in A375P, cabotegravir lowered cell viability to 50.9% at 6 µM and 38.9% at 12 µM (S.D. ± 1.7 and 6.4, respectively). Doravirine reduced cell viability to 56.8% at 10 µM and 51.7% at 20 µM (S.D. ± 2.6 and 3.3). In FO-1P cells, cabotegravir diminished cell viability to 62.5% at 6 µM and 60.1% at 12 µM (S.D. ± 0.6 and 3.2), while doravirine decreased the survival rate to 81.7% at 10 µM and 80% at 20 µM (S.D. ± 2.6 and 6.0) (Figure 1). Interestingly, both antiretroviral drugs remain effective in resistant cell populations, with a particularly strong effect observed in A375DR cells, in which cabotegravir decreased cell survival to 40.9% at 6 µM and 40.5% at 12 µM (S.D. ± 5.1 and 6.2, respectively). Similarly, doravirine reduced cell survival to 56.9% at 10 µM and 40.5% at 20 µM (S.D. ± 4.4 and 5.4) (Figure 2). Although the viability of A375AR and FO-1R was also significantly affected, the effect was less pronounced. Specifically, cabotegravir reduced A375AR cell survival to 82.4% at 6 µM and 77.8% at 12 µM (S.D. ± 5.5 and 2.8, respectively), whereas doravirine decreased cell viability to 77% at 10 µM and 74.5% at 20 µM (S.D. ± 4.8 and 2.2). In FO-1DR cells, cabotegravir reduced viability to 66.6% at 6 µM and 63.7% at 12 µM (S.D. ± 7.5 and 8.4, respectively); meanwhile, doravirine reduced the survival rate to 71% at 10 µM and 63.7% at 20 µM (S.D. ± 8.2 and 5.0). In FO-1AR cells, cabotegravir reduced viability to 67.2% at 6 µM and 61.8% at 12 µM (S.D. ± 3.2 and 2.0), while doravirine reduced cell viability to 63.6% at 10 µM and 55.5% at 20 µM (S.D. ± 1.0 and 2.8) (Figure 2).

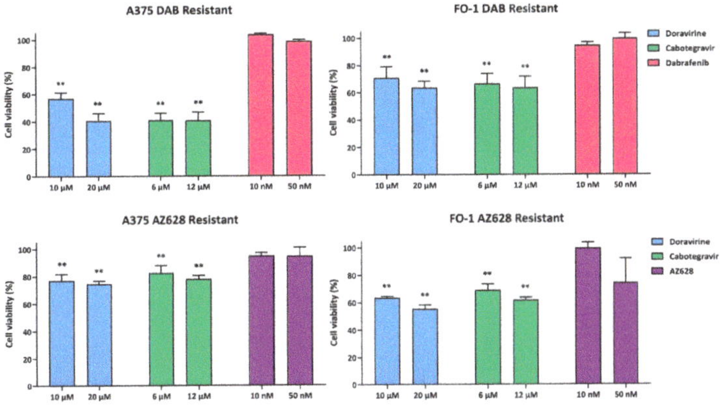

Figure 2. Cell viability of dabrafenib- or AZ628-resistant cell populations after antiretroviral treatments. Cell viability was assessed using the DAPI fluorometric assay after 72 h of treatment with either doravirine, cabotegravir, dabrafenib or AZ628 in A375R, and FO-1R cell lines. Data were acquired by calculating the mean ± S.D. of values from four independent experiments, each conducted in eight technical replicates, and then compared with the untreated control. Statistical significance was indicated as ** $p < 0.01$.

2.3. *Administration of Antiretroviral Drugs and RAF Inhibitors Affect HERV-K Pol and Env Gene Expression*

As we recently reported [20], doravirine and cabotegravir were shown to reduce the expression of human endogenous retrovirus-K (*HERV-K*) genes, *Pol* and *Env*, in A375P and FO-1P cell lines.

In the present work, we examine the effects of dabrafenib and AZ628 on *Pol* and *Env* gene expression in both parental and resistant cell lines.

As shown in Figure 3, real-time PCR assays demonstrate that treatment with both dabrafenib and AZ628 at a concentration of 50 nM resulted in a significant increase in *Pol* gene expression in A375P and FO-1P cells. However, the *Env* gene expression showed a noticeable, though not statistically significant, increase in the same parental cells (Figure 3, Top). Accordingly, the baseline expression of both *Pol* and *Env* genes increased following the development of RAFi resistance in the untreated control cells (Figure 3, Bottom). This suggests a potential involvement of *HERV-K* gene reactivation in the progression and worsening of the melanoma phenotype.

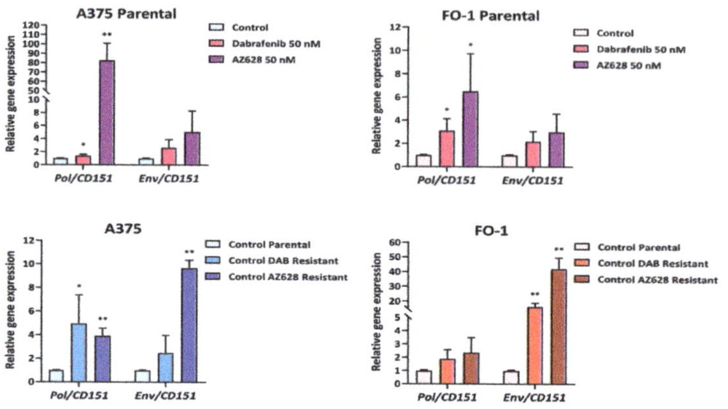

Figure 3. Relative expression of HERV-K *Pol* and *Env* genes in parental and RAFi-resistant cell populations after treatment with RAF inhibitors. Cells were treated with dabrafenib (50 nM) or AZ628 (50 nM) for 24 h. The mRNA expression levels of treated samples were measured by RT-PCR and compared with untreated cells of each population. The bars represent the mean values ± standard deviation (S.D.) of four independent experiments, each conducted in triplicates. All comparisons were made against each control sample after normalization with CD151 expression. Statistical significance was indicated as * $p < 0.05$; ** $p < 0.01$.

Moreover, in both A375DR and FO-1DR, a further increase in *Env* gene expression was observed after the administration of 50 nM dabrafenib (Figure 4). Meanwhile, in AZ628-resistant cell lines, a significant increase in both *Pol* and *Env* gene expression was detected after AZ628 treatment in FO-1AR cells, with no significant changes observed in A375AR cells (Figure 4).

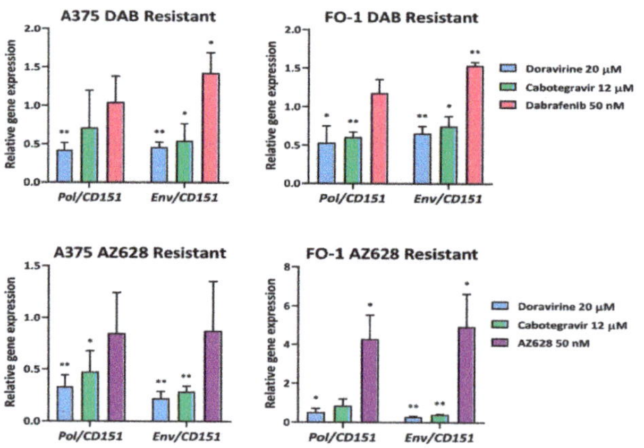

Figure 4. Relative expression of HERV-K *Pol* and *Env* genes in different RAFi-resistant cell populations. Cells were treated with doravirine (20 μM), cabotegravir (12 μM), dabrafenib (50 nM) or AZ628 (50 nM) for 24 h. The mRNA expression levels of treated samples were measured by RT-PCR and compared with untreated cells of each population. The bars represent the mean values ± standard deviation (S.D.) of four independent experiments, each conducted in triplicates. All comparisons were made against each control sample after normalization with CD151 expression. Statistical significance was indicated as * $p < 0.05$; ** $p < 0.01$.

Since RAF inhibitors appear to generally reactivate HERV-K gene expression in both parental and resistant cell populations, we used real-time PCR assays to evaluate whether the antiretroviral drugs doravirine and cabotegravir could reduce *HERV-K* gene expression levels in RAFi-resistant cell lines. Following treatment with 20 μM doravirine or 12 μM cabotegravir in A375R and FO-1R cell lines, a general reduction in *HERV-K* gene expression was observed across all four resistant cell populations, despite some variability (Figure 4). These findings suggest that the antiretroviral drugs remain effective even in the context of elevated *HERV-K* expression associated with RAF-inhibitor resistance.

2.4. Molecular Characterization of Melanoma Cells Resistant to Dabrafenib or AZ628

We first characterized the phenotypes of A375R and FO-1R by evaluating the expression levels of proteins involved in proliferative signaling, cell cycle, and cell death. These data were compared to those obtained from A375P and FO-1P cells, respectively. All the cell populations were treated for 72 h with the highest concentration previously tested on the parental cells (50 nM of either dabrafenib or AZ628).

In both parental cell lines, immunoblot analysis showed that treatment with dabrafenib or AZ628 significantly reduced the expression of BRAF1 and CRAF, as well as the effector kinases ERKs, both in their phosphorylated (activated) forms, and total protein levels (Figure 5). Additionally, two cell surface tyrosine kinase receptors constitutively expressed in melanoma cells, AXL (tyrosine-protein kinase receptor UFO) and c-Met (mesenchymal–epithelial transition factor) [23], were also downregulated by either dabrafenib or AZ628 in the parental cell populations (Figure 5).

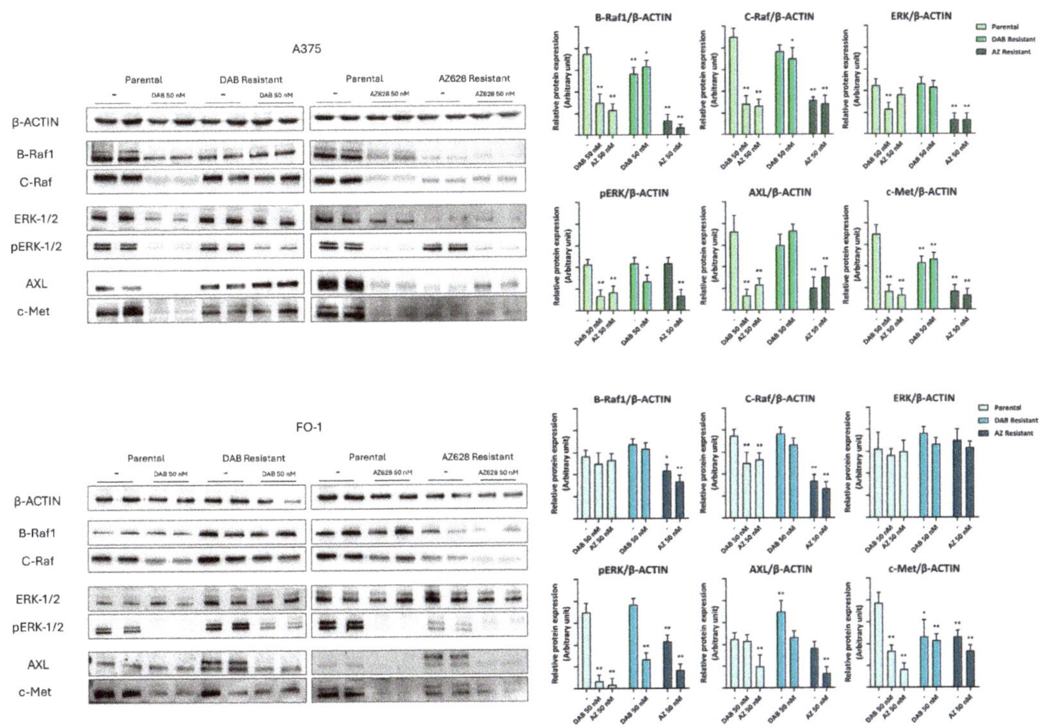

Figure 5. Representative immunoblots show the effects of RAF inhibitors on the expression of oncoproteins regulating MAPK pathway. Dabrafenib (50 nM) or AZ628 (50 nM) treatment regulate B-Raf1(B-V-raf murine sarcoma viral oncogene), C-Raf (C-V-raf murine sarcoma viral oncogene), ERK (extracellular signal-regulated kinases), pERK, AXL (tyrosine-protein kinase receptor UFO), and c-Met

(mesenchymal–epithelial transition factor) protein expressions in both parental and resistant cell populations. The histograms represent the mean values ± S.D. of protein expression levels measured by densitometry deriving from three independent experiments and normalized to β-actin expression. All comparisons were made relative to each control sample after data normalization. Statistical significance was indicated as * $p < 0.05$; ** $p < 0.01$.

Notably, in A375DR and FO-1DR cells, the expression levels of all these proteins returned to high levels, and further treatment with 50 nM dabrafenib was completely ineffective. These malignant features correlate with cell cycle reactivation in A375DR and FO-1DR cells, whether treated with dabrafenib or not. Indeed, the phosphorylation levels of retinoblastoma protein (pRb) and M-phase inducer phosphatase 3 (pCDC25C), as well as the total expression of cyclin D1 and cyclin A2, were reduced only in parental cells, but not in A375DR or FO-1DR cells, following dabrafenib treatment (Figure 6).

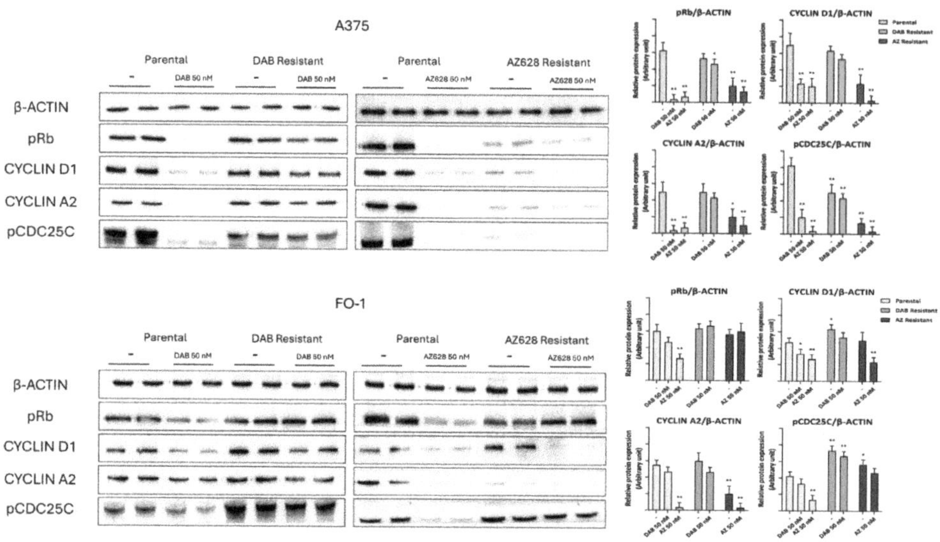

Figure 6. Representative immunoblots show the effects of RAF inhibitors on the expression of proteins regulating cell cycle. Dabrafenib (50 nM) or AZ628 (50 nM) treatment downregulates cell cycle regulatory proteins in both parental and resistant cell populations. pRb (phosphorylated form of retinoblastoma protein), pCDC25C (phosphorylated form of M-phase inducer phosphatase 3). The histograms represent the mean values ± S.D. of protein expression levels measured by densitometry deriving from three independent experiments and normalized to β-actin expression. All comparisons were made relative to each control sample after data normalization. Statistical significance was indicated as * $p < 0.05$; ** $p < 0.01$.

We also examined the expression levels of proteins involved in the regulation of cell death, focusing on apoptosis and ferroptosis. The expression of cleaved poly (ADP-ribose) polymerase (cPARP), a substrate cleaved by effector caspases 3 and 7, increases during apoptosis [24]. The mitochondrial carrier homolog 2 (MTCH2) protein, which facilitates the recruitment of pro-apoptotic proteins to the mitochondria, is essential for apoptosis induction, as deletion of the MTCH2 gene impairs this process [25]. In parental cells, cPARP levels increased following treatment with both RAF inhibitors, confirming their pro-apoptotic effect (Figure 7). In A375DR and FO-1DR cells, cPARP expression remained higher in both untreated or dabrafenib-treated conditions than in each corresponding parental untreated cell populations and was comparable to the levels observed in dabrafenib-treated parental cells (Figure 7). However, the elevated apoptosis levels in dabrafenib resistant cells were not explained by changes in the expression of anti-apoptotic proteins Bcl-2 (B-cell lymphoma 2) and Bcl-xL (B-cell lymphoma-extra-large), or the pro-apoptotic protein Bax (Bcl-2-like protein 4).

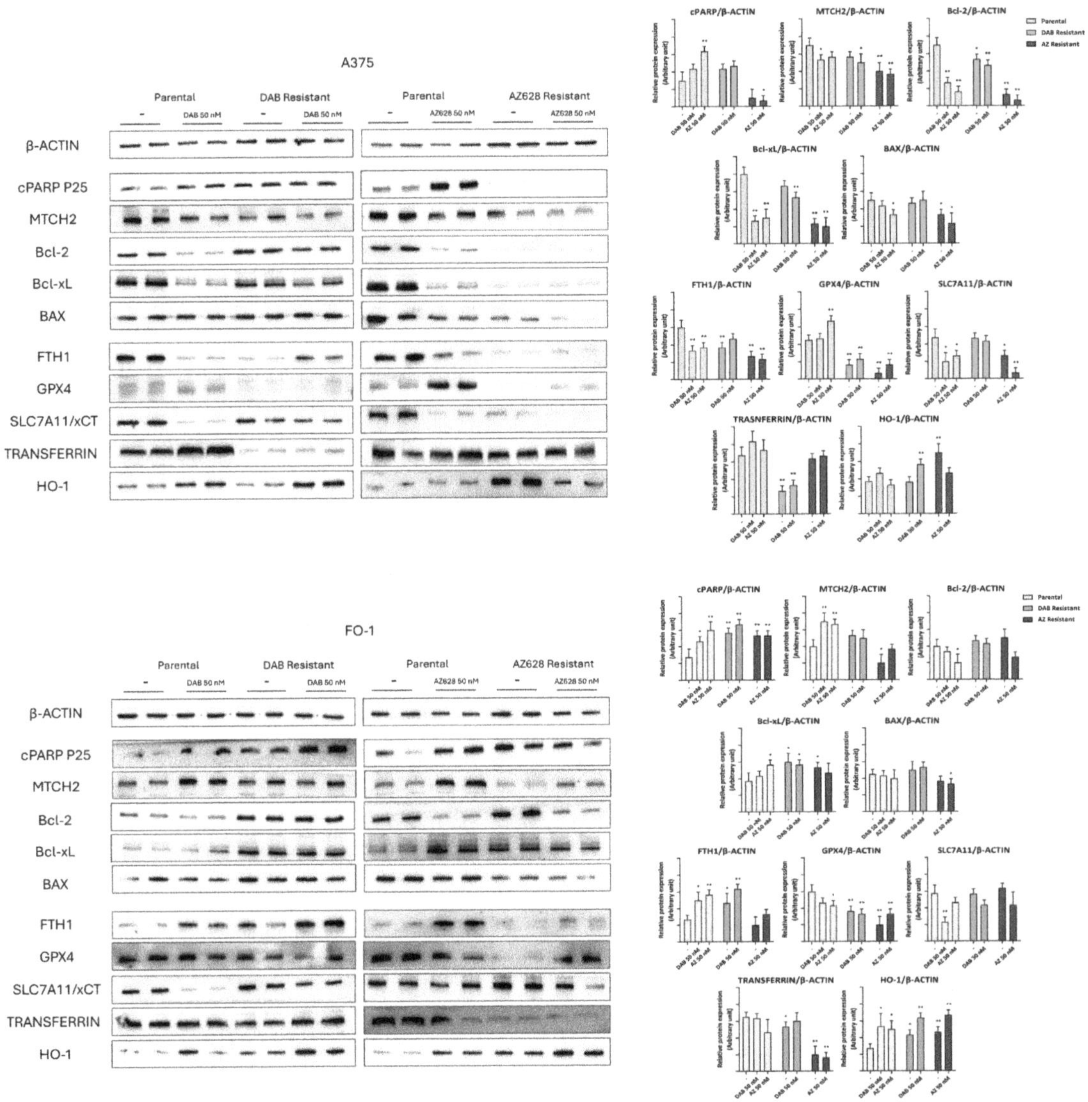

Figure 7. Representative immunoblots show the effects of RAF inhibitors on the expression of proteins regulating cell death in parental and resistant cell populations. Dabrafenib induced apoptosis in the parental melanoma cells as well as in A375DR, FO-1DR and FO-1AR, as suggested by the high expression of the cleaved form of poly (ADP-ribose) polymerase (cPARP). Ferroptosis is induced in all parental cells lines and in A375AR cell population, as suggested by a decrease in ferritin (FTH1), cystine-glutamate antiporter (SLC7A11) and/or glutathione peroxidase 4 (GPX4) expression and increased transferrin or heme oxygenase-1 (HO-1). The histograms represent the mean values ± S.D. of protein expression levels measured by densitometry deriving from three independent experiments and normalized to β-actin expression. All comparisons were made relative to each control sample after data normalization. Statistical significance was indicated as * $p < 0.05$; ** $p < 0.01$.

The propensity of A375P cells to undergo ferroptosis increased following treatment with dabrafenib, as indicated by elevated expression of transferrin and HO-1 (heme oxygenase-1), both of which contribute to augmented intracellular iron levels. This increase was associated with decreased levels of FTH1 (ferritin heavy chain 1) and reductions in GPX4 (glutathione peroxidase 4) and SLC7A11 (cystine-glutamate antiporter, also known as xCT). In contrast, A375DR cells exhibited a reduced likelihood of undergoing ferroptosis, as evidenced by lower transferrin levels and elevated SLC7A11 expression (Figure 7). Conversely, FO-1P cells treated with dabrafenib showed a lower propensity for ferroptosis, maintaining high levels of GPX4 and FTH1. Although FO-1DR cells displayed high levels of transferrin and HO-1, they appear protected from ferroptosis by elevated levels of SLC7A11, GPX4, and FTH1 (Figure 7).

A distinct phenotype was observed in A375AR cells. This population, resistant to the pan-Raf inhibitor AZ628, exhibited consistently low levels of signaling kinases (BRAF1, CRAF, ERKs, AXL, and c-Met), both in the presence and absence of the drug in the culture medium (Figure 5). Correspondently, the expression of cell cycle regulatory proteins (pRb, pCDC25C, cyclin D1, and cyclin A2) was similarly reduced, suggesting a very low proliferation rate (Figure 6).

While A375P cells treated with AZ628 showed increased cPARP expression, A375AR cells displayed nearly undetectable levels of cPARP, regardless of the presence of AZ628 in the culture medium. A375P cells treated with AZ628 were susceptible to cell death through ferroptosis, as evidenced by high transferrin expression and lower levels of SLC7A11 and FTH1 compared to untreated A375P cells (Figure 7). The propensity for ferroptosis appeared even more pronounced in A375AR cells, where HO-1 expression increased, while GPX4, SLC7A11, and FTH1 were significantly downregulated (Figure 7).

The FO-1AR cell population differs from A375AR in terms of total ERK expression and, consequently, in the expression of cell cycle-activating proteins, the expression levels of which remain elevated (Figures 5 and 6). Furthermore, FO-1AR cells showed a lower propensity for ferroptosis but exhibited higher levels of apoptosis compared to A375AR (Figure 7).

2.5. Doravirine and Cabotegravir Inhibit Cell Cycle Progression and Induce Apoptosis in RAFi-Resistant Cell Populations

We investigated the molecular effects of antiretroviral drugs on RAFi-resistant cell populations, focusing specifically on apoptosis and cell cycle regulation.

After 72 h of treatment with doravirine (20 μM) in A375R and FO-1R cells, we observed an increase in cPARP expression levels. In contrast, cabotegravir (12 μM) elevated cPARP levels only in the FO-1R cell population (Figure 8).

$P27^{Kip1}$ and $P16^{Ink4a}$, both negative regulators of cyclin-dependent kinases (CDKs), inhibit cell proliferation when highly expressed. Immunoblot analysis revealed that $P27^{Kip1}$ levels increased in FO-1R and A375AR cells, while $P16^{Ink4a}$ expression was elevated only in A375DR and FO-1DR cells (Figure 8).

Our results demonstrate that both doravirine and cabotegravir can regulate the cell cycle and enhance apoptosis in RAFi-resistant melanoma cells.

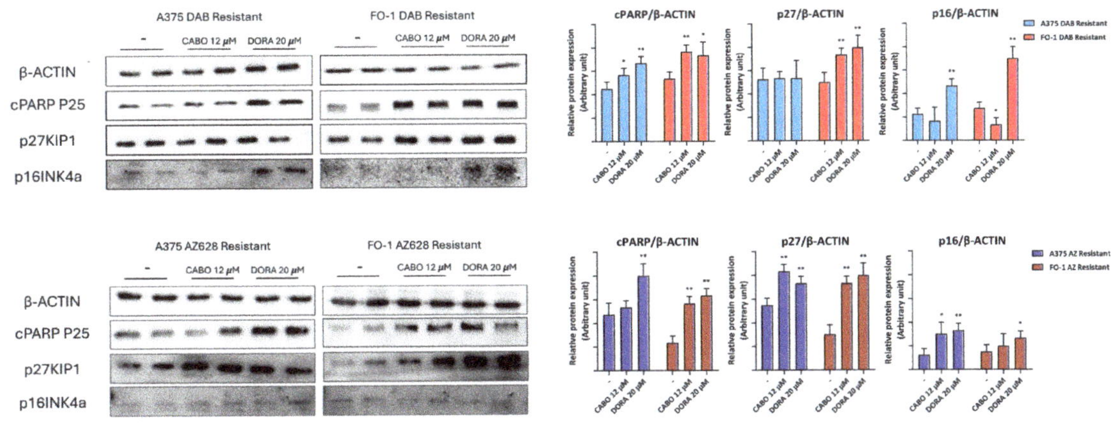

Figure 8. Representative immunoblots show the effects of antiretroviral drugs on the expression of proteins regulating cell cycle and apoptosis in resistant cell populations. Cabotegravir (CABO) and doravirine (DORA) induced apoptosis in FO-1R cells, while doravirine also induced apoptosis in A375R cell populations, as indicated by the high expression of cPARP. The expression of tumor suppressor protein p27 increased in FO-1R and in A375AR cell populations when treated with either cabotegravir or doravirine. The expression of tumor suppressor protein p16 increased only in dabrafenib-resistant cell populations. The histograms represent the mean values ± S.D. of protein expression levels measured by densitometry deriving from three independent experiments and normalized to β-actin expression. All comparisons were made relative to each control sample after data normalization. Statistical significance was indicated as * $p < 0.05$; ** $p < 0.01$.

2.6. RAF-Inhibitors and Antiretroviral Drugs Affect the Ability of Parental and Resistant Cell Lines to Form Colonies in Soft Agar

We aimed to evaluate the ability of RAF inhibitors and antiretroviral drugs to inhibit anchorage-independent cell growth in both parental and resistant cell populations using a soft agar colony formation assay.

Dabrafenib and AZ628, administered at 50 nM, strongly inhibited the anchorage-independent growth of the A375P and FO-1P cell lines, as expected. Interestingly, treatments with both RAF inhibitors of the A375DR, FO-1DR and FO-1AR cell populations conserved a significative reduction in both the size and number of colonies (Figure 9).

Our previous findings [20] indicated that cabotegravir and doravirine were effective in reducing the formation of soft agar colonies in A375P and FO-1P cells. In this work, we investigated their effectiveness in RAF-inhibitor-resistant cell populations. The treatment with 20 μM doravirine or 12 μM cabotegravir effectively decreased the number and size of the colonies in the FO-1R cell lines and almost completely prevented colony formation in A375DR cells. In contrast, A375AR cells exhibited low and slow growth even in untreated conditions, making the reduction in colony number with doravirine not significative. Cabotegravir, however, appeared to have a significative impact on growth in an anchorage-independent manner; meanwhile, AZ628 seems to not affect the growth much at all (Figure 9).

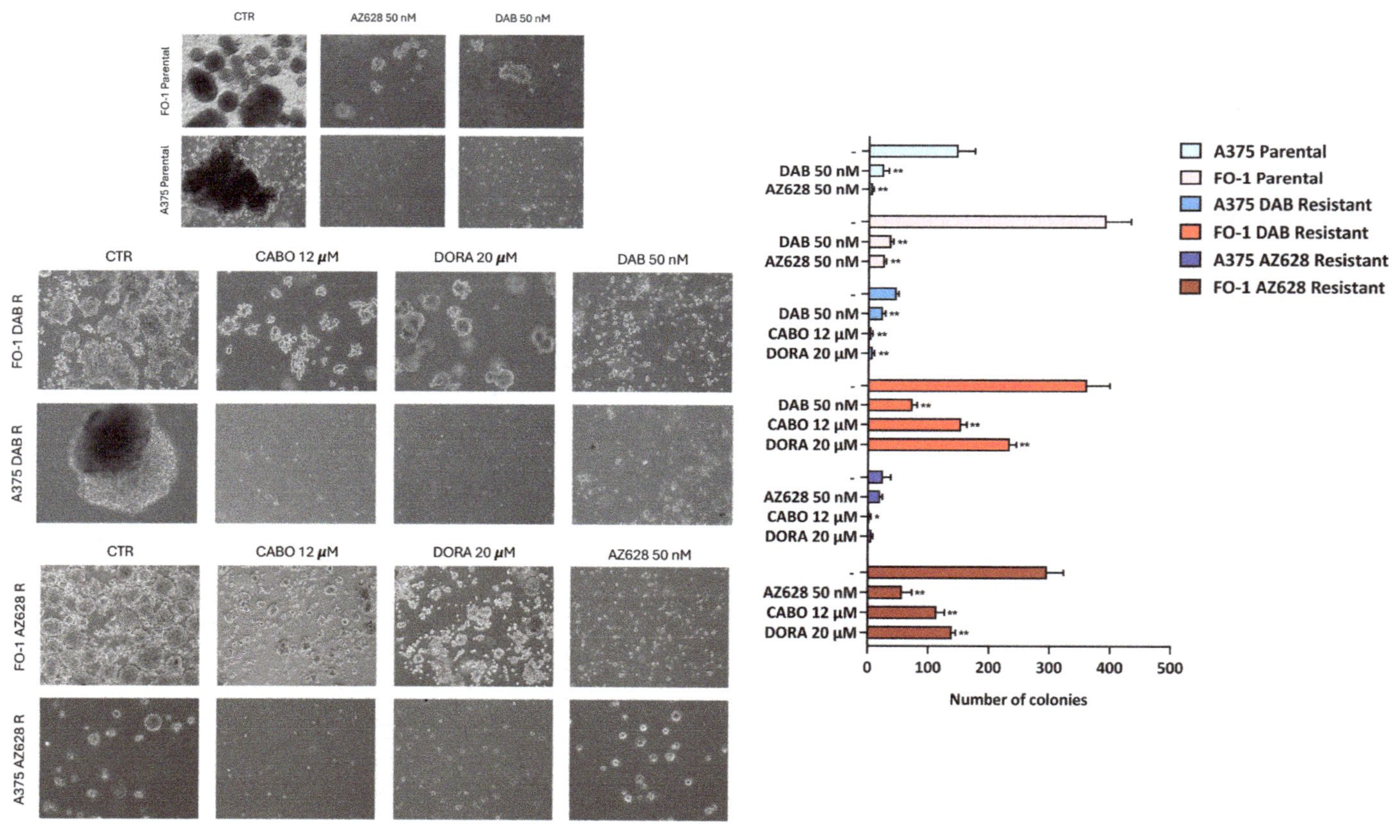

Figure 9. Effects of RAF inhibitors and antiretroviral drugs in soft agar colony formation in melanoma parental and resistant cell populations. The images shown are representative examples from experiments illustrating colony formation in soft agar. The histograms show the quantification of colony numbers for each treatment, based on data from three independent experiments, each performed in duplicate. Microscopic images depict the size and density of colonies (5× magnification, inverted microscopy, Axio Vert A1, Zeiss, Oberkochen, Germany). All comparisons were made against each respective control sample. Statistical significance was indicated as * $p < 0.05$; ** $p < 0.01$.

3. Discussion

Melanoma is a malignant tumor with a global presence, known for its rapid growth, early metastasis, recurrence, and poor prognosis [26]. Despite significant advancements in melanoma treatment, many patients have developed resistance to current therapies, highlighting the need for more effective options [2]. Melanoma's aggressiveness is largely attributed to significant intra-tumoral heterogeneity, which contributes to treatment resistance and a high potential for spread [27]. The tumor's heterogeneity is driven by transcriptionally distinct melanoma cell phenotypes, which can reprogram to adapt to different stages of progression and treatment exposure [27].

BRAF mutations, which occur in approximately 40–60% of melanoma cases, lead to the constitutive activation of MAPK pathway driving uncontrolled cell division and contributing to melanoma initiation and progression [28,29]. In vitro cellular models are valuable tools for mimicking and studying resistance mechanisms. Understanding the molecular transformations that occur in cells developing resistance to RAF inhibitors can guide the development of therapies to overcome this resistance and improve clinical outcomes.

Firstly, we examined the baseline phenotype of two BRAF-mutated human melanoma cell lines (A375P and FO-1P) and assessed the molecular signature changes after 4–5 months of treatment with increasing concentrations of the second-generation BRAF inhibitor dabrafenib and of the third-generation pan-RAF inhibitor AZ628.

As expected, both A375P and FO-1P cell lines were initially sensitive to the cytostatic/cytotoxic effects of the targeted drugs at the concentrations of 10 and 50 nM (Figure 1). However, prolonged treatment of the parental cells with either drug applied selective pressure, allowing the cells to survive at significantly higher concentrations, up to 5 μM. This indicates that, over the course of 4–5 months, both cell lines exhibit plasticity and can adapt to new conditions, developing drug-resistant phenotypes. Vitality assays, measuring fluorescence emission following DAPI staining, revealed that dabrafenib- or AZ628-treatment of A375R and FO-1R cells did not significantly reduce cell viability compared to untreated resistant-control cells, further confirming the development of drug resistance (Figure 2).

Therefore, we investigated the molecular signatures of A375R and FO-1R cells in comparison to their respective parental populations. Additionally, since the two targeted drugs have different mechanisms of action, we can simultaneously examine whether cell adaptation to each RAFi leads to distinct phenotypes.

Immunoblot analysis revealed that cell-cycle-regulating proteins (pRb, pCDC25C, cyclin D1, and cyclin A2), as markers of cell proliferation, were significantly downregulated by both targeted drugs in A375P and FO-1P cells, as expected (Figure 6). While A375DR and FO-1DR fully restored their ability to proliferate in the presence and absence of dabrafenib, FO-1AR only partially restored this ability, and A375AR remained in a state where cell cycle progression was completely hindered (Figure 6).

To further investigate the mechanisms underlying RAF inhibitor resistance, we focused on the oncoproteins that drive melanoma cell growth. BRAF overexpression or alternative splicing may contribute to BRAFi resistance [30,31]. Reactivation of ERKs can also occur through enhanced RAF dimerization, a key mechanism of resistance to RAFi in melanoma [32], as well as the abnormal expression of other RAF isoforms, such as CRAF and ARAF [14,33].

Consequently, we measured the expression levels of key proteins, including BRAF1, CRAF, and ERKs in both parental and resistant cell populations (Figure 5). Both RAF inhibitors downregulated the MAPK signaling pathway in parental cell lines and affected the total amount of ERK proteins in addition to their activation (Figure 5).

Receptor tyrosine kinases (RTKs) can function as upstream activators of the MAPK/ERK signaling pathway, and their increased expression has previously been observed in BRAFi-resistant cell lines [34–36]. Abnormal expression of RTKs has been shown to contribute to melanoma development and progression [23]. AXL enhances melanoma aggressiveness by activating the AKT (protein kinase B), p38 kinase, and MAPK signaling pathways [37]. The hepatocyte growth factor/MET pathway also plays a key role in melanoma development, progression, and therapeutic resistance [38].

The expression of two tyrosine kinase receptors, AXL and c-Met, was lower in parental populations treated with RAF inhibitors (Figure 5), reducing tumor aggressiveness when the cells were still sensitive. Resistant cells displayed distinct phenotypes after prolonged treatment with the BRAFi dabrafenib or the pan-RAF inhibitor AZ628. In dabrafenib-resistant cells, RTKs, MAPKs, and cell-cycle-regulating factors are reactivated, exhibiting a very high proliferative phenotype driven by the elevated expression of oncoproteins involved in growth signaling pathways. Other studies have reported that cells resistant to BRAF inhibitors, such as vemurafenib or dabrafenib, undergo metabolic reprogramming and reactivate several kinase pathways [16]. These cells also exhibit cell cycle deregulation [15]. Our findings in dabrafenib-resistant cells (A375DR and FO-1DR) are consistent with these previous reports. Conversely, in AZ628-resistant cell populations, these pathways remained almost inactive (Figures 5, 6 and 10). A375AR melanoma cells, characterized by slow-cycling or growth arrest and a senescent-like appearance, represent a different tumor signature (Figure 10). Although this phenotype is less aggressive, it requires alternative strategies, distinct from those targeting highly proliferative tumor cells, which instead leave the slow-cycling cancer cells unaffected [39].

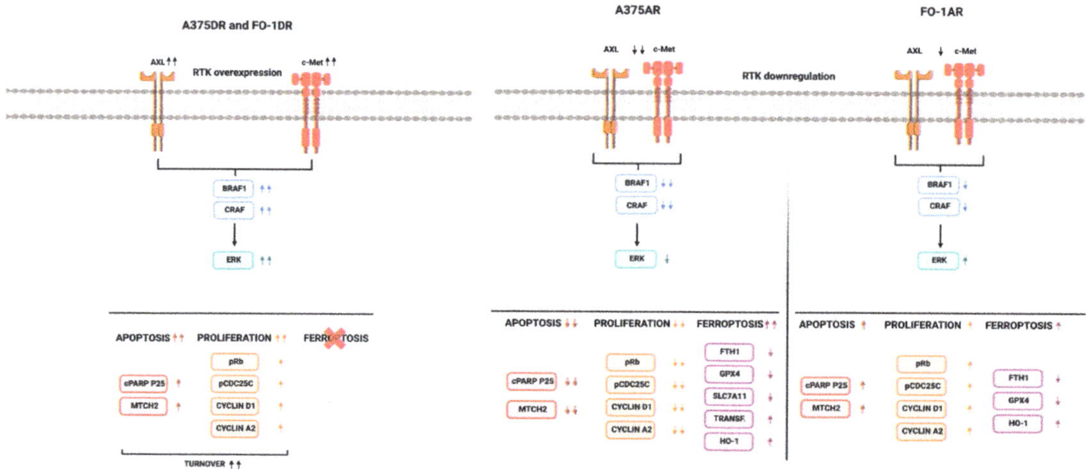

Figure 10. Characterization of phenotypes in melanoma cell populations resistant to dabrafenib or AZ628. This figure illustrates various features of melanoma cell populations with respect to signaling pathways, cell cycle regulation, and susceptibility to cell death. Receptor tyrosine kinase (RTK): including tyrosine-protein kinase receptor UFO (AXL) and mesenchymal–epithelial transition factor (c-Met). RAS/RAF/MAPK signaling pathway: detailing expression levels of V-raf murine sarcoma viral oncogenes (RAF) including BRAF and CRAF isoforms, as well as total extracellular signal-regulated kinases (ERK) expression. Pro-proliferative proteins: including phosphorylation levels of retinoblastoma protein (pRb) and M-phase inducer phosphatase 3 (pCDC25C), along with cyclin D1 and cyclin A2 expression. Apoptosis markers: displaying levels of cleaved poly (ADP-ribose) polymerase (cPARP) and mitochondrial carrier homolog 2 (MTCH2). Ferroptosis markers: highlighting the expression of transferrin and heme oxygenase-1 (HO-1), both of which contribute to increased intracellular iron. Levels of ferritin heavy chain 1 (FTH1), glutathione peroxidase 4 (GPX4), and cystine-glutamate antiporter (SLC7A11) are also presented.

The dysregulated expression of oncoproteins in the growth signaling pathway, which affects cell cycle regulation, should be assessed through the diverse functionalities of the two drugs. Notably, a major issue with second-generation BRAF inhibitors, such as dabrafenib, is that they are ATP-competitive and specifically target BRAF-mutated monomers and homodimers. However, they can induce a 'paradoxical effect' in non-tumor cells of melanoma patients, activating the MAPK pathway, which leads to cell proliferation and an increased risk of secondary malignancies [7]. In contrast, as above described, third-generation inhibitors also target CRAF in both monomeric and heterodimeric forms through an allosteric, non-competitive mechanism [7]. Only dabrafenib-resistant cells showed re-expression of BRAF along with CRAF expression. These events facilitate the bypass of BRAF inhibition by promoting the formation of BRAF-CRAF heterodimers. Conversely, the pan-RAFi AZ628 permanently blocks both CRAF or BRAF-CRAF activity. Accordingly, some studies reported that AZ628 has a superior ability to block the MAPK signaling pathway compared to the second-generation BRAFi vemurafenib [40,41], as well as a high binding affinity to other intracellular targets involved in proliferation and migration pathways [42].

Considering these different factors, it is crucial to investigate the propensity to cell death across all cell populations. Cleaved PARP expression is a key indicator that the execution phase of apoptosis has begun [24]. After 72 h of treatment with either dabrafenib or AZ628, cPARP levels increased in all sensitive parental cell lines (Figure 7), highlighting the potent cytotoxic effects of RAF inhibitors. Unexpectedly, only A375AR cells completely suppressed apoptosis. Conversely, dabrafenib-resistant cells (A375DR and FO-1DR) and FO-1AR maintained high levels of cPARP, both in the presence and absence of the drug, suggesting that some cells continued to undergo apoptosis after acquiring resistance (Figures 7 and 10). To explore the regulation of this process, we measured the expression of proteins involved in apoptotic cell death [43], including the antiapoptotic proteins Bcl2 and Bcl-xL, and the proapoptotic proteins Bax and MTCH2. It was found that in resistant melanoma cell lines, the expression of the proapoptotic proteins BAX and MTCH2 were negatively or not correlated to cPARP levels. Additionally, the same cell population exhibited a positive correlation between the expression of the antiapoptotic proteins Bcl2 or Bcl-xL and cPARP. Strikingly, studies in the literature have also reported similarly contradictory findings in various tumors, including melanoma [44–46]. However, our immunoblots suggest that additional proteins or mechanisms may be involved.

If the plasticity and dedifferentiation of melanoma cells promote resistance to targeted therapies, the newly acquired phenotype might also render the cells more susceptible to other vulnerabilities. Therefore, we investigated whether melanoma cells can undergo ferroptosis, a non-apoptotic form of cell death triggered by iron. Ferroptosis is induced by an increase in intracellular free iron, which can occur due to high transferrin uptake, heme oxygenase 1 (HO-1) induction, and/or low expression of ferritin (FTH1), a protein that sequesters iron in its cage [47,48]. Free iron can induce lipid peroxidation and cell death, but only if its damaging effects are not counteracted by specific intracellular antioxidant systems, such as glutathione peroxidase 4 (GPX4) activity and the availability of glutathione, which is highly dependent on the cystine transporter SLC7A11 [49,50].

In general, our immunoblot data suggest that A375 cell line is more susceptible to ferroptosis than FO-1 cells (Figures 7 and 10). Specifically, A375P cells treated with both RAF inhibitors and FO-1P cells treated with dabrafenib exhibited protein expression signatures indicative of ferroptosis, including high levels of transferrin and HO-1, along with low expression of SLC7A11 and GPX4/FTH1 (Figure 7). In contrast, FO-1DR cells appeared to be the most resistant population to ferroptosis, while A375DR cells showed only weak signs of susceptibility to this type of cell death. However, AZ628-resistant cells, particularly A375AR, seemed prone to ferroptosis (Figures 7 and 10). Notably, the A375AR population displayed a low proliferative and low apoptotic phenotype but showed a strong propensity to ferroptosis, with high expression of transferrin and HO-1, and very low expression of FTH1, GPX4, and SLC7A11.

In summary, the differences in RAF-inhibitor-resistant cells are dependent on the type of RAFi used to induce resistance. Dabrafenib-resistant cells are highly proliferative, with a high propensity for apoptosis, but not for ferroptosis, and can be hindered by blocking cell cycle progression (Figure 10). In contrast, AZ628-resistant cells, particularly the A375AR population, exhibit a low proliferative rate and low apoptosis but have a high propensity for ferroptosis (Figure 10). These cells can be targeted with inducers of either apoptosis or ferroptosis.

We and others have previously demonstrated that some antiretroviral drugs, typically used to combat retroviruses, with a particular focus on HIV infection, can reduce melanoma aggressiveness by inhibiting the expression of human endogenous retrovirus (HERV-K) [20,51]. Moreover, several studies have reported the antitumor effects of antiretroviral drugs in other malignancies as well [52–58]. In this work, we confirmed the ability of doravirine and cabotegravir to reduce cell viability in parental cells, as previously reported [20], and we analyzed their activity on resistant cell populations. While cabotegravir appears equally effective against both A375P and FO-1P cells, doravirine shows greater efficacy in A375P compared to FO-1P, consistent with our previous findings [20] (Figure 1). In cell populations that have acquired resistance to RAFi, both doravirine and cabotegravir remain effective, particularly in A375DR cells, where they reduced cell viability more than in A375P cells (Figure 2). Furthermore, both antiretroviral drugs significantly reduced the number of colonies in soft agar, suggesting that they retain the ability to inhibit cell growth in an anchorage-independent manner (Figure 9).

According to the literature, RAFi resistance is associated with a more aggressive tumor phenotype [59]. Moreover, as highlighted by Serafino et al. [60], the activation of human endogenous retroviral genes may contribute to the worsening of the melanoma phenotype in patients. Our real-time-PCR data showed that both dabrafenib and AZ628 reactivated the expression of *HERV-K Pol* and *Env* genes compared to untreated parental cells (Figure 3). These results highlight the need for further investigation into HERV-K gene expression levels in resistant cell populations.

A general reduction in HERV-K gene expression was observed in all four resistant cell lines following treatment with either antiretroviral drug (Figure 4). This suggests that the decrease in HERV-K gene expression may contribute to the antimelanoma effects of antiretroviral drugs, even in the context of RAF inhibitor resistance, which reactivates HERV-K *Pol* and *Env* expression.

At the molecular level, antiretroviral drugs may influence the expression of key regulatory proteins involved in the cell cycle and cell death. In our previous study, cabotegravir demonstrated pro-apoptotic activity in FO-1P cells after 48 h of treatment [20]. In FO-1 cells resistant to RAFi, cabotegravir induced cPARP expression after 72 h of treatment, confirming its cytotoxic effects in these resistant cell lines as well (Figure 8). Although doravirine did not induce apoptotic cell death in A375P and FO-1P cells after 48 h of treatment [20], it led to an increase in cPARP expression across all RAFi-resistant cell populations after 72 h (Figure 8). Notably, in the same cell populations, doravirine showed stronger inhibition of HERV-K *Pol* and *Env* expression compared to cabotegravir (Figure 4). Additionally, doravirine effectively reactivated apoptosis in the A375AR cell population, where long-term AZ628 treatment had previously suppressed apoptotic activity (Figure 8).

A substantial reduction in the expression of $p16^{Ink4a}$ and $p27^{Kip1}$ has been observed with melanoma progression [61]. These proteins act as tumor suppressors by inhibiting CDKs, which play a crucial role in regulating cell cycle checkpoint transitions [62,63]. Doravirine significantly increased $p16^{Ink4a}$ expression in dabrafenib-resistant cells (A375DR and FO-1DR), indicating a potential reduction in cell growth within these highly proliferative resistant populations (Figure 8). Additionally, both doravirine and cabotegravir elevated $P27^{Kip1}$ expression in FO-1DR cells as well as in AZ628-resistant cells (A375AR and FO-1AR).

In summary, antiretroviral drugs may influence both apoptosis and cell proliferation in RAFi-resistant melanoma cell lines, partly by targeting cell cycle regulation and promoting apoptotic cell death.

4. Materials and Methods

4.1. Cell Cultures

The A375 (CRL-1619) and FO-1 (CRL-12177) melanoma cell lines were obtained from ATCC (Manassas, VA, USA) and cultured at 37 °C in a humidified atmosphere containing 5% CO_2. The culture medium used was high-glucose Dulbecco's Modified Eagle's Medium (DMEM, Gibco, BRL Invitrogen Corp., Carlsbad, CA, USA), supplemented with 10% heat-inactivated fetal bovine serum (FBS, Euroclone S.p.A, Pero, Milan, Italy) and 1% antibiotic–antimycotic solution (Gibco, BRL Invitrogen Corp., Carlsbad, CA, USA).

4.2. Cell Viability Assay (DAPI Staining and Measure of Fluorescence)

4′,6-diamidino-2-phenylindole dihydrochloride (DAPI) is a fluorescent compound that exhibits multiple binding modes to DNA [22,64] and is transferred to descendant cells during proliferation.

Melanoma cells were plated in 96-well black plates with clear bottoms (LUMOX multiwell, Sarstedt AG & Co. KG, Nümbrecht, Germany). The following cell lines were used: A375P, A375DR, and A375AR melanoma cells (1.45×10^3 cells/well); and FO-1P, FO-1DR, and FO-1AR melanoma cells (1.75×10^3 cells/well).

The next day, the cells were treated with antiretroviral drugs or the kinase inhibitors dabrafenib (GSK2118436, Selleckchem, Huston, TX, USA) or AZ628 (Merck, Milan, Italy) for 72 h. After the treatment period, the medium was removed by vacuum, and the cells were fixed by adding 50 µL/well of 4% (*w/v*) paraformaldehyde (PFA) (AppliChem, Monza, Italy). After 10 min of incubation, the PFA was removed by vacuum, and the wells were washed three times for 10 min each with 1× Dulbecco's Phosphate-Buffered Saline (DPBS) (Gibco, BRL Invitrogen Corp., Carlsbad, CA, USA) on a shaker.

Subsequently, 50 µL/well of DAPI (1:1000 dilution, Thermofisher Scientific, Milan, Italy) was added, and the plates were incubated at room temperature (RT) for 15 min in the dark on a shaker. The DAPI was then removed by vacuum, and the wells were washed three times for 10 min each with 1× DPBS, again in the dark.

Finally, fluorescence intensity was measured at an excitation wavelength of 350 nm and an emission wavelength of 461 nm using a TECAN NanoQuant Infinite M200 Pro plate reader (Tecan Group Ltd., Männedorf, Switzerland). Each experimental condition was performed in 8 replicates.

4.3. RNA Extraction, Reverse Transcription, and Real-Time PCR

A375P, A375R, FO-1P, and FO-1R cell lines were seeded in 6 mm petri dishes at the following densities: A375P and FO-1P 100×10^3 cells/dish; A375DR, FO-1DR, and FO-1AR 150×10^3 cells/dish; A375AR 180×10^3 cells/dish. Upon reaching 80% confluence, all cell lines were treated with either 20 µM doravirine, 12 µM cabotegravir (Merck, Milan, Italy), 50 nM dabrafenib (GSK2118436, Selleckchem, Huston, TX, USA) or 50 nM AZ628 (Merck, Milan, Italy). After 24 h of treatment, total RNA was extracted for gene expression analysis using TRIzol Reagent (Thermofisher Scientific, Milan, Italy), following the manufacturer's protocol. RNA quantification was performed using a Tecan NanoQuant Infinite M200 Pro plate reader (Tecan Group Ltd., Männedorf, Switzerland), and RNA quality was assessed via 1% agarose gel electrophoresis.

A total of 1000 ng of RNA was reverse transcribed using the SensiFAST cDNA Synthesis Kit (Bioline, Trento, Italy) in accordance with the manufacturer's instructions. Following reverse transcription, the expression levels of HERV-K genes (*Pol, Env*) were measured using Real-Time Polymerase Chain Reaction (RT-PCR). Normalization was carried out using Cluster of Differentiation 151 protein (*CD151*), which was identified as the most stable gene under our experimental conditions.

The primers used for amplification were as follows:
CD151: (Fw) 5′-CTACGCCTACTACCAGCAGC-3′
(Rv) 5′-CGGAACCACTCACTGTCTCG-3′
Pol: (Fw) 5′-CCACTGTAGAGCCTCCTAAACCC-3′

(Rv) 5′-GCTGGTATAGTAAAGGCAAATTTTTC-3′
Env: (Fw) 5′-GCCATCCACCAAGAAAGCA-3′
(Rv) 5′-AACTGCGTCAGCTCTTTAGTTGT-3′

Real-Time PCR was performed using the Bio-Rad CFX Connect Real-Time System and the SensiFAST SYBR No-ROX Kit (Bioline, Trento, Italy). The amplification protocol consisted of an initial polymerase activation step at 95 °C for 2 min, followed by 40 cycles of denaturation at 95 °C for 5 s and primer annealing/polymerization at 60 °C for 20 s. Each measurement was performed in triplicate in at least four independent experiments.

4.4. Colony Formation Assay in Soft Agar

The ability of FO-1P, A375P, A375R, and FO-1R melanoma cells to grow in an anchorage-independent manner was evaluated using a colony formation assay in soft agar, as described previously [65]. First, the bottom layer of 6-well plates was prepared with 1% low-gelling temperature agarose (Sigma-Merck, Milan, Italy) dissolved in 2× DMEM, 20% FBS, and 2% antibiotic–antimycotic solution. A second layer, consisting of 0.6% low-gelling temperature agarose dissolved in the same medium, was added on top. This layer contained treated or untreated melanoma cells (A375P, and FO-1P 12 × 10^3 cells/well; A375R 20 × 10^3 cells/well; FO-1R 10 × 10^3 cells/well).

Fresh medium (200 μL) was added to each well twice a week. After 15–21 days, colony formation was assessed using an inverted microscope (Axio Vert A1, Zeiss, Oberkochen, Germany).

4.5. Total Protein Extraction

Cells were seeded in 35 mm petri dishes at the following densities: A375P 40 × 10^3 cells/dish; FO-1P 50 × 10^3 cells/dish; A375DR and FO-1R 60 × 10^3 cells/dish; A375AR 80 × 10^3 cells/dish. After 24 h, cells were treated with each drug or left untreated as a control. After 72 h of treatment, the cells were scraped using warm 1× sample buffer (2% SDS, 10% glycerol, 50 mM Tris-HCl, 1.75% β-mercaptoethanol, and bromophenol blue), boiled at 98 °C and then put in ice for 10 min. The total protein extracts were stored at −80 °C for subsequent analysis.

4.6. Immunoblot Analysis

Protein extracts were separated by electrophoresis on 10 to 15% polyacrylamide SDS-PAGE gels and then transferred onto polyvinylidene difluoride (PVDF) membranes (Merck-Millipore, Milan, Italy). Membranes were blocked at room temperature (RT) for 1 h in TBST buffer (10 mM Tris-HCl, pH 7.5, 100 mM NaCl, 0.1% Tween 20) containing 5% milk. Following blocking, the membranes were incubated overnight at 4 °C on a shaker in a 5% BSA solution containing the following primary antibodies: Transferrin (A1448), Ferritin heavy chain (A19544), cleaved PARP-P25 (A19612), CDKN1B/p27KIP1 (A19095), CDKN2A/p16INK4a (A11651), Cyclin A2 (A19036), Bcl-xL (A0209), Heme Oxygenase 1 (A19062), ERK 1/2 (A16686), pERK 1/2 (AP0974), SLC7A11/xCT (A2413), C-Raf (A19638) from ABclonal (Woburn, MA, USA); Cyclin D1 (GTX634347), MTCH2 (GTX130324), β-actin (GTX124214), p21 Cip (GTX29543), CDC25C phospho Ser216 (GTX128153), BAX (GTX109683), c-Met (GTX100637), B-Raf1 (GTX100913) from Genetex (Alton Parkway, Irvine, CA, USA); Bcl-2 (#15071), pRb (#8516) from Cell Signaling Technology (Danvers, MA, USA) and AXL (13196-1-AP), GPX4 (67763-1) from ProteinTech (Manchester, UK).

After primary antibody incubation, the membranes were washed three times for 10 min each with TBST buffer, followed by a 1 h incubation with horseradish peroxidase-conjugated secondary antibodies (anti-rabbit or anti-mouse) from Cell Signaling Technology (Danvers, MA, USA). The membranes were then washed again three times for 10 min each with TBST. Protein expression levels were normalized to β-actin unless otherwise specified. Immunodetection was performed using an ECL detection kit (Cyanagen, Bologna, Italy), and chemiluminescence signals were visualized using a ChemiDoc system (Bio-Rad, Hercules, CA, USA).

4.7. Statistical Analysis

Data are presented as mean ± standard deviation (S.D.). Statistical differences were analyzed using GraphPad Prism software, version 8.0.2, employing an unpaired two-tailed Student's *t*-test, unless otherwise specified. A *p*-value of less than 0.05 (*) or less than 0.01 (**) was considered statistically significant. Each experiment was performed with a minimum of three independent biological replicates. Normal data distribution was verified using the Shapiro–Wilk test.

5. Conclusions

RAF inhibitor therapy creates resistance in vitro and in vivo. Targeting other molecular pathways may provide therapeutic benefits when RAF inhibitors lose effectiveness. Our work demonstrates that antiretroviral drugs, doravirine and cabotegravir, not only induce apoptosis but also modulate the expression of cell cycle regulators in RAFi-resistant melanoma cells. These antiretrovirals, which have been used long-term with minimal side effects for AIDS treatment, show promise in inhibiting tumor growth in RAFi-resistant cell lines, suggesting their potential utility in slowing melanoma progression after RAFi resistance. We assume that these findings should be validated in preclinical studies.

Author Contributions: Conceptualization, M.M. and V.Z.; methodology, V.Z., A.C. and C.P.; investigation, V.Z., A.C. and C.P.; resources, M.M., F.B. and S.D.B.; data curation, A.C. and C.P.; writing—original draft preparation, M.M. and V.Z.; writing—review and editing, M.M., F.B., V.Z. and S.D.B.; supervision, M.M.; funding acquisition, M.M. and F.B. All authors have read and agreed to the published version of the manuscript.

Funding: This research received no external funding.

Institutional Review Board Statement: Not applicable.

Informed Consent Statement: Not applicable.

Data Availability Statement: Data contained within the article are recorded using instruments in our labs. These instruments are not connected to the internet; however, further inquiries can be directed to the corresponding author.

Acknowledgments: We thank Raffaella Pacchiana for her technical assistance. This paper and the associated research were conducted as part of the Excellence Project 2023–2027 within the Department of Neuroscience, Biomedicine, and Movement Sciences of the University of Verona, Italy.

Conflicts of Interest: The authors declare no conflicts of interest.

References

1. Arnold, M.; Singh, D.; Laversanne, M.; Vignat, J.; Vaccarella, S.; Meheus, F.; Cust, A.E.; de Vries, E.; Whiteman, D.C.; Bray, F. Global Burden of Cutaneous Melanoma in 2020 and Projections to 2040. *JAMA Dermatol.* **2022**, *158*, 495–503. [CrossRef] [PubMed]
2. Gagliardi, M.; Saverio, V.; Monzani, R.; Ferrari, E.; Piacentini, M.; Corazzari, M. Ferroptosis: A New Unexpected Chance to Treat Metastatic Melanoma? *Cell Cycle* **2020**, *19*, 2411–2425. [CrossRef] [PubMed]
3. Cancer Genome Atlas Network Genomic Classification of Cutaneous Melanoma. *Cell* **2015**, *161*, 1681–1696. [CrossRef] [PubMed]
4. Gray-Schopfer, V.; Wellbrock, C.; Marais, R. Melanoma Biology and New Targeted Therapy. *Nature* **2007**, *445*, 851–857. [CrossRef] [PubMed]
5. Leonardi, G.C.; Falzone, L.; Salemi, R.; Zanghì, A.; Spandidos, D.A.; Mccubrey, J.A.; Candido, S.; Libra, M. Cutaneous Melanoma: From Pathogenesis to Therapy (Review). *Int. J. Oncol.* **2018**, *52*, 1071–1080. [CrossRef]
6. Conner, S.R.; Scott, G.; Aplin, A.E. Adhesion-Dependent Activation of the ERK1/2 Cascade Is by-Passed in Melanoma Cells. *J. Biol. Chem.* **2003**, *278*, 34548–34554. [CrossRef]
7. Singh, A.K.; Sonawane, P.; Kumar, A.; Singh, H.; Naumovich, V.; Pathak, P.; Grishina, M.; Khalilullah, H.; Jaremko, M.; Emwas, A.-H.; et al. Challenges and Opportunities in the Crusade of BRAF Inhibitors: From 2002 to 2022. *ACS Omega* **2023**, *8*, 27819–27844. [CrossRef]
8. Ballantyne, A.D.; Garnock-Jones, K.P. Dabrafenib: First Global Approval. *Drugs* **2013**, *73*, 1367–1376. [CrossRef]
9. Karoulia, Z.; Wu, Y.; Ahmed, T.A.; Xin, Q.; Bollard, J.; Krepler, C.; Wu, X.; Zhang, C.; Bollag, G.; Herlyn, M.; et al. An Integrated Model of RAF Inhibitor Action Predicts Inhibitor Activity against Oncogenic BRAF Signaling. *Cancer Cell* **2016**, *30*, 485–498. [CrossRef]

10. Karoulia, Z.; Gavathiotis, E.; Poulikakos, P.I. New Perspectives for Targeting RAF Kinase in Human Cancer. *Nat. Rev. Cancer* **2017**, *17*, 676–691. [CrossRef]
11. Cotto-Rios, X.M.; Agianian, B.; Gitego, N.; Zacharioudakis, E.; Giricz, O.; Wu, Y.; Zou, Y.; Verma, A.; Poulikakos, P.I.; Gavathiotis, E. Inhibitors of BRAF Dimers Using an Allosteric Site. *Nat. Commun.* **2020**, *11*, 4370. [CrossRef] [PubMed]
12. Wang, J.-Q.; Teng, Q.-X.; Lei, Z.-N.; Ji, N.; Cui, Q.; Fu, H.; Lin, L.; Yang, D.-H.; Fan, Y.-F.; Chen, Z.-S. Reversal of Cancer Multidrug Resistance (MDR) Mediated by ATP-Binding Cassette Transporter G2 (ABCG2) by AZ-628, a RAF Kinase Inhibitor. *Front. Cell Dev. Biol.* **2020**, *8*, 601400. [CrossRef] [PubMed]
13. McDermott, U.; Sharma, S.V.; Dowell, L.; Greninger, P.; Montagut, C.; Lamb, J.; Archibald, H.; Raudales, R.; Tam, A.; Lee, D.; et al. Identification of Genotype-Correlated Sensitivity to Selective Kinase Inhibitors by Using High-Throughput Tumor Cell Line Profiling. *Proc. Natl. Acad. Sci. USA* **2007**, *104*, 19936–19941. [CrossRef] [PubMed]
14. Montagut, C.; Sharma, S.V.; Shioda, T.; McDermott, U.; Ulman, M.; Ulkus, L.E.; Dias-Santagata, D.; Stubbs, H.; Lee, D.Y.; Singh, A.; et al. Elevated CRAF as a Potential Mechanism of Acquired Resistance to BRAF Inhibition in Melanoma. *Cancer Res.* **2008**, *68*, 4853–4861. [CrossRef]
15. Dulgar, O.; Kutuk, T.; Eroglu, Z. Mechanisms of Resistance to BRAF-Targeted Melanoma Therapies. *Am. J. Clin. Dermatol.* **2021**, *22*, 1–10. [CrossRef]
16. Datta, K.K.; Kore, H.; Gowda, H. Multi-Omics Analysis Delineates Resistance Mechanisms Associated with BRAF Inhibition in Melanoma Cells. *Exp. Cell Res.* **2024**, *442*, 114215. [CrossRef] [PubMed]
17. Johnson, D.B.; Menzies, A.M.; Zimmer, L.; Eroglu, Z.; Ye, F.; Zhao, S.; Rizos, H.; Sucker, A.; Scolyer, R.A.; Gutzmer, R.; et al. Acquired BRAF Inhibitor Resistance: A Multicenter Meta-Analysis of the Spectrum and Frequencies, Clinical Behaviour, and Phenotypic Associations of Resistance Mechanisms. *Eur. J. Cancer* **2015**, *51*, 2792–2799. [CrossRef]
18. Raineri, A.; Fasoli, S.; Campagnari, R.; Gotte, G.; Menegazzi, M. Onconase Restores Cytotoxicity in Dabrafenib-Resistant A375 Human Melanoma Cells and Affects Cell Migration, Invasion and Colony Formation Capability. *Int. J. Mol. Sci.* **2019**, *20*, 5980. [CrossRef]
19. Alonso-Marañón, J.; Villanueva, A.; Piulats, J.M.; Martínez-Iniesta, M.; Solé, L.; Martín-Liberal, J.; Segura, S.; Pujol, R.M.; Iglesias, M.; Bigas, A.; et al. Combination of Chemotherapy with BRAF Inhibitors Results in Effective Eradication of Malignant Melanoma by Preventing ATM-Dependent DNA Repair. *Oncogene* **2021**, *40*, 5042–5048. [CrossRef]
20. Zanrè, V.; Bellinato, F.; Cardile, A.; Passarini, C.; Monticelli, J.; Di Bella, S.; Menegazzi, M. Lamivudine, Doravirine, and Cabotegravir Downregulate the Expression of Human Endogenous Retroviruses (HERVs), Inhibit Cell Growth, and Reduce Invasive Capability in Melanoma Cell Lines. *Int. J. Mol. Sci.* **2024**, *25*, 1615. [CrossRef]
21. Sinibaldi-Vallebona, P.; Lavia, P.; Garaci, E.; Spadafora, C. A Role for Endogenous Reverse Transcriptase in Tumorigenesis and as a Target in Differentiating Cancer Therapy. *Genes. Chromosomes Cancer* **2006**, *45*, 1–10. [CrossRef] [PubMed]
22. Atale, N.; Gupta, S.; Yadav, U.C.S.; Rani, V. Cell-Death Assessment by Fluorescent and Nonfluorescent Cytosolic and Nuclear Staining Techniques. *J. Microsc.* **2014**, *255*, 7–19. [CrossRef]
23. De Tomi, E.; Campagnari, R.; Orlandi, E.; Cardile, A.; Zanrè, V.; Menegazzi, M.; Gomez-Lira, M.; Gotte, G. Upregulation of miR-34a-5p, miR-20a-3p and miR-29a-3p by Onconase in A375 Melanoma Cells Correlates with the Downregulation of Specific Onco-Proteins. *Int. J. Mol. Sci.* **2022**, *23*, 1647. [CrossRef]
24. Taylor, R.C.; Cullen, S.P.; Martin, S.J. Apoptosis: Controlled Demolition at the Cellular Level. *Nat. Rev. Mol. Cell Biol.* **2008**, *9*, 231–241. [CrossRef]
25. Zaltsman, Y.; Shachnai, L.; Yivgi-Ohana, N.; Schwarz, M.; Maryanovich, M.; Houtkooper, R.H.; Vaz, F.M.; De Leonardis, F.; Fiermonte, G.; Palmieri, F.; et al. MTCH2/MIMP Is a Major Facilitator of tBID Recruitment to Mitochondria. *Nat. Cell Biol.* **2010**, *12*, 553–562. [CrossRef]
26. Shalata, W.; Attal, Z.G.; Solomon, A.; Shalata, S.; Abu Saleh, O.; Tourkey, L.; Abu Salamah, F.; Alatawneh, I.; Yakobson, A. Melanoma Management: Exploring Staging, Prognosis, and Treatment Innovations. *Int. J. Mol. Sci.* **2024**, *25*, 5794. [CrossRef] [PubMed]
27. Diazzi, S.; Tartare-Deckert, S.; Deckert, M. The Mechanical Phenotypic Plasticity of Melanoma Cell: An Emerging Driver of Therapy Cross-Resistance. *Oncogenesis* **2023**, *12*, 7. [CrossRef]
28. Wilson, T.R.; Fridlyand, J.; Yan, Y.; Penuel, E.; Burton, L.; Chan, E.; Peng, J.; Lin, E.; Wang, Y.; Sosman, J.; et al. Widespread Potential for Growth-Factor-Driven Resistance to Anticancer Kinase Inhibitors. *Nature* **2012**, *487*, 505–509. [CrossRef] [PubMed]
29. Benedusi, M.; Lee, H.; Lim, Y.; Valacchi, G. Oxidative State in Cutaneous Melanoma Progression: A Question of Balance. *Antioxidants* **2024**, *13*, 1058. [CrossRef]
30. Poulikakos, P.I.; Persaud, Y.; Janakiraman, M.; Kong, X.; Ng, C.; Moriceau, G.; Shi, H.; Atefi, M.; Titz, B.; Gabay, M.T.; et al. RAF Inhibitor Resistance Is Mediated by Dimerization of Aberrantly Spliced BRAF(V600E). *Nature* **2011**, *480*, 387–390. [CrossRef]
31. Shi, H.; Moriceau, G.; Kong, X.; Lee, M.-K.; Lee, H.; Koya, R.C.; Ng, C.; Chodon, T.; Scolyer, R.A.; Dahlman, K.B.; et al. Melanoma Whole-Exome Sequencing Identifies (V600E)B-RAF Amplification-Mediated Acquired B-RAF Inhibitor Resistance. *Nat. Commun.* **2012**, *3*, 724. [CrossRef]
32. Moriceau, G.; Hugo, W.; Hong, A.; Shi, H.; Kong, X.; Yu, C.C.; Koya, R.C.; Samatar, A.A.; Khanlou, N.; Braun, J.; et al. Tunable-Combinatorial Mechanisms of Acquired Resistance Limit the Efficacy of BRAF/MEK Cotargeting but Result in Melanoma Drug Addiction. *Cancer Cell* **2015**, *27*, 240–256. [CrossRef] [PubMed]

33. Zhang, F.; Tang, X.; Fan, S.; Liu, X.; Sun, J.; Ju, C.; Liang, Y.; Liu, R.; Zhou, R.; Yu, B.; et al. Targeting the P300/NONO Axis Sensitizes Melanoma Cells to BRAF Inhibitors. *Oncogene* **2021**, *40*, 4137–4150. [CrossRef] [PubMed]
34. Shaffer, S.M.; Dunagin, M.C.; Torborg, S.R.; Torre, E.A.; Emert, B.; Krepler, C.; Beqiri, M.; Sproesser, K.; Brafford, P.A.; Xiao, M.; et al. Rare Cell Variability and Drug-Induced Reprogramming as a Mode of Cancer Drug Resistance. *Nature* **2017**, *546*, 431–435. [CrossRef]
35. Müller, J.; Krijgsman, O.; Tsoi, J.; Robert, L.; Hugo, W.; Song, C.; Kong, X.; Possik, P.A.; Cornelissen-Steijger, P.D.M.; Geukes Foppen, M.H.; et al. Low MITF/AXL Ratio Predicts Early Resistance to Multiple Targeted Drugs in Melanoma. *Nat. Commun.* **2014**, *5*, 5712. [CrossRef] [PubMed]
36. Kot, M.; Simiczyjew, A.; Wądzyńska, J.; Ziętek, M.; Matkowski, R.; Nowak, D. Characterization of Two Melanoma Cell Lines Resistant to BRAF/MEK Inhibitors (Vemurafenib and Cobimetinib). *Cell Commun. Signal* **2024**, *22*, 410. [CrossRef] [PubMed]
37. Sensi, M.; Catani, M.; Castellano, G.; Nicolini, G.; Alciato, F.; Tragni, G.; De Santis, G.; Bersani, I.; Avanzi, G.; Tomassetti, A.; et al. Human Cutaneous Melanomas Lacking MITF and Melanocyte Differentiation Antigens Express a Functional Axl Receptor Kinase. *J. Investig. Dermatol.* **2011**, *131*, 2448–2457. [CrossRef]
38. Zhou, Y.; Song, K.Y.; Giubellino, A. The Role of MET in Melanoma and Melanocytic Lesions. *Am. J. Pathol.* **2019**, *189*, 2138–2148. [CrossRef]
39. Ahn, A.; Chatterjee, A.; Eccles, M.R. The Slow Cycling Phenotype: A Growing Problem for Treatment Resistance in Melanoma. *Mol. Cancer Ther.* **2017**, *16*, 1002–1009. [CrossRef]
40. Hatzivassiliou, G.; Song, K.; Yen, I.; Brandhuber, B.J.; Anderson, D.J.; Alvarado, R.; Ludlam, M.J.C.; Stokoe, D.; Gloor, S.L.; Vigers, G.; et al. RAF Inhibitors Prime Wild-Type RAF to Activate the MAPK Pathway and Enhance Growth. *Nature* **2010**, *464*, 431–435. [CrossRef]
41. Whittaker, S.R.; Theurillat, J.-P.; Van Allen, E.; Wagle, N.; Hsiao, J.; Cowley, G.S.; Schadendorf, D.; Root, D.E.; Garraway, L.A. A Genome-Scale RNA Interference Screen Implicates NF1 Loss in Resistance to RAF Inhibition. *Cancer Discov.* **2013**, *3*, 350–362. [CrossRef] [PubMed]
42. Dong, X.; Zhang, K.; Yi, S.; Wang, L.; Wang, X.; Li, M.; Liang, S.; Wang, Y.; Zeng, Y. Multi-Omics Profiling Combined with Molecular Docking Reveals Immune-Inflammatory Proteins as Potential Drug Targets in Colorectal Cancer. *Biochem. Biophys. Res. Commun.* **2024**, *739*, 150598. [CrossRef] [PubMed]
43. Valentini, E.; Di Martile, M.; Brignone, M.; Di Caprio, M.; Manni, I.; Chiappa, M.; Sergio, I.; Chiacchiarini, M.; Bazzichetto, C.; Conciatori, F.; et al. Bcl-2 Family Inhibitors Sensitize Human Cancer Models to Therapy. *Cell Death Dis.* **2023**, *14*, 441. [CrossRef] [PubMed]
44. Guttà, C.; Rahman, A.; Aura, C.; Dynoodt, P.; Charles, E.M.; Hirschenhahn, E.; Joseph, J.; Wouters, J.; de Chaumont, C.; Rafferty, M.; et al. Low Expression of Pro-Apoptotic Proteins Bax, Bak and Smac Indicates Prolonged Progression-Free Survival in Chemotherapy-Treated Metastatic Melanoma. *Cell Death Dis.* **2020**, *11*, 124. [CrossRef]
45. Hantusch, A.; Rehm, M.; Brunner, T. Counting on Death-Quantitative Aspects of Bcl-2 Family Regulation. *FEBS J.* **2018**, *285*, 4124–4138. [CrossRef]
46. Kale, J.; Osterlund, E.J.; Andrews, D.W. BCL-2 Family Proteins: Changing Partners in the Dance towards Death. *Cell Death Differ.* **2018**, *25*, 65–80. [CrossRef]
47. Tsoi, J.; Robert, L.; Paraiso, K.; Galvan, C.; Sheu, K.M.; Lay, J.; Wong, D.J.L.; Atefi, M.; Shirazi, R.; Wang, X.; et al. Multi-Stage Differentiation Defines Melanoma Subtypes with Differential Vulnerability to Drug-Induced Iron-Dependent Oxidative Stress. *Cancer Cell* **2018**, *33*, 890–904.e5. [CrossRef]
48. Cardile, A.; Passarini, C.; Zanrè, V.; Fiore, A.; Menegazzi, M. Hyperforin Enhances Heme Oxygenase-1 Expression Triggering Lipid Peroxidation in BRAF-Mutated Melanoma Cells and Hampers the Expression of Pro-Metastatic Markers. *Antioxidants* **2023**, *12*, 1369. [CrossRef]
49. Khorsandi, K.; Esfahani, H.; Ghamsari, S.K.-; Lakhshehei, P. Targeting Ferroptosis in Melanoma: Cancer Therapeutics. *Cell Commun. Signal* **2023**, *21*, 337. [CrossRef]
50. Ta, N.; Jiang, X.; Zhang, Y.; Wang, H. Ferroptosis as a Promising Therapeutic Strategy for Melanoma. *Front. Pharmacol.* **2023**, *14*, 1252567. [CrossRef]
51. Giovinazzo, A.; Balestrieri, E.; Petrone, V.; Argaw-Denboba, A.; Cipriani, C.; Miele, M.T.; Grelli, S.; Sinibaldi-Vallebona, P.; Matteucci, C. The Concomitant Expression of Human Endogenous Retroviruses and Embryonic Genes in Cancer Cells under Microenvironmental Changes Is a Potential Target for Antiretroviral Drugs. *Cancer Microenviron.* **2019**, *12*, 105–118. [CrossRef] [PubMed]
52. Maze, E.A.; Agit, B.; Reeves, S.; Hilton, D.A.; Parkinson, D.B.; Laraba, L.; Ercolano, E.; Kurian, K.M.; Hanemann, C.O.; Belshaw, R.D.; et al. Human Endogenous Retrovirus Type K Promotes Proliferation and Confers Sensitivity to Antiretroviral Drugs in Merlin-Negative Schwannoma and Meningioma. *Cancer Res.* **2022**, *82*, 235–247. [CrossRef]
53. Paskas, S.; Mazzon, E.; Basile, M.S.; Cavalli, E.; Al-Abed, Y.; He, M.; Rakocevic, S.; Nicoletti, F.; Mijatovic, S.; Maksimovic-Ivanic, D. Lopinavir-NO, a Nitric Oxide-Releasing HIV Protease Inhibitor, Suppresses the Growth of Melanoma Cells in Vitro and in Vivo. *Investig. New Drugs* **2019**, *37*, 1014–1028. [CrossRef] [PubMed]
54. Jiang, W.; Mikochik, P.J.; Ra, J.H.; Lei, H.; Flaherty, K.T.; Winkler, J.D.; Spitz, F.R. HIV Protease Inhibitor Nelfinavir Inhibits Growth of Human Melanoma Cells by Induction of Cell Cycle Arrest. *Cancer Res.* **2007**, *67*, 1221–1227. [CrossRef]

55. Landriscina, M.; Fabiano, A.; Altamura, S.; Bagalà, C.; Piscazzi, A.; Cassano, A.; Spadafora, C.; Giorgino, F.; Barone, C.; Cignarelli, M. Reverse Transcriptase Inhibitors Down-Regulate Cell Proliferation in Vitro and in Vivo and Restore Thyrotropin Signaling and Iodine Uptake in Human Thyroid Anaplastic Carcinoma. *J. Clin. Endocrinol. Metab.* **2005**, *90*, 5663–5671. [CrossRef]
56. Brzozowski, Z.; Saczewski, F.; Neamati, N. Synthesis, Antitumor and Anti-HIV Activities of Benzodithiazine-Dioxides. *Bioorg Med. Chem.* **2006**, *14*, 2985–2993. [CrossRef]
57. Mangiacasale, R.; Pittoggi, C.; Sciamanna, I.; Careddu, A.; Mattei, E.; Lorenzini, R.; Travaglini, L.; Landriscina, M.; Barone, C.; Nervi, C.; et al. Exposure of Normal and Transformed Cells to Nevirapine, a Reverse Transcriptase Inhibitor, Reduces Cell Growth and Promotes Differentiation. *Oncogene* **2003**, *22*, 2750–2761. [CrossRef] [PubMed]
58. Yang, Y.; Dong, S.; You, B.; Zhou, C. Dual Roles of Human Endogenous Retroviruses in Cancer Progression and Antitumor Immune Response. *Biochim. Biophys. Acta Rev. Cancer* **2024**, *1879*, 189201. [CrossRef]
59. Luebker, S.A.; Koepsell, S.A. Diverse Mechanisms of BRAF Inhibitor Resistance in Melanoma Identified in Clinical and Preclinical Studies. *Front. Oncol.* **2019**, *9*, 268. [CrossRef]
60. Serafino, A.; Balestrieri, E.; Pierimarchi, P.; Matteucci, C.; Moroni, G.; Oricchio, E.; Rasi, G.; Mastino, A.; Spadafora, C.; Garaci, E.; et al. The Activation of Human Endogenous Retrovirus K (HERV-K) Is Implicated in Melanoma Cell Malignant Transformation. *Exp. Cell Res.* **2009**, *315*, 849–862. [CrossRef]
61. Sanki, A.; Li, W.; Colman, M.; Karim, R.Z.; Thompson, J.F.; Scolyer, R.A. Reduced Expression of P16 and P27 Is Correlated with Tumour Progression in Cutaneous Melanoma. *Pathology* **2007**, *39*, 551–557. [CrossRef] [PubMed]
62. Sa, G.; Guo, Y.; Stacey, D.W. The Regulation of S Phase Initiation by p27Kip1 in NIH3T3 Cells. *Cell Cycle* **2005**, *4*, 618–627. [CrossRef] [PubMed]
63. Monahan, K.B.; Rozenberg, G.I.; Krishnamurthy, J.; Johnson, S.M.; Liu, W.; Bradford, M.K.; Horner, J.; Depinho, R.A.; Sharpless, N.E. Somatic P16(INK4a) Loss Accelerates Melanomagenesis. *Oncogene* **2010**, *29*, 5809–5817. [CrossRef] [PubMed]
64. Eriksson, S.; Kim, S.K.; Kubista, M.; Nordén, B. Binding of 4′,6-Diamidino-2-Phenylindole (DAPI) to AT Regions of DNA: Evidence for an Allosteric Conformational Change. *Biochemistry* **1993**, *32*, 2987–2998. [CrossRef]
65. Cardile, A.; Zanrè, V.; Campagnari, R.; Asson, F.; Addo, S.S.; Orlandi, E.; Menegazzi, M. Hyperforin Elicits Cytostatic/Cytotoxic Activity in Human Melanoma Cell Lines, Inhibiting Pro-Survival NF-κB, STAT3, AP1 Transcription Factors and the Expression of Functional Proteins Involved in Mitochondrial and Cytosolic Metabolism. *Int. J. Mol. Sci.* **2023**, *24*, 1263. [CrossRef]

International Journal of
Molecular Sciences

MDPI

Article

Quercetin Impairs the Growth of Uveal Melanoma Cells by Interfering with Glucose Uptake and Metabolism

Aysegül Tura *, Viktoria Herfs, Tjorge Maaßen, Huaxin Zuo, Siranush Vardanyan, Michelle Prasuhn, Mahdy Ranjbar, Vinodh Kakkassery and Salvatore Grisanti

Department of Ophthalmology, University of Lübeck, Ratzeburger Allee 160, 23562 Luebeck, Germany; v.herfs@gmx.de (V.H.); tjorge.maassen@web.de (T.M.); zuohuaxin@163.com (H.Z.); sirivardanyan@gmail.com (S.V.); michelle.prasuhn@uksh.de (M.P.); vinodh.kakkassery@uni-luebeck.de (V.K.); salvatore.grisanti@uksh.de (S.G.)

* Correspondence: ayseguel.tura@uni-luebeck.de; Tel.: +49-451-500-43987

Abstract: Monosomy 3 in uveal melanoma (UM) increases the risk of lethal metastases, mainly in the liver, which serves as the major site for the storage of excessive glucose and the metabolization of the dietary flavonoid quercetin. Although primary UMs with monosomy 3 exhibit a higher potential for basal glucose uptake, it remains unknown as to whether glycolytic capacity is altered in such tumors. Herein, we initially analyzed the expression of n = 151 genes involved in glycolysis and its interconnected branch, the "pentose phosphate pathway (PPP)", in the UM cohort of The Cancer Genome Atlas Study and validated the differentially expressed genes in two independent cohorts. We also evaluated the effects of quercetin on the growth, survival, and glucose metabolism of the UM cell line 92.1. The rate-limiting glycolytic enzyme *PFKP* was overexpressed whereas the *ZBTB20* gene (locus: 3q13.31) was downregulated in the patients with metastases in all cohorts. Quercetin was able to impair proliferation, viability, glucose uptake, glycolysis, ATP synthesis, and PPP rate-limiting enzyme activity while increasing oxidative stress. UMs with monosomy 3 display a stronger potential to utilize glucose for the generation of energy and biomass. Quercetin can prevent the growth of UM cells by interfering with glucose metabolism.

Keywords: uveal melanoma; glycolysis; pentose phosphate pathway; quercetin; glucose uptake; proliferation; oxidative stress

1. Introduction

Despite the advances in the local control of primary uveal melanoma (UM), approximately half of UM patients develop metastases, mainly in the liver, which sadly results in a very short average survival time of less than six months [1–3]. The risk of metastasis is particularly high for primary UM cells that exhibit the loss of one copy of chromosome 3 (monosomy 3) [4,5]. Similarly, the presence of monosomy 3 in the metastasized UMs has been associated with more rapid disease progression [6]. However, the molecular mechanisms and pathophysiological factors that give rise to aggressive UM metastases remain incompletely understood, which impedes the development of efficient therapies.

Interestingly, UM patients exhibited an insulin-resistant serum profile with a slight but significant increase in their fasting glucose levels compared to age-matched controls [7]. Moreover, the basal level of glucose uptake in UM cells may be influenced by chromosome 3 status, as suggested by the increased metabolic activity of monosomy 3 tumors in fluorodeoxyglucose positron emission tomography scans [8,9]. We have also recently reported the upregulation of the high-affinity glucose transporter GLUT1 in primary UMs with monosomy 3, possibly as a compensation for the very-low-affinity glucose transporter GLUT2 [10], which is encoded by the *SLC2A2* gene on chromosome 3 [11]. These findings therefore highlight hyperglycemia and the increased potency for glucose influx as novel pathophysiological factors that may aggravate the course of UM. Yet, it is still not well known as to how glucose is mainly processed inside UM cells and whether the presence of monosomy 3 confers a growth advantage through the modulation of glucose metabolism to address cellular demands more efficiently.

Proliferating cells need to have high biosynthetic activity to increase their biomass and replicate their genome. The cells should therefore maintain the influx of oxygen and nutrients at a sufficient rate to generate energy in the form of adenosine triphosphate (ATP) and conduct biosynthetic reactions. However, the rapidly proliferating solid malignancies may overgrow their blood supply, with them becoming progressively deprived of oxygen and nutrients. Cancer cells adapt to such conditions by preferentially executing glycolysis instead of oxidative phosphorylation even in the presence of oxygen, which is known as the Warburg effect [12–18].

The production of ATP via glycolysis may initially appear to be an inefficient form of metabolism due to the lower energetic yield obtained from each glucose molecule compared to oxidative phosphorylation [15,17,18]. However, glycolysis can be completed at a rate that may be up to 100 times faster than oxidative phosphorylation [19]. Glycolysis can therefore enable the rapid production of sufficient ATP as long as the cells are provided abundantly with glucose [17]. In addition, glycolysis generates metabolic intermediates that can be diverted into the "pentose-phosphate-pathway" (PPP) in a reversible manner for the production of biosynthetic materials depending on cellular needs [17].

The PPP is divided into branches that produce the nucleotide precursor ribose-5-phosphate and the cofactor NADPH, which serves as a reducing agent during the biosynthesis of lipids and amino acids. NADPH also enables the regeneration of glutathione, which is essential for protection against the reactive oxygen species that are mainly produced during oxidative phosphorylation [17,19–21]. Tumor cells may exploit these pathways as suggested by the overexpression of the rate-limiting enzymes of glycolysis and the PPP in malignant diseases such as lung, liver, colorectal, prostate, breast, and cervical cancer [17,20,21]. Despite the association between several glycolysis-associated genes and poor survival in UM [22–24], it is not known whether the potential for the glycolytic switch is altered in monosomy 3 tumors and whether the glycolysis–PPP axis in UM cells can be modulated by natural compounds.

Flavonoids are bioactive plant molecules that are present in a wide variety of foods and drinks such as fruits, vegetables, herbs, spices, teas, and wine. Quercetin is the most abundant dietary flavonoid, with many of its natural sources being included in the Mediterranean diet [25,26]. Quercetin is able to exert beneficial effects against inflammation, insulin resistance, and hyperglycemia in animal models [27,28]. Quercetin also demonstrated promising anti-carcinogenic potential by suppressing the metastatic activities of various tumor cells [25,26,29–31] while protecting normal cells from the side effects of chemotherapy and radiotherapy in preclinical studies [29,31]. The cytotoxic effect of quercetin was higher in the aggressive tumor cells compared to the slowly growing ones [30]. In addition, quercetin was able to inhibit aerobic glycolysis in diverse tumor cells [18,32,33] and suppress the self-renewal capacity of cancer stem cells [31]. Despite its well-established antioxidant effect, quercetin can also function as a pro-oxidant at high concentrations by depleting the glutathione reserves in cancer cells [18,34]. However, it remains unknown whether quercetin can suppress the growth of UM cells.

In this study, we initially determined the expression profile of the major genes involved in glycolysis and the PPP in the UM cohort of The Cancer Genome Atlas (TCGA) Study and validated the differentially expressed genes in two independent, publicly available cohorts. We also analyzed the growth, survival, and glucose metabolism of the UM cell line 92.1 in response to quercetin.

2. Results

2.1. Expression of the Genes Involved in Glycolysis and the PPP with Regard to Monosomy 3 Status and Metastases in the UM-Cohort of the TCGA Study

We initially assembled a list of $n = 151$ human genes that are involved in glycolysis and the PPP using the Gene Ontology (GO) and Reactome databases. The gene list also included the "lactate (transmembrane) transport" (Supplementary Table S1).

In the UM cohort of the TCGA study, a total of $n = 67$ genes (44.4%) were differentially expressed with regard to the copy number of chromosome 3, with $n = 27$ genes (17.9%) retaining significance after multiple hypothesis testing (Supplementary Table S2). Among the latter group, $n = 5$ genes were also significantly associated with the development of metastases (p-adjusted < 0.05, Figure 1A, Supplementary Table S2). The genes that were upregulated in the monosomy 3/metastatic tumors (*PFKP*, *NUP88*) exhibited an average fold change (FC) of 2.06 ± 0.82, whereas the downregulated genes (*INSR*, *RBKS*, and *ZBTB20*) differed by an average of -1.87 ± 0.44-fold (Figure 1B).

An unbiased gene set enrichment was performed for the differentially expressed genes. The most relevant biological processes, pathways, and phenotypes involved the "positive regulation of the glycolytic and purine nucleotide metabolic pathways", "phosphofructokinase activity", "insulin-like growth factor II/I/AMP binding", "Pentose phosphate/HIF-1/AMPK pathways", "galactose, fructose, and mannose metabolism", "insulin receptor substrate activation", "signal attenuation/insulin receptor recycling", and "diabetes (type 2)" (Figure 1C).

2.2. Validation of the Differentially Expressed Genes

Validation of differential gene expression was performed using the normalized microarray data of two independent studies which are publicly available in the Gene Expression Omnibus (GEO) database. The first study involved the total RNA isolated from the primary tumors of $n = 63$ UM patients ($n = 24$ females; $n = 39$ males) with an average age of 61.0 ± 12.3 years (GEO accession number: GSE22138). Systemic metastases developed in $n = 35$ of these patients (55.6%). The second microarray study included the primary tumors of $n = 57$ patients with $n = 25$ females and $n = 32$ males. Metastases were detected in 56.1% ($n = 32$) of these patients (GEO accession number: GSE44295).

Expression of the *PFKP* and *ZBTB20* genes was significantly altered with regard to the metastases in the validation cohorts. *PFKP* (locus: 10p15.2) was positively associated with the development of metastases, whereas the *ZBTB20* gene (locus: 3q13.31) was downregulated in the metastatic tumors (p-raw < 0.05, Figure 2A).

Further analysis of the validated genes revealed significant associations between the expression of *PFKP* or *ZBTB20* and the survival rate and multiple prognostic factors in the UM cohort of the TCGA study. The upregulation of *PFKP* and the downregulation of *ZBTB20* were correlated with shorter overall and disease-specific survival, an epithelioid morphology, heavy pigmentation, and the presence of closed loops. *PFKP* was also positively associated with tumor diameter and extrascleral extension whereas the tumors with *ZBTB20* deficiency exhibited a more diffuse rather than focal pattern of macrophage infiltration (Figure 2B,C).

2.3. Anti-Proliferative and Pro-Oxidant Effects of Quercetin on the Cultured UM Cells

Based on the findings of our gene expression analysis, which highlighted glucose metabolism as a crucial factor that may be involved in the aggressive growth of UM cells, we next focused on the inhibitory potential of quercetin on metabolic activity, proliferation, survival, and redox state in the UM cell line 92.1. Incubation of the 92.1 cells with quercetin for three days induced a significant, dose-dependent reduction in the number of metabolically active cells, with an IC50 of quercetin at 44.05 µM (Figure 3A,B, $p < 0.001$ for all groups, Kruskal–Wallis test). This effect was associated with the down-regulation of the proliferation marker Ki67 and a 69% decline in the incorporation of BrdU in response to 50 µM quercetin compared to the solvent control (Figure 3C,D, $p < 0.05$ for all groups, Kruskal–Wallis test). Incubation with 50 μM quercetin also reduced the ratio of live/dead cells by approximately 36% (Figure 3E,F, $p < 0.01$ for all groups, one-way analysis of variance) and increased the accumulation of reactive oxygen species (ROS) by two-fold (Figure 3G,H, $p = 0.049$, Mann–Whitney U test) compared to the solvent control.

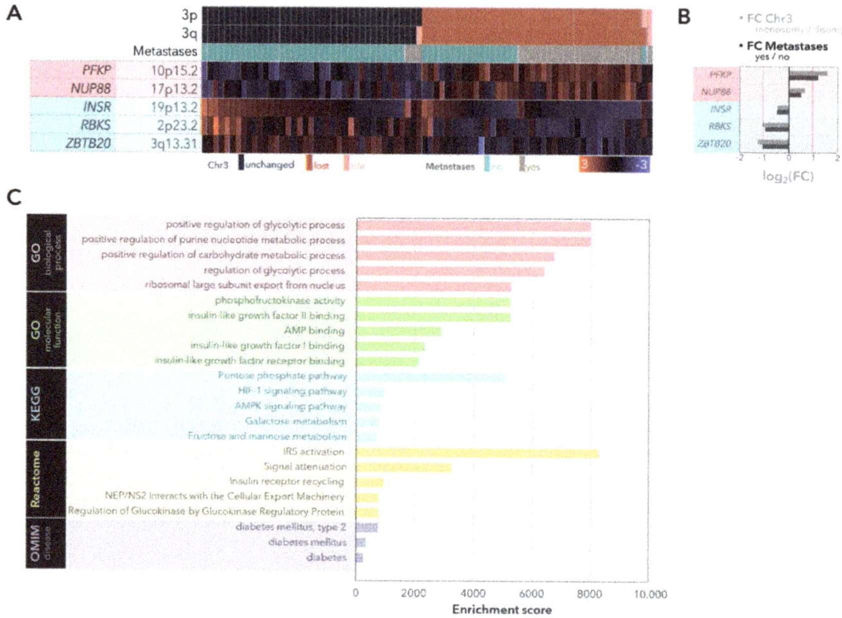

Figure 1. Differentially expressed genes in the monosomy 3 and metastatic tumors of the TCGA-UM cohort (n = 80 patients). (**A**) The tumor samples were aligned according to the copy numbers of chromosome 3p and 3q (dark blue: normal, red: loss) as well as the metastatic status in the uppermost three rows. The expression heatmap was constructed using the z-scores, with red and blue indicating mRNA levels that were up to three standard deviations above or below the mean (black), respectively. The gene symbols and loci are stated on the left. All of the genes had an adjusted p-value < 0.05 with regard to the copy number of chromosome 3 and metastases. n/a: Not available. (**B**) Fold changes (FC) of median gene expression in the monosomy 3 tumors and patients with metastases. The up- and downregulated genes are highlighted with a red or blue background, respectively. The red lines indicate an FC of |2|. Chr3: Chromosome 3. (**C**) Gene set enrichment analysis demonstrating the biological pathways and phenotypes that were over-represented among the differentially expressed genes. All of the p-values and false discovery rates were <0.05. For simplicity, the five most enriched processes or pathways were demonstrated for the Gene Ontology (GO), KEGG, and Reactome databases.

2.4. Suppression of Glucose Uptake and Metabolism in the UM Cells in Response to Quercetin

Having determined the optimal concentration of quercetin for the suppression of metabolic activity in the 92.1 cells, we next evaluated the outcomes of quercetin treatment on different aspects of glucose metabolism, such as glucose intake, glycolytic rate, ATP production, PPP activity, and glutathione levels. Incubation of the 92.1 cells with 50 μM quercetin made it possible to significantly reduce the uptake of the fluorescent glucose analog 6-NBDG by approximately 32–36% compared to the solvent or untreated controls ($p = 0.041$, Kruskal–Wallis test, Figure 4A,B). Quercetin could also suppress the glycolytic rate by approximately 45–48% within 3 h and ATP production by 21–25% after 2 days compared to the untreated and solvent controls ($p = 0.010$ and $p = 0.009$, respectively, one-way analysis of variance, Figure 4C,D). The activity of the glucose-6-phosphate dehydrogenase (G6PDH), which serves as the rate-limiting enzyme of the PPP [17,20,21], underwent an approximately 20–22% decrease in response to 50 μM quercetin compared to the untreated and solvent controls after 11–13 h ($p < 0.05$, Mann–Whitney U test with respect to the untreated or solvent controls, Figure 4E). We also observed a slight but significant decline of 8.4% in the levels of total glutathione after incubation with 50 μM quercetin for 7–10 h compared to the untreated or solvent controls ($p < 0.05$, Mann–Whitney U test, Figure 4F).

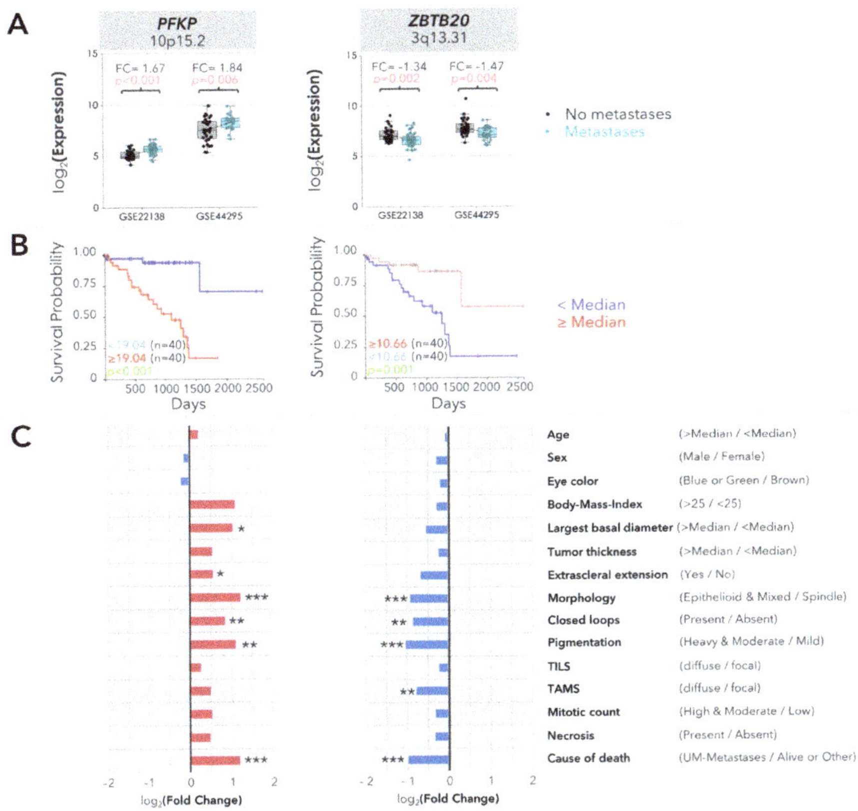

Figure 2. Validation of gene expression in two independent cohorts and the correlation of validated genes with prognostic factors. (**A**) The expression of *PFKP* and *ZBTB20* with regard to the metastases in the GSE22138 and GSE44295 cohorts is presented as boxplots. The mean values are connected by the sloped lines. For the GSE22138 cohort, the average expression of all of the available isoforms is presented (n = 2 isoforms for *PFKP*; n = 12 isoforms for *ZBTB20*). FC: fold change of median gene expression in the patients with metastases. The raw p-values were determined using the Mann–Whitney U test. Gene loci were indicated underneath the gene symbols. (**B**) The probability of overall survival with regard to the expression of *PFKP* and *ZBTB20* in the primary UMs of the TCGA cohort is demonstrated by the Kaplan–Meier curves. The median gene expression was taken as the cut-off value. p-values were determined via the log-rank test. (**C**) Expression of *PFKP* and *ZBTB20* with regard to the clinical and histopathological factors in the UM cohort of the TCGA study is presented as bar charts. The fold change of median gene expression in the subgroup with the unfavorable condition was calculated based on the classification of the prognostic factors according to the categories indicated in parentheses. The $\log_2$(Fold Change) values above or below 0 were depicted in pink or blue, respectively. TILS: tumor-infiltrating lymphocytes, TAMS: tumor-activated macrophages. The raw p-values were determined using the Mann–Whitney U test. * $p < 0.05$, ** $p < 0.005$, and *** $p < 0.001$.

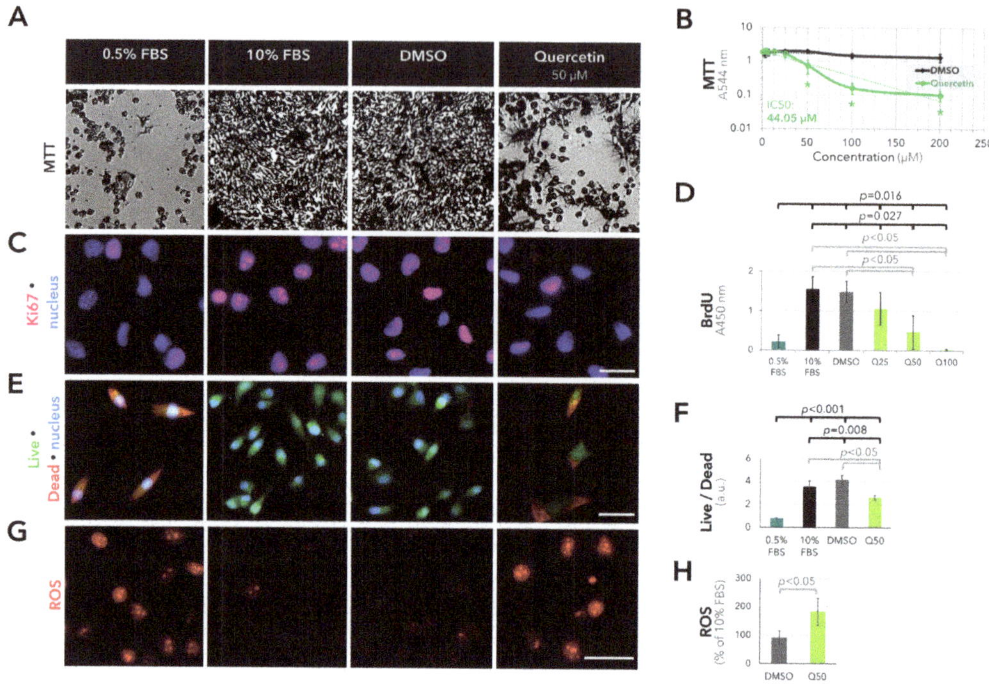

Figure 3. Quercetin suppresses the viability and proliferation of UM cells by increasing oxidative stress. (**A**) Representative light microscopy images of the UM cells after 3-day incubation with the substances indicated above followed by the MTT dye. A group of cells were incubated in culture medium with 0.5% fetal bovine serum (FBS) as the positive control for growth factor deprivation. A separate group of cells were incubated with the solvent of quercetin (dimethylsulfoxide; DMSO) at the same volume required for the administration of quercetin. (**B**) Quantification of the MTT assay (mean $\pm$ standard deviation (SD) of n = 4–5 independent experiments). The exponential trendlines were fitted and indicated in a dashed pattern in dark gray or green for DMSO or quercetin, respectively. Quercetin exhibited an IC50 of approximately 44.05 µM that was calculated from its respective trendline. * $p < 0.05$ for the pairwise comparison of the quercetin treatment to the corresponding solvent control, Mann–Whitney U test. (**C**) Representative images of immunofluorescence staining for the proliferation marker Ki67 (red) after 3 days. Nuclei were counterstained with DAPI (blue). Scale bar = 25 µm. (**D**) BrdU-assay demonstrating the dose-dependent anti-proliferative effect of quercetin after 3 days (mean $\pm$ SD of n = 3 independent experiments). p-values were determined through the use of the Mann–Whitney U or Kruskal–Wallis tests for pairwise or collective comparisons, respectively. (**E**) Representative images of the live/dead assay after 3 days. Scale bar = 50 µm. (**F**) Ratio of the live/dead intensity (mean $\pm$ SD of n = 3 wells from a representative experiment). p-values were assessed using the two-sided t-test or one-way analysis of variance for pairwise or collective comparisons, respectively. (**G**) Representative images demonstrating the accumulation of reactive oxygen species (ROS) in the cells treated with 50 µM quercetin for 12–13 h. Scale bar = 50 µm. (**H**) Quantification of the ROS intensity (mean $\pm$ SD of n = 3 independent experiments, Mann–Whitney U test).

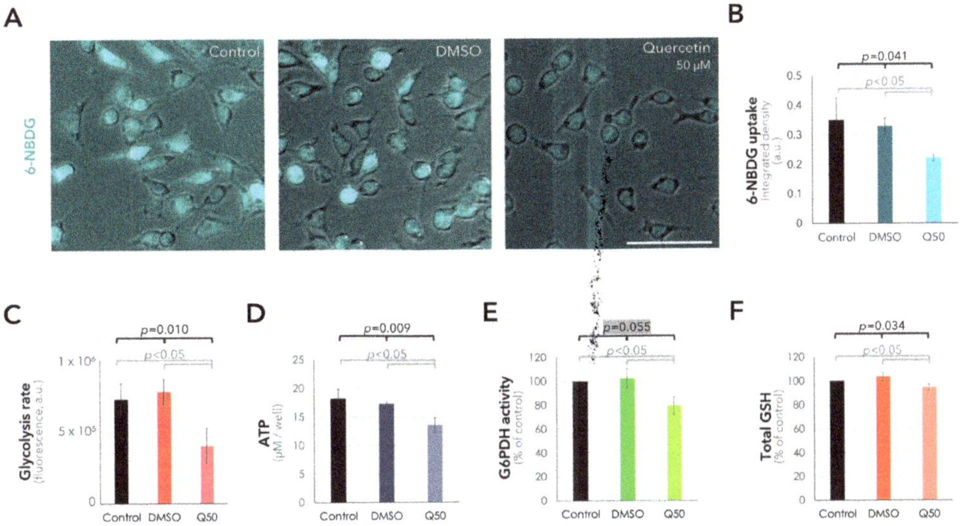

Figure 4. Quercetin interferes with glucose uptake and metabolism in the UM cells. (**A**) Representative images demonstrating the uptake of the fluorescent glucose analog 6-NBDG in the cells incubated with the normal medium alone (control) and with the supplementation of 50 µM quercetin or its solvent DMSO. The overlay images of fluorescence and phase-contrast microscopy are presented to demonstrate the cell boundaries. Scale bar = 100 µm. (**B**) Quantification of 6-NBDG uptake (mean ± SD of n = 3–4 independent experiments, a.u.: arbitrary units, Q50: 50 µM quercetin,). (**C**) Quantification of the fluorometric glycolysis assay, demonstrating the significant reduction in the glycolytic rate in response to quercetin after 3 h (mean ± SD of n = 3 independent experiments). (**D**) The luminescent ATP-assay, demonstrating the reduction in ATP levels in the cells incubated with 50 µM quercetin for 2 days (mean ± SD of n = 3 independent experiments). (**E**) Activity of the glucose-6-phosphate dehydrogenase (G6PDH), which functions as the rate-limiting enzyme of the PPP [17,20,21], as determined by a colorimetric assay after exposing the cells for 11–13 h to the indicated treatments (mean ± SD of n = 3 independent experiments). G6PDH activity was normalized to the amount of total protein extracted from each group. The insignificant p-value above 0.05 is highlighted with a gray background. (**F**) Quantification of the total glutathione (GSH) levels after 7–10 h (mean ± SD of n = 3 independent experiments). In panels (**B–E**), all of the pairwise comparisons were evaluated via the Mann–Whitney U test whereas the collective comparisons of the three subgroups were performed with the Kruskal–Wallis test (**B**,**E**,**F**) or one-way analysis of variance (**C**,**D**).

2.5. Outcomes of Quercetin Treatment on the Expression of the PFKP and ZBTB20 Proteins in the UM Cells

To elucidate whether the validated, glucose-related genes are involved in the suppressive effects of quercetin on glucose metabolism, we also analyzed the expression of the PFKP and ZBTB20 proteins via immunocytochemistry and blotting in the UM cells that were incubated with or without 50 µM quercetin or DMSO for 1 day. Our results demonstrated uniform expression of both proteins regardless of the treatment, suggesting that quercetin does not exert a significant influence on the levels of these proteins (Figure 5).

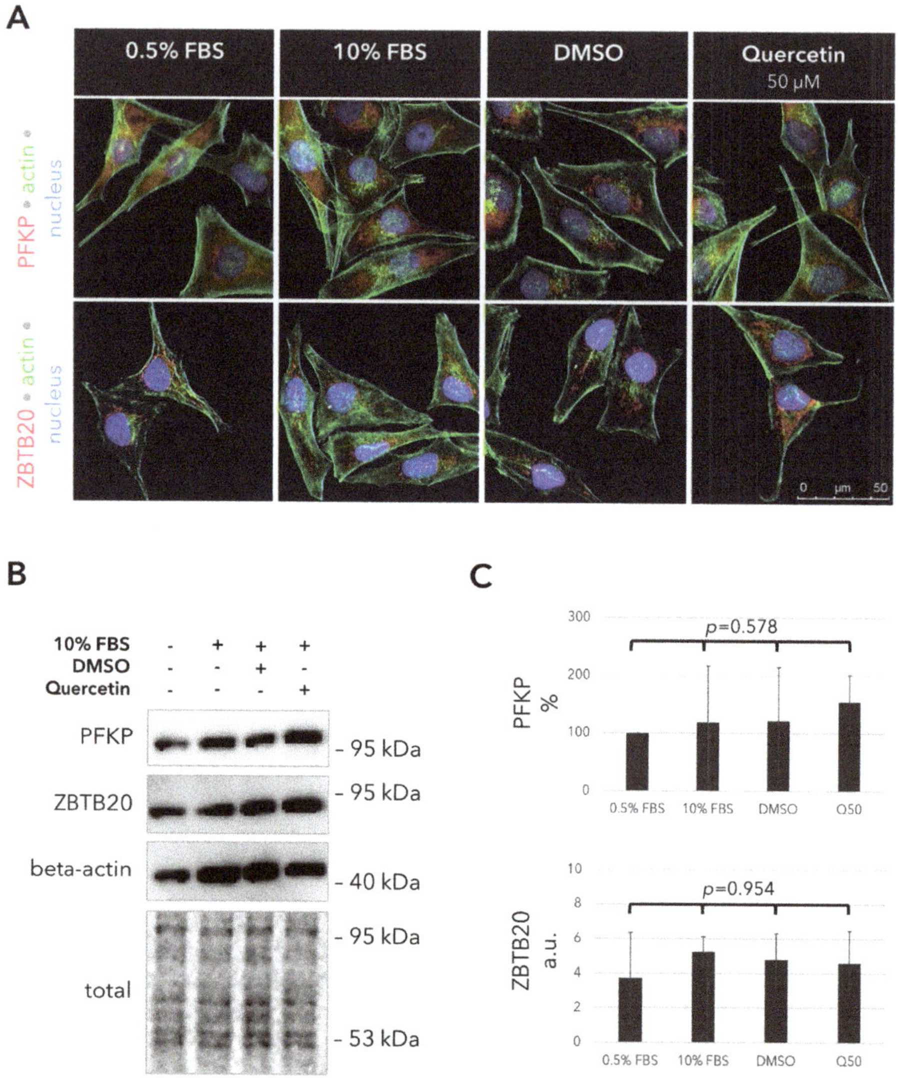

Figure 5. Expression of the PFKP and ZBTB20 proteins in response to quercetin after 1 day. (**A**) Representative images of the fluorescent immunostainings for PFKP and ZBTB20 (red). The actin filaments were visualized via Alexa 488-phalloidin staining (green). Nuclei were counterstained with DAPI (blue). (**B**) Immunoblotting for PFKP and ZBTB20. Quercetin was administered at a concentration of 50 µM. Membranes were probed for beta-actin as a loading control. The total amount of protein in each well is also depicted for a more comprehensive evaluation of sample loading. kDa: Kilodalton. (**C**) Quantification of the PFKP and ZBTB20 levels in the immunoblots, which were normalized to the total protein loadings in each well. The PFKP levels are stated as the percentage of the 0.5% FBS group. a.u.: arbitrary units. Data represent the mean ± standard deviation of $n = 3$ independent experiments. p-values were evaluated with the Kruskal–Wallis test for the simultaneous comparison of all subgroups.

3. Discussion

The prevention of lethal UM metastases remains an unresolved clinical need, which sadly leaves affected patients with a very short survival time of several months. In this study, we provide the first evidence that primary UMs with higher metastatic potential exhibit a greater glycolytic gene expression profile, whereas the incubation of the UM cell line 92.1 with the dietary flavonoid quercetin could suppress cell growth by interfering with glucose uptake and metabolism.

Our gene expression analysis demonstrated the overexpression of *PFKP* in the aggressive UM samples from three independent cohorts, whereas the *ZBTB20* gene was significantly downregulated in the tumors that developed metastases. The *PFKP* gene on chromosome 10p15.2 encodes the platelet isoform of phosphofructokinase, which serves as the most important rate-limiting enzyme of glycolysis by catalyzing the irreversible phosphorylation of fructose-6-phosphate to fructose-1,6-biphosphate [35,36]. Moreover, the silencing of *PFKP* resulted in a reduction in PPP activity and nucleotide biosynthesis in renal cancer cells [36]. The overexpression of *PFKP* may therefore be providing the UMs with monosomy 3 a growth advantage by channeling the glucose metabolites towards glycolysis or the PPP depending on the metabolic demands and cellular priorities. The phosphofructokinase isoforms are also upregulated in diverse tumors and regarded as potential therapeutic targets [35–37]. Enhanced glycolytic metabolism was also detected in the T cells with deficiency in the transcriptional repressor ZBTB20 [38], which is encoded by a gene on chromosome 3q13.31. However, there is conflicting evidence regarding the function of ZBTB20 in tumorigenesis, with the overexpression of this protein noted in hepatocellular carcinoma [39]. ZBTB20 could also promote the invasion of various tumor cells, including glioblastoma and breast and gastric cancers [40–42]. Further research is therefore required to elucidate the functional consequences of *ZBTB20* downregulation in UMs with monosomy 3. Interestingly, the silencing of *Zbtb20* was associated with a slight increase in the expression of phosphofructokinase in mouse liver cells, which failed to reach significance [43]. It would therefore be interesting to analyze whether the deficiency in *ZBTB20* mRNA promotes the overexpression of *PFKP* in UM cells or whether the upregulation of *PFKP* is a response to the higher rate of glucose influx into monosomy 3 tumors.

Our preliminary findings also demonstrate the anti-proliferative and toxic effects of the dietary flavonoid quercetin in the UM cell line 92.1 via interference with glucose metabolism. For instance, the extent of glucose uptake was lowered by approximately 25–30%, whereas the rate of glycolysis underwent an almost 50% reduction in response to quercetin. The more profound inhibitory effect of quercetin on the latter event suggests that this flavonoid may be interfering with certain glycolytic enzymes or their regulators. However, we did not observe a significant change in the expression of the PFKP and ZBTB20 proteins in response to quercetin. It therefore remains to be determined whether the activity rather than the total levels of these proteins or other glycolytic enzymes is influenced by quercetin in UM cells. The suppressive effects of quercetin on glucose metabolism also deserve further analysis with regard to the paralogous genes *GNAQ* or *GNA11*, which undergo activating mutations in 80–90% of UMs [44,45]. The somatic mutations in *GNAQ/GNA11*, which usually occur in a mutually exclusive pattern, can initiate UM tumorigenesis via the constitutive activation of the alpha-subunits of the heterotrimeric G proteins Gq or G11, respectively [44,45]. Remarkably, oncogenic Gq/G11 signaling was recently reported as the major driver of metabolic reprogramming in UM cells via the promotion of glucose uptake, glycolysis, and mitochondrial respiration [45]. Since 92.1 cells harbor the Q209L-activating mutation in *GNAQ* [46], it would be very interesting to evaluate the inhibitory potential of quercetin on the aberrant Gq signaling in UM in future studies.

Our study entails several limitations, such as the administration of quercetin at the single dose of 50 μM in the majority of our experiments. Although this dosage was selected as the optimal concentration based on the screening of metabolic activity via the MTT assay, it may not have been sufficient to interfere with all of the cellular events that we analyzed at the same efficacy. Moreover, the incubation period with quercetin varied from 30 min to three days among the different assays, which complicated the interpretation of the treatment outcomes. Three-day incubation was preferred to evaluate the long-term effects of quercetin on metabolic activity, proliferation, and survival. For the remaining assays, we incubated the cells for shorter periods based on the assay principle and/or previous data regarding the influence of quercetin on the cellular event of interest. For instance, the glucose uptake and glycolytic rate were evaluated through exposure of the cells to the test conditions for 30 min or 3 h, respectively, based on the recommendations of the assay manufacturers. To analyze G6PDH activity, glutathione reserves, and ROS accumulation, we preferred the incubation periods of 7–13 h based on a previous study, which reported the time-dependent effects of quercetin on glutathione levels in human aortic endothelial cells. In the aforementioned work, quercetin resulted in a temporal increase in the ratio of total glutathione (GSH) to the oxidized form (GSSG), which reached a peak after 6 h despite the significant decrease in the levels of both the total and oxidized glutathione [47]. Regarding the ATP reserves, we selected an incubation time of 2 days to gain insight into the energetic status of UM cells after long-term exposure to quercetin. For this assay, we also needed to normalize the results based on the amount of cellular material, which deviated substantially among the treatment groups owing to differences in the proliferation and survival rate over extended periods. However, we could not evaluate the protein concentration of the cellular lysates as a control for equal cellular material due to the interference of the lysis buffer of the ATP assay with the protein quantification reagents, as stated by the manufacturer. We therefore quantified the number of cells in each group for the normalization of the ATP levels. Based on these factors, we considered the incubation period of 2 days more appropriate to reduce the confounding effects of proliferation and survival in the ATP assay while providing the cells sufficient time to respond to the test conditions. A further limitation of our study is the utilization of a single cell line. Future studies with validated UM cell lines from different donors as well as normal control cells such as choroidal melanocytes, fibroblasts, or normal skin cells would therefore provide deeper insight into the therapeutic potential and safety of quercetin for the management of UM. The time- and dose-dependent effects of quercetin treatment on different aspects of glucose metabolism also deserve further investigation.

Quercetin is usually available as glycosylated isoforms which are conjugated to sugars like glucose or rutinose. Earlier studies have reported that quercetin glycosides can compete with glucose to pass through the energy-dependent or -independent glucose transporters SGLT-1 or GLUT1, respectively, interfering with glucose influx [48,49]. The free, aglycone form of quercetin, which we used in our study, could also reduce glucose uptake in Caco-2 cells, although to a lesser extent compared to the glycosylated isoforms [50]. It would therefore be very interesting to determine the glucose transporters that are targeted by the quercetin aglycone in UM cells in future studies, with particular focus on the GLUT family of energy-independent transporters [11,51].

Our findings further demonstrate a reduction in ATP production of approximately 22% in response to quercetin. The magnitude of this effect also remained lower than the 50% decrease in the glycolytic rate, suggesting that the quercetin-treated UM cells may be switching to mitochondrial metabolism to compensate for the energy shortage. However, an earlier study reported that UM cells with monosomy 3 exhibit a higher capacity for mitochondrial function [52]. A certain level of mitochondrial respiration could also promote the growth of UM cells [53]. Although these findings may initially appear to contradict our results, hyperactivity of mitochondria for prolonged periods can intensify oxidative stress [54]. This may also account for the almost two-fold increase in the levels of reactive oxygen species, which mainly arise as by-products of oxidative phosphorylation, in the quercetin-treated UM cells in our study. Although low concentrations of reactive oxygen species may promote cell proliferation by acting as second messengers, the massive accumulation of oxidative stress may overwhelm the repair capacity of cells, resulting in growth arrest or cell death [55]. Interestingly, the reactive oxygen species and mitochondrial activity were diminished in mesothelioma cells or human fibroblasts, respectively, with the inactivating mutations of the tumor suppressor *BAP1* [56,57]. Deficiency in BAP1, which is encoded by a gene on chromosome 3, is a significant prognostic factor which is associated with a higher metastatic risk in UM patients [5]. The influence of BAP1 depletion and quercetin treatment on the mitochondrial activity of UM cells therefore merits future investigation.

In our study, the activity of G6PDH, which serves as the rate-limiting enzyme of the PPP [17,20,21,58], underwent an approximately 30% decline in response to quercetin. Interference with PPP activity may also account for the mild but significant decrease of approximately 8.4% in the levels of total glutathione after quercetin treatment. The PPP plays a fundamental role in the cellular defense against oxidative stress by enabling the production of the co-factor NADPH, which acts as a reducing agent for the regeneration of glutathione [58]. However, NADPH can also be produced by alternative mechanisms that are mainly catalyzed by mitochondrial enzymes [59]. This compensation may therefore account for the modest inhibitory effect of quercetin on the levels of total glutathione as opposed to PPP activity, which deserves further examination.

In our present work, the effective dosage of quercetin on the 92.1 cell line was relatively high, with an IC50 of 44.1 µM. This concentration was in accordance with the findings of earlier studies, which reported the anticarcinogenic effects of quercetin at the optimal doses of approximately 20–160 µM in diverse tumor cell lines derived from ovarian, breast, and hepatocellular carcinomas [60–62]. In our study, quercetin was administered in RPMI-1640 medium, which is hyperglycemic with a glucose concentration of 11 mM. To simulate an insulin-resistant rather than a diabetic environment, UM cells can be maintained under milder or transiently hyperglycemic conditions. To mimic the regular intake of a quercetin-rich diet in vitro, UM cells can also be exposed to lower doses of quercetin for longer periods in future studies.

The bioavailability of quercetin has remained a concern due to the low solubility and absorption of this flavonoid. After ingestion, the lipophilic aglycone form of quercetin can diffuse passively from the intestinal lumen through the enterocytes, with it being absorbed into the hepatic portal vein. In contrast, the lipophobic glycosides of quercetin need to be converted to the aglycone form in the intestinal lumen or enterocytes before being absorbed into the hepatic portal vein. The quercetin aglycone then undergoes further metabolization in the liver before being distributed to other body tissues [63]. Interestingly, the hepatic portal vein may also serve as the major entry route of the disseminated UM cells into the liver, because the liver receives the majority of its blood supply via this vessel [64]. The regular intake of a quercetin-rich diet would therefore increase the abundance of this flavonoid in the portal vein and liver, which may create a less permissive microenvironment for the hepatic micrometastasis of UM.

To enhance the bioavailability of quercetin, this flavonoid can also be administered as a dietary supplement, which usually range between doses of 150 and 5000 mg [63]. The intake of 150–730 mg quercetin aglycone per day could indeed significantly reduce the blood pressure of hypertensive individuals [65]. A supplement of up to 5000 mg of quercetin per day for 4 weeks was also reported to be safe without adverse effects in clinical studies [63,66]. Assuming the complete absorption and metabolization of the ingested quercetin (molecular weight: 302.236 g/mole), the daily intake of 76 mg of quercetin would be necessary to reach a plasma concentration of 50 µM in a total blood volume of 5 L. It may therefore be feasible to reach the optimal concentration of quercetin through dietary supplements, which needs to be verified in future studies with animal models of UM metastasis.

4. Materials and Methods

4.1. Analysis of Gene Expression

The list of genes involved in glycolysis and/or the PPP was constructed using the Gene Ontology (http://geneontology.org/) and Reactome (https://reactome.org/) databases (accessed on 21 April 2021). The mRNA expression data of the UM cohort of the TCGA study were downloaded from the Xena platform of the University of California, Santa Cruz (https://xena.ucsc.edu/; accessed on 23 April 2021). Validation of gene expression was performed using the normalized microarray data of two independent studies available in the GEO database (https://www.ncbi.nlm.nih.gov/geo/; accession numbers: GSE22138 and GSE44295; accessed on 10 May 2021). Gene expression was presented in log_2-converted values. Fold changes were calculated from the mean expression values. Heatmaps were generated using the z-scores of gene expression. Kaplan–Meier curves were constructed using the UCSC Xena platform. The unbiased analysis of gene set enrichment was performed by using the Enrichr database [67].

4.2. Cell Culture and Test Substances

The UM cell line 92.1 was kindly provided by Prof. Martine J. Jager (Leiden University Medical Center, Leiden, the Netherlands), in whose laboratory this cell line was established [68]. The 92.1 cells were authenticated by the profiling of short tandem repeats in previous studies [46,69] and harbor the Q209L-activating mutation in *GNAQ* [46,69]. The cells were grown under normoxic conditions at 37 °C with 5% CO_2 in RPMI-1640 medium supplemented with 10% fetal bovine serum (FBS), 2 mM L-glutamine, 100 units/mL penicillin, and 100 µg/mL streptomycin (Life Technologies, Darmstadt, Germany) and passaged weekly via trypsinization.

Quercetin aglycone (Sigma-Aldrich, Darmstadt, Germany) was reconstituted in DMSO at 50 mM, stored as aliquots at −20 °C under light protection, and diluted in the culture medium at the indicated concentrations for the subsequent assays. The solvent controls were incubated with the culture medium that was supplemented with DMSO at the same volumes of quercetin. An additional group of cells were incubated in a low-serum medium with 0.5% FBS as a control for growth factor deprivation.

4.3. Immunocytochemistry

The cells were seeded into 8-well polycycloalkanes slides (Sarstedt, Nümbrecht, Germany) at a concentration of 10,000 cells/well, allowed to attach overnight, incubated with the test substances for 3 days at 37 °C with 5% CO_2, fixed with 2% paraformaldehyde in phosphate-buffered saline (PBS) for 10 min followed by 4% paraformaldehyde–PBS for 10 min, rinsed three times in PBS, and kept in the blocking buffer (3% bovine serum albumin in 10 mM Tris-HCl (pH = 7.5), 120 mM KCl, 20 mM NaCl, 5 mM ethylenediaminetetraacetic acid, and 0.1% Triton X-100) for 30 min. The cells were incubated with the rabbit primary antibodies against Ki67 (Abcam, Cambridge, UK, 1:1000 dilution in blocking buffer), PFKP (Proteintech Germany GmbH, St. Planegg-Martinsried, Germany; 1:200 dilution in blocking buffer), or ZBTB20 (Proteintech Germany GmbH, 1:200 dilution in blocking buffer) overnight at 4 °C followed by the Cy3-conjugated secondary anti-rabbit antibodies (Jackson Immunoresearch, Cambridgeshire, UK, catalog number: 111-165-003, 3.75 µg/mL in blocking buffer) for 1 h at room temperature and protected from light. In the samples that were processed for the detection of PFKP or ZBTB20, actin filaments were stained with Alexa 488-phalloidin (Invitrogen, Thermo Fisher Scientific, Waltham, MA, USA; 240 units/mL in blocking buffer) for 30 min. The nuclei were counterstained with 0.5 µg/mL 4′,6-diamidino-2-phenylindole (DAPI, 0.5 µg/mL in PBS) for 10 min, with the rinsing of cells three times in PBS after each step. The cells were mounted in Mowiol and stored at 4 °C. Images were acquired with a monochrome digital camera (DFC 350 FX; Leica Microsystems, Wetzlar, Germany) that was attached to a fluorescence microscope (Leica DMI 6000B) by using Leica Application Software (Advanced Fluorescence 2.3.0, build 5131) and the following filter sets: A4 (excitation: 360/40 nm; emission: 470/40 nm); L5 (excitation: 460/40 nm; emission: 527/30 nm); and Y3 (excitation: 545/30 nm; emission: 610/75 nm).

4.4. MTT Assay and IC50 Calculation

The cells were seeded into 96-well plates (5000 cells per well), allowed to attach overnight at 37 °C, and incubated with the test substances in triplicate for three days at 37 °C. The MTT dye solution was added at a final concentration of 0.5 mg/mL into each well except for the background controls, and the cells were incubated further for 3 h at 37 °C. The formazan crystals were solubilized by DMSO, and the absorption at 544 nm was measured with a spectrophotometer (FLUOstar Optima, BMG Labtech GmbH, Ortenberg, Germany). The mean absorbance was calculated for each group after background substraction.

For the calculation of IC50, a scatter plot was constructed with the concentrations of the test substances versus the absorbance values on the x- versus y-axes, respectively, by using Windows Excel (Version 2402). The y-axis was converted into the logarithmic scale. The IC50 of quercetin was calculated from the function of the exponential trendline that was fitted onto the respective curve.

4.5. Live/Dead Assay

The cells were seeded into flat-based 96-well plates with black polystyrene frames (Lumox® multiwell, Sarstedt, Germany) at a concentration of 8000 cells/well, allowed to attach overnight at 37 °C, and incubated with the test substances in quadruplicates for three days at 37 °C. The cells were then washed twice with PBS and incubated for 45 min at room temperature with the mixture of Calcein-AM and propidium iodide (ABP Biosciences, Beltville, MD, USA), which were diluted in PBS at the final concentrations of 2 µM and 4 µM, respectively. A single well per each group was left in PBS as the background control. The fluorescence intensities were measured by using a fluorometer (FLUOstar Optima) at the following wavelength settings: Calcein-AM—excitation: 485 nm, emission: 520 nm, and gain: 1100; propidium iodide—excitation: 544 nm, emission: 590 nm, and gain: 2300. The mean fluorescence in each group was calculated after substracting the corresponding background signals, and the ratio of the Calcein-AM/propidium iodide intensities was taken as the live/dead index per group. Prior to fluorescence microscopy, the nuclei were counterstained with 10 µg/mL DAPI in PBS for 10 min. Images of the cells were acquired by using an inverted fluorescence microscope (Leica DMI 6000B) by using the filter sets as described in the Immunocytochemistry section above.

4.6. BrdU Assay

The cells were seeded into 96-well plates at a concentration of 8000 cells/well, allowed to attach overnight, and incubated with the test substances for 3 days at 37 °C with 5% CO_2. Incorporation of BrdU into the DNA was measured with a colorimetric detection kit (Abcam, Berlin, Germany) by following the manufacturer's instructions. The cells were exposed to the BrdU reagent during the final 24 h of incubation. The cells that were incubated without the BrdU reagent served as the negative control. The absorbance values were read at 450 nm with a spectrophotometric microplate reader (FLUOstar Optima). The mean absorbance for each group was determined after subtracting the mean value of the negative control.

4.7. Measurement of Reactive Oxygen Species

The cells were seeded into flat-based 96-well plates with black polystyrene walls (Lumox® multiwell, Sarstedt, Germany) at a concentration of 30,000 cells/well, allowed to attach overnight at 37 °C and treated with the test substances in triplicate for 12–13 h at 37 °C with 5% CO_2. The cells were then incubated for 30 min at 37 °C with the MitoROS™ 580 reagent that was diluted in the assay buffer following the manufacturer's instructions (AAT Bioquest, Pleasanton, CA, USA). A single well per each group was left in normal test medium as the background control. The fluorescence intensities were measured from the well bottom by using a fluorometer (SpectraMax i3x; Molecular Devices, Munich, Germany) at an excitation of 540 nm and an emission of 590 nm, with a cutoff at 570 nm. For the normalization of cell numbers in each well, the cells were fixed with 4% paraformaldehyde in PBS for 10 min, washed twice briefly in PBS, counterstained with 0.5 µg/mL DAPI in PBS for 10 min, and rinsed twice in PBS. The fluorescence signals of the nuclear stainings were measured from the well bottom by using a fluorometer (SpectraMax i3x) at the excitation/emission values of 360/470 nm. For each group, the mean fluorescence values were calculated after substracting the corresponding background signals, and the intensity of the MitoROS signals was divided by the intensity of the respective nuclear staining for normalization based on the cell number. Images of the cells were acquired with the use of an inverted fluorescence miscroscope (Leica DMI 6000B) by using the A4 and Y3 filter sets as described in the Immunocytochemistry section above.

4.8. Glucose Uptake

The cells were seeded into 24-well plates at a concentration of 20,000 cells/well and allowed to attach overnight at 37 °C with 5% CO_2. The cells were then rinsed twice with serum- and glucose-free RPMI-1640 medium and incubated for 30 min at 37 °C with the test substances in glucose-free RPMI-1640. Afterward, 6-NBDG was introduced into the culture medium at a final concentration of 300 μM, except for the negative control group, and the cells were further incubated for 30 min, followed by two brief rinses in PBS. The cells were then visualized immediately via fluorescence and phase-contrast microscopy (Leica DMI 6000B). Quantification of the integrated density was performed in a minimum of $n = 201$ cells/group using Fiji software (version 1.53t) [70]. For this purpose, the cell contours were circumscribed on the phase-contrast images. The mean intensity was determined by redirecting the measurements to the fluorescence images. The mean intensity of the negative control group was subtracted from the mean intensity of each cell, which was then multiplied with the cellular area for calculation of the integrated density.

4.9. Glycolysis Assay

The cells were seeded into flat-based 96-well plates with black, polystyrene walls (Lumox® multiwell, Sarstedt, Germany) at a concentration of 60,000 cells/well and allowed to attach overnight at 37 °C with 5% CO_2. The glycolytic rate was measured by using a fluorometric assay that was based on extracellular acidification following the manufacturer's instructions (Abcam, catalog number: ab197244). Prior to the test, CO_2 was removed by incubating the plate in a humidified, CO_2-free incubator at 37 °C for 3 h to minimize background acidification. The cells were then treated with the test substances that were diluted in the respiration buffer of the assay in duplicate for 3 h at 37 °C without CO_2 in a temperature-controlled fluorometer (SpectraMax i3x; Molecular Devices). The negative control of each group was incubated without the glycolysis assay reagent. The fluorescence intensity was measured at an excitation of 380 nm and an emission of 615 nm. The mean intensity of each group was calculated after background subtraction.

4.10. ATP Assay

The cells were seeded into 96-well plates at a density of 30,000 cells/well (100 μL/well), allowed to attach overnight, and incubated with the test substances in triplicate for 2 days. ATP levels were measured by using a luminescence assay as instructed by the manufacturer (Abcam, ab113849). As a control for equal cellular material, phase contrast images of the center of each well were acquired prior to cell lysis using an inverse microscope (Leica) at 50× magnification, and cell density was quantified by using Fiji software. The contents of each well were transferred into an opaque, white 96-well microplate, and luminescence was measured using a multi-mode microplate reader (SpectraMax i3x). After background subtraction, the mean ATP concentration of each group was normalized to the cell density of the corresponding group.

4.11. G6PDH Activity

The cells were seeded into 12-well plates at a concentration of 200,000 cells/well, allowed to attach overnight at 37 °C with 5% CO_2, and incubated with the test substances for 11–13 h. G6PDH activity was measured by using a colorimetric assay in duplicate for each group following the manufacturer's instructions (Cell Biolabs Inc., San Diego, CA, USA, catalog number: MET-5081). The background control of each group was treated without the G6PDH substrate. Absorbance at 450 nm was measured using a multi-mode microplate reader (SpectraMax i3x). After background subtraction, the mean G6PDH activity of each group was normalized to the total protein concentration of the corresponding cellular lysate that was determined by the bicinchoninic acid (BCA) assay (Thermo Fisher Scientific).

4.12. *Total Glutathione Assay*

The cells were seeded into 96-well plates at a density of 10,000 cells/well (100 µL/well), allowed to attach overnight, and incubated with the test substances in duplicate for 7–10 h. The wells without cells served as the background control. The total glutathione levels were measured by using a luminescence assay following the manufacturer's instructions (Promega, Walldorf, Germany, V6611). The contents of each well were transferred into an opaque, white 96-well plate, and luminescence was measured by using a multi-mode microplate reader (SpectraMax i3x).

4.13. *Immunoblotting*

The cells that were grown in 6-well-plates were washed twice with ice-cold PBS, kept on ice, and lysed in ice-cold cell lysis buffer (50 mmol/L Tris-HCl, pH 7.4, 150 mmol/L NaCl, 2 mmol/L EDTA, 1% NP-40 [*v*/*v*], 0.1% SDS, 0.5% sodium deoxycholate, and 50 mmol/L NaF, supplemented with protease and phosphatase inhibitors (Sigma-Aldrich, Munich, Germany; 1:100 each) immediately before use) for 15 min under gentle agitation on a shaker. Lysates were cleared by centrifugation at 12,000× *g*, 4 °C for 20 min (Sigma 2-16PK; Hettich, Tuttlingen, Germany). The supernatants were collected and stored at −80 °C. Protein concentration was determined by the BCA assay (Thermo Fisher Scientific). Samples were denatured at 95–99 °C for 5 min and run in 4–10% TGX stain-free polyacrylamide gels (Bio-Rad, Munich, Germany) under denaturing and non-reducing conditions with 15 µg of protein/well. Protein loading in the gels was visualized using ChemiDoc MP stain-free imaging (Bio-Rad) through activation with ultraviolet light for 5 min. The gels were then equilibrated in blotting buffer (48 mmol/L Tris, 39 mmol/L glycine, 10% methanol [*v*/*v*], and 0.04% SDS [*w*/*v*]) for 10 min and transferred onto methanol-activated polyvinylidene fluoride (PVDF) membranes via semi-dry blotting (Biotec-Fischer, Reiskirchen, Germany) at a constant current of 0.8 mA/cm^2 for 1 h. Protein transfer onto the membranes was visualized through the use of the ChemiDoc MP stain-free system. Membranes were blocked in 5% non-fat dry milk in Tris-buffered saline solution with 0.1% Tween-20 (TBST) for 1 h under gentle agitation and incubated with a mixture of the rabbit primary antibodies against ZBTB20 (Proteintech, 1:1000) and beta-actin (Abcam, 1:1000) that were diluted in TBST with 0.5% non-fat dry milk followed by the HRP-conjugated goat anti-rabbit secondary antibodies (Jackson Immunoresearch, Cambridgeshire, UK, 1:5000 in blocking buffer) for 1 h at room temperature. Signal detection was performed with the Super Enhanced Chemiluminescence Kit (ABP Biosciences, Rockville, MD, USA) using the ChemiDoc MP system. After stripping the membranes at 37 °C for 15 min as instructed by the manufacturer (Thermo Fisher Scientific), the blots were reprobed with the primary rabbit antibodies against PFKP (Proteintech, 1:2000), followed by the abovementioned secondary antibodies and signal detection.

4.14. *Statistical Analysis*

Data were analyzed using NCSS statistical software (Version 2021; NCSS, Kaysville, UT, USA) on Windows 10. The correlation between gene expression and the copy number of chromosome 3 was assessed through the use of the Pearson and Spearman tests. The normality of distribution and equality of variances were verified through the use of the Shapiro–Wilk and Brown–Forsythe tests, respectively. The association between binary factors and continuous variables was evaluated through the use of the non-paired two-sided *t*-test, assuming equal variance, or the Mann–Whitney U test with normal approximation. The categorical variables with three or more subgroups were analyzed using one-way analysis of variance or the Kruskal–Wallis test, with tie correction for the latter performed when necessary. Bonferroni correction was applied for multiple hypothesis testing. p-values less than 0.05 were considered as significant.

5. Conclusions

In conclusion, we report for the first time that aggressive UM cells with monosomy 3 exhibit a more glycolytic gene expression profile, which may confer these cells with a growth advantage by enabling the efficient usage of glucose for the production of energy or biomass depending on cellular priorities. Our preliminary findings also highlight the therapeutic potential of quercetin as a novel, affordable, and immediately available therapy approach to prevent the growth of UM cells by interfering with the glucose metabolism of these tumors. The anti-carcinogenic potential and safety of quercetin in UM therefore deserves further investigation in future studies by analyzing a wider range of quercetin concentrations for different cellular events and including multiple melanoma cell lines as well as normal melanocytes or skin cells as controls.

Supplementary Materials: The following supporting information can be downloaded at: https://www.mdpi.com/article/10.3390/ijms25084292/s1.

Author Contributions: Conceptualization, A.T. and S.G.; methodology, A.T., V.H., H.Z., T.M. and S.V.; software, A.T., V.H., H.Z., T.M. and S.V.; validation, A.T., V.H., H.Z. and S.V.; formal analysis, A.T., V.H. and H.Z.; investigation, A.T., V.H., H.Z., T.M. and S.V.; resources, S.G.; data curation, A.T. and V.H.; writing—original draft preparation, A.T., T.M., H.Z. and S.G.; writing—review and editing, M.P., M.R. and V.K.; visualization, A.T., V.H., H.Z. and S.V.; supervision, A.T. and S.G.; project administration, S.G.; funding acquisition, S.G. All authors have read and agreed to the published version of the manuscript.

Funding: This research was funded by the Werner und Klara Kreitz-Stiftung, Germany, grant number F279097.

Institutional Review Board Statement: Not applicable.

Informed Consent Statement: Not applicable.

Data Availability Statement: Publicly available datasets were analyzed in this study. The gene expression data of the UM cohort of the TCGA study were downloaded from the University of California, Santa Cruz Xena databank (https://xenabrowser.net/) (accessed on 23 April 2021). The validation cohorts can be accessed from the Gene Expression Omnibus databank (https://www.ncbi.nlm.nih.gov/geo/; accession numbers GSE22138 and GSE44295) (accessed on 10 May 2021).

Conflicts of Interest: A.T. received financial support from Novartis Pharma, Germany. The funder had no role in the design of the study; in the collection, analysis, or interpretation of the data; in the writing of the manuscript; or in the decision to publish the results. The remaining authors declare no conflicts of interest.

References

1. Blum, E.S.; Yang, J.; Komatsubara, K.M.; Carvajal, R.D. Clinical Management of Uveal and Conjunctival Melanoma. *Oncology* **2016**, *30*, 29–32, 34–43, 48. [PubMed]
2. Nichols, E.E.; Richmond, A.; Daniels, A.B. Tumor Characteristics, Genetics, Management, and the Risk of Metastasis in Uveal Melanoma. *Semin. Ophthalmol.* **2016**, *31*, 304–309. [CrossRef] [PubMed]
3. Jager, M.J.; Shields, C.L.; Cebulla, C.M.; Abdel-Rahman, M.H.; Grossniklaus, H.E.; Stern, M.H.; Carvajal, R.D.; Belfort, R.N.; Jia, R.; Shields, J.A.; et al. Uveal Melanoma. *Nat. Rev. Dis. Primers* **2020**, *6*, 24. [CrossRef] [PubMed]
4. Prescher, G.; Bornfeld, N.; Hirche, H.; Horsthemke, B.; Jöckel, K.H.; Becher, R. Prognostic Implications of Monosomy 3 in Uveal Melanoma. *Lancet* **1996**, *347*, 1222–1225. [PubMed]
5. Kaliki, S.; Shields, C.L.; Shields, J.A. Uveal Melanoma: Estimating Prognosis. *Indian J. Ophthalmol.* **2015**, *63*, 93–102. [CrossRef]
6. Abdel-Rahman, M.H.; Cebulla, C.M.; Verma, V.; Christopher, B.N.; Carson, W.E., 3rd; Olencki, T.; Davidorf, F.H. Monosomy 3 Status of Uveal Melanoma Metastases Is Associated with Rapidly Progressive Tumors and Short Survival. *Exp. Eye Res.* **2012**, *100*, 26–31. [CrossRef] [PubMed]
7. Sevim, D.G.; Kiratli, H. Serum Adiponectin, Insulin Resistance, and Uveal Melanoma: Clinicopathological Correlations. *Melanoma Res.* **2016**, *26*, 164–172. [CrossRef] [PubMed]

8. McCannel, T.A.; Reddy, S.; Burgess, B.L.; Auerbach, M. Association of Positive Dual-Modality Positron Emission Tomography/Computed Tomography Imaging of Primary Choroidal Melanoma with Chromosome 3 Loss and Tumor Size. *Retina* **2010**, *30*, 146–151. [CrossRef] [PubMed]
9. Papastefanou, V.P.; Islam, S.; Szyszko, T.; Grantham, M.; Sagoo, M.S.; Cohen, V.M. Metabolic Activity of Primary Uveal Melanoma on PET/CT Scan and Its Relationship with Monosomy 3 and Other Prognostic Factors. *Br. J. Ophthalmol.* **2014**, *98*, 1659–1665. [CrossRef]
10. Maaßen, T.; Vardanyan, S.; Brosig, A.; Merz, H.; Ranjbar, M.; Kakkassery, V.; Grisanti, S.; Tura, A. Monosomy-3 Alters the Expression Profile of the Glucose Transporters GLUT1-3 in Uveal Melanoma. *Int. J. Mol. Sci.* **2020**, *21*, 9345. [CrossRef]
11. Mueckler, M.; Thorens, B. The SLC2 (GLUT) Family of Membrane Transporters. *Mol. Asp. Med.* **2013**, *34*, 121–138. [CrossRef] [PubMed]
12. Ward, P.S.; Thompson, C.B. Metabolic Reprogramming: A Cancer Hallmark Even Warburg Did Not Anticipate. *Cancer Cell* **2012**, *21*, 297–308. [CrossRef] [PubMed]
13. Bronkhorst, I.H.; Jager, M.J. Inflammation in Uveal Melanoma. *Eye* **2013**, *27*, 217–223. [CrossRef] [PubMed]
14. Kozal, K.; Jóźwiak, P.; Krześlak, A. Contemporary Perspectives on the Warburg Effect Inhibition in Cancer Therapy. *Cancer Control.* **2021**, *28*, 10732748211041243. [CrossRef] [PubMed]
15. Kubicka, A.; Matczak, K.; Łabieniec-Watała, M. More Than Meets the Eye Regarding Cancer Metabolism. *Int. J. Mol. Sci.* **2021**, *22*, 9507. [CrossRef] [PubMed]
16. Liu, C.; Jin, Y.; Fan, Z. The Mechanism of Warburg Effect-Induced Chemoresistance in Cancer. *Front. Oncol.* **2021**, *11*, 698023. [CrossRef] [PubMed]
17. Jiang, P.; Du, W.; Wu, M. Regulation of the Pentose Phosphate Pathway in Cancer. *Protein Cell* **2014**, *5*, 592–602. [CrossRef] [PubMed]
18. Reyes-Farias, M.; Carrasco-Pozo, C. The Anti-Cancer Effect of Quercetin: Molecular Implications in Cancer Metabolism. *Int. J. Mol. Sci.* **2019**, *20*, 3177. [CrossRef] [PubMed]
19. Liberti, M.V.; Locasale, J.W. The Warburg Effect: How Does It Benefit Cancer Cells? *Trends Biochem. Sci.* **2016**, *41*, 211–218. [CrossRef]
20. Ge, T.; Yang, J.; Zhou, S.; Wang, Y.; Li, Y.; Tong, X. The Role of the Pentose Phosphate Pathway in Diabetes and Cancer. *Front. Endocrinol.* **2020**, *11*, 365. [CrossRef]
21. Stincone, A.; Prigione, A.; Cramer, T.; Wamelink, M.M.; Campbell, K.; Cheung, E.; Olin-Sandoval, V.; Grüning, N.M.; Krüger, A.; Tauqeer Alam, M.; et al. The Return of Metabolism: Biochemistry and Physiology of the Pentose Phosphate Pathway. *Biol. Rev. Camb. Philos. Soc.* **2015**, *90*, 927–963. [CrossRef] [PubMed]
22. Liu, Y.; Huo, Y.; Wang, D.; Tai, Y.; Li, J.; Pang, D.; Zhang, Y.; Zhao, W.; Du, N.; Huang, Y. MiR-216a-5p/Hexokinase 2 Axis Regulates Uveal Melanoma Growth through Modulation of Warburg Effect. *Biochem. Biophys. Res. Commun.* **2018**, *501*, 885–892. [CrossRef]
23. Bao, R.; Surriga, O.; Olson, D.J.; Allred, J.B.; Strand, C.A.; Zha, Y.; Carll, T.; Labadie, B.W.; Bastos, B.R.; Butler, M.; et al. Transcriptional Analysis of Metastatic Uveal Melanoma Survival Nominates NRP1 as a Therapeutic Target. *Melanoma Res.* **2021**, *31*, 27–37. [CrossRef] [PubMed]
24. Liu, J.; Lu, J.; Li, W. A Comprehensive Prognostic and Immunological Analysis of a Six-Gene Signature Associated with Glycolysis and Immune Response in Uveal Melanoma. *Front. Immunol.* **2021**, *12*, 738068. [CrossRef] [PubMed]
25. Kashyap, D.; Mittal, S.; Sak, K.; Singhal, P.; Tuli, H.S. Molecular Mechanisms of Action of Quercetin in Cancer: Recent Advances. *Tumour Biol.* **2016**, *37*, 12927–12939. [CrossRef] [PubMed]
26. Khan, F.; Niaz, K.; Maqbool, F.; Ismail Hassan, F.; Abdollahi, M.; Nagulapalli Venkata, K.C.; Nabavi, S.M.; Bishayee, A. Molecular Targets Underlying the Anticancer Effects of Quercetin: An Update. *Nutrients* **2016**, *8*, 529. [CrossRef]
27. Yi, H.; Peng, H.; Wu, X.; Xu, X.; Kuang, T.; Zhang, J.; Du, L.; Fan, G. The Therapeutic Effects and Mechanisms of Quercetin on Metabolic Diseases: Pharmacological Data and Clinical Evidence. *Oxid. Med. Cell. Longev.* **2021**, *2021*, 6678662. [CrossRef] [PubMed]
28. Hosseini, A.; Razavi, B.M.; Banach, M.; Hosseinzadeh, H. Quercetin and Metabolic Syndrome: A Review. *Phytother. Res.* **2021**, *35*, 5352–5364. [CrossRef] [PubMed]
29. Brito, A.F.; Ribeiro, M.; Abrantes, A.M.; Pires, A.S.; Teixo, R.J.; Tralhão, J.G.; Botelho, M.F. Quercetin in Cancer Treatment, Alone or in Combination with Conventional Therapeutics? *Curr. Med. Chem.* **2015**, *22*, 3025–3039. [CrossRef]
30. Sak, K. Site-Specific Anticancer Effects of Dietary Flavonoid Quercetin. *Nutr. Cancer* **2014**, *66*, 177–193. [CrossRef]
31. Sak, K.; Everaus, H. Role of Flavonoids in Future Anticancer Therapy by Eliminating the Cancer Stem Cells. *Curr. Stem Cell Res. Ther.* **2015**, *10*, 271–282. [CrossRef] [PubMed]
32. Umar, S.M.; Kashyap, A.; Kahol, S.; Mathur, S.R.; Gogia, A.; Deo, S.V.S.; Prasad, C.P. Prognostic and Therapeutic Relevance of Phosphofructokinase Platelet-Type (PFKP) in Breast Cancer. *Exp. Cell Res.* **2020**, *396*, 112282. [CrossRef] [PubMed]
33. Wu, H.; Pan, L.; Gao, C.; Xu, H.; Li, Y.; Zhang, L.; Ma, L.; Meng, L.; Sun, X.; Qin, H. Quercetin Inhibits the Proliferation of Glycolysis-Addicted HCC Cells by Reducing Hexokinase 2 and Akt-MTOR Pathway. *Molecules* **2019**, *24*, 1993. [CrossRef] [PubMed]
34. Gibellini, L.; Pinti, M.; Nasi, M.; De Biasi, S.; Roat, E.; Bertoncelli, L.; Cossarizza, A. Interfering with ROS Metabolism in Cancer Cells: The Potential Role of Quercetin. *Cancers* **2010**, *2*, 1288–1311. [CrossRef] [PubMed]

35. Li, X.B.; Gu, J.D.; Zhou, Q.H. Review of Aerobic Glycolysis and Its Key Enzymes—New Targets for Lung Cancer Therapy. *Thorac Cancer* **2015**, *6*, 17–24. [CrossRef] [PubMed]
36. Wang, J.; Zhang, P.; Zhong, J.; Tan, M.; Ge, J.; Tao, L.; Li, Y.; Zhu, Y.; Wu, L.; Qiu, J.; et al. The Platelet Isoform of Phosphofructokinase Contributes to Metabolic Reprogramming and Maintains Cell Proliferation in Clear Cell Renal Cell Carcinoma. *Oncotarget* **2016**, *7*, 27142–27157. [CrossRef] [PubMed]
37. Al Hasawi, N.; Alkandari, M.F.; Luqmani, Y.A. Phosphofructokinase: A Mediator of Glycolytic Flux in Cancer Progression. *Crit. Rev. Oncol. Hematol.* **2014**, *92*, 312–321. [CrossRef] [PubMed]
38. Sun, Y.; Preiss, N.K.; Valenteros, K.B.; Kamal, Y.; Usherwood, Y.K.; Frost, H.R.; Usherwood, E.J. Zbtb20 Restrains CD8 T Cell Immunometabolism and Restricts Memory Differentiation and Antitumor Immunity. *J. Immunol.* **2020**, *205*, 2649–2666. [CrossRef] [PubMed]
39. Wang, Q.; Tan, Y.X.; Ren, Y.B.; Dong, L.W.; Xie, Z.F.; Tang, L.; Cao, D.; Zhang, W.P.; Hu, H.P.; Wang, H.Y. Zinc Finger Protein ZBTB20 Expression Is Increased in Hepatocellular Carcinoma and Associated with Poor Prognosis. *BMC Cancer* **2011**, *11*, 271. [CrossRef]
40. Liu, J.; Jiang, J.; Hui, X.; Wang, W.; Fang, D.; Ding, L. Mir-758-5p Suppresses Glioblastoma Proliferation, Migration and Invasion by Targeting ZBTB20. *Cell. Physiol. Biochem.* **2018**, *48*, 2074–2083. [CrossRef]
41. Fan, D.; Qiu, B.; Yang, X.J.; Tang, H.L.; Peng, S.J.; Yang, P.; Dong, Y.M.; Yang, L.; Bao, G.Q.; Zhao, H.D. LncRNA SNHG8 Promotes Cell Migration and Invasion in Breast Cancer Cell through MiR-634/ZBTB20 Axis. *Eur. Rev. Med. Pharmacol. Sci.* **2020**, *24*, 11639–11649. [PubMed]
42. Zhang, Y.; Zhou, X.; Zhang, M.; Cheng, L.; Zhang, Y.; Wang, X. ZBTB20 Promotes Cell Migration and Invasion of Gastric Cancer by Inhibiting IκBα to Induce NF-KB Activation. *Artif. Cells Nanomed. Biotechnol.* **2019**, *47*, 3862–3872. [CrossRef] [PubMed]
43. Liu, G.; Zhou, L.; Zhang, H.; Chen, R.; Zhang, Y.; Li, L.; Lu, J.Y.; Jiang, H.; Liu, D.; Qi, S.; et al. Regulation of Hepatic Lipogenesis by the Zinc Finger Protein Zbtb20. *Nat. Commun.* **2017**, *8*, 14824. [CrossRef] [PubMed]
44. Silva-Rodríguez, P.; Fernández-Díaz, D.; Bande, M.; Pardo, M.; Loidi, L.; Blanco-Teijeiro, M.J. GNAQ and GNA11 Genes: A Comprehensive Review on Oncogenesis, Prognosis and Therapeutic Opportunities in Uveal Melanoma. *Cancers* **2022**, *14*, 3066. [CrossRef] [PubMed]
45. Onken, M.D.; Noda, S.E.; Kaltenbronn, K.M.; Frankfater, C.; Makepeace, C.M.; Fettig, N.; Piggott, K.D.; Custer, P.L.; Ippolito, J.E.; Blumer, K.J. Oncogenic Gq/11 Signaling Acutely Drives and Chronically Sustains Metabolic Reprogramming in Uveal Melanoma. *J. Biol. Chem.* **2022**, *298*, 101495. [CrossRef] [PubMed]
46. Griewank, K.G.; Yu, X.; Khalili, J.; Sozen, M.M.; Stempke-Hale, K.; Bernatchez, C.; Wardell, S.; Bastian, B.C.; Woodman, S.E. Genetic and Molecular Characterization of Uveal Melanoma Cell Lines. *Pigment. Cell Melanoma Res.* **2012**, *25*, 182–187. [CrossRef] [PubMed]
47. Li, C.; Zhang, W.J.; Choi, J.; Frei, B. Quercetin Affects Glutathione Levels and Redox Ratio in Human Aortic Endothelial Cells not Through Oxidation but Formation and Cellular Export of Quercetin-Glutathione Conjugates and Upregulation of Glutamate-Cysteine Ligase. *Redox Biol.* **2016**, *9*, 220–228. [CrossRef] [PubMed]
48. Ader, P.; Blöck, M.; Pietzsch, S.; Wolffram, S. Interaction of Quercetin Glucosides with the Intestinal Sodium/Glucose Co-Transporter (SGLT-1). *Cancer Lett.* **2001**, *162*, 175–180. [CrossRef] [PubMed]
49. Strobel, P.; Allard, C.; Perez-Acle, T.; Calderon, R.; Aldunate, R.; Leighton, F. Myricetin, Quercetin and Catechin-Gallate Inhibit Glucose Uptake in Isolated Rat Adipocytes. *Biochem. J.* **2005**, *386 Pt 3*, 471–478. [CrossRef]
50. Zhang, H.; Hassan, Y.I.; Liu, R.; Mats, L.; Yang, C.; Liu, C.; Tsao, R. Molecular Mechanisms Underlying the Absorption of Aglycone and Glycosidic Flavonoids in a Caco-2 BBe1 Cell Model. *ACS Omega* **2020**, *5*, 10782–10793. [CrossRef]
51. Ismail, A.; Tanasova, M. Importance of GLUT Transporters in Disease Diagnosis and Treatment. *Int. J. Mol. Sci.* **2022**, *23*, 8698. [CrossRef] [PubMed]
52. Chattopadhyay, C.; Oba, J.; Roszik, J.; Marszalek, J.R.; Chen, K.; Qi, Y.; Eterovic, K.; Robertson, A.G.; Burks, J.K.; McCannel, T.A.; et al. Elevated Endogenous SDHA Drives Pathological Metabolism in Highly Metastatic Uveal Melanoma. *Investig. Ophthalmol. Vis. Sci.* **2019**, *60*, 4187–4195. [CrossRef] [PubMed]
53. Giallongo, S.; Di Rosa, M.; Caltabiano, R.; Longhitano, L.; Reibaldi, M.; Distefano, A.; Lo Re, O.; Amorini, A.M.; Puzzo, L.; Salvatorelli, L.; et al. Loss of MacroH2A1 Decreases Mitochondrial Metabolism and Reduces the Aggressiveness of Uveal Melanoma Cells. *Aging* **2020**, *12*, 9745–9760. [CrossRef] [PubMed]
54. Mor, D.E.; Murphy, C.T. Mitochondrial Hyperactivity as a Potential Therapeutic Target in Parkinson's Disease. *Transl. Med. Aging* **2020**, *4*, 117–120. [CrossRef] [PubMed]
55. Day, R.M.; Suzuki, Y.J. Cell proliferation, reactive oxygen and cellular glutathione. *Dose Response* **2006**, *3*, 425–442. [CrossRef] [PubMed]
56. Hebert, L.; Bellanger, D.; Guillas, C.; Campagne, A.; Dingli, F.; Loew, D.; Fievet, A.; Jacquemin, V.; Popova, T.; Jean, D.; et al. Modulating BAP1 expression affects ROS homeostasis, cell motility and mitochondrial function. *Oncotarget* **2017**, *8*, 72513–72527. [CrossRef] [PubMed]
57. Bononi, A.; Yang, H.; Giorgi, C.; Patergnani, S.; Pellegrini, L.; Su, M.; Xie, G.; Signorato, V.; Pastorino, S.; Morris, P.; et al. Germline BAP1 Mutations Induce a Warburg Effect. *Cell Death Differ.* **2017**, *24*, 1694–1704. [CrossRef] [PubMed]
58. Patra, K.C.; Hay, N. The Pentose Phosphate Pathway and Cancer. *Trends Biochem. Sci.* **2014**, *39*, 347–354. [CrossRef] [PubMed]

59. Lewis, C.A.; Parker, S.J.; Fiske, B.P.; McCloskey, D.; Gui, D.Y.; Green, C.R.; Vokes, N.I.; Feist, A.M.; Vander Heiden, M.G.; Metallo, C.M. Tracing Compartmentalized NADPH Metabolism in the Cytosol and Mitochondria of Mammalian Cells. *Mol. Cell* **2014**, *55*, 253–263. [CrossRef]
60. Vafadar, A.; Shabaninejad, Z.; Movahedpour, A.; Fallahi, F.; Taghavipour, M.; Ghasemi, Y.; Akbari, M.; Shafiee, A.; Hajighadimi, S.; Moradizarmehri, S.; et al. Quercetin and Cancer: New Insights into Its Therapeutic Effects on Ovarian Cancer Cells. *Cell Biosci.* **2020**, *10*, 32. [CrossRef]
61. Srivastava, S.; Somasagara, R.R.; Hegde, M.; Nishana, M.; Tadi, S.K.; Srivastava, M.; Choudhary, B.; Raghavan, S.C. Quercetin, a Natural Flavonoid Interacts with DNA, Arrests Cell Cycle and Causes Tumor Regression by Activating Mitochondrial Pathway of Apoptosis. *Sci. Rep.* **2016**, *6*, 24049. [CrossRef]
62. Wu, L.; Li, J.; Liu, T.; Li, S.; Feng, J.; Yu, Q.; Zhang, J.; Chen, J.; Zhou, Y.; Ji, J.; et al. Quercetin Shows Anti-Tumor Effect in Hepatocellular Carcinoma LM3 Cells by Abrogating JAK2/STAT3 Signaling Pathway. *Cancer Med.* **2019**, *8*, 4806–4820. [CrossRef]
63. Dabeek, W.M.; Marra, M.V. Dietary Quercetin and Kaempferol: Bioavailability and Potential Cardiovascular-Related Bioactivity in Humans. *Nutrients* **2019**, *11*, 2288. [CrossRef]
64. Eipel, C.; Abshagen, K.; Vollmar, B. Regulation of Hepatic Blood Flow: The Hepatic Arterial Buffer Response Revisited. *World J. Gastroenterol.* **2010**, *16*, 6046–6057. [CrossRef] [PubMed]
65. Egert, S.; Bosy-Westphal, A.; Seiberl, J.; Kürbitz, C.; Settler, U.; Plachta-Danielzik, S.; Wagner, A.E.; Frank, J.; Schrezenmeir, J.; Rimbach, G.; et al. Quercetin Reduces Systolic Blood Pressure and Plasma Oxidised Low-Density Lipoprotein Concentrations in Overweight Subjects with a High-Cardiovascular Disease Risk Phenotype: A Double-Blinded, Placebo-Controlled Cross-over Study. *Br. J. Nutr.* **2009**, *102*, 1065–1074. [CrossRef] [PubMed]
66. Lu, N.T.; Crespi, C.M.; Liu, N.M.; Vu, J.Q.; Ahmadieh, Y.; Wu, S.; Lin, S.; McClune, A.; Durazo, F.; Saab, S.; et al. A Phase I Dose Escalation Study Demonstrates Quercetin Safety and Explores Potential for Bioflavonoid Antivirals in Patients with Chronic Hepatitis C. *Phytother. Res.* **2016**, *30*, 160–168. [CrossRef] [PubMed]
67. Chen, E.Y.; Tan, C.M.; Kou, Y.; Duan, Q.; Wang, Z.; Meirelles, G.V.; Clark, N.R.; Ma'ayan, A. Enrichr: Interactive and Collaborative HTML5 Gene List Enrichment Analysis Tool. *BMC Bioinform.* **2013**, *14*, 128. [CrossRef]
68. De Waard-Siebinga, I.; Blom, D.J.; Griffioen, M.; Schrier, P.I.; Hoogendoorn, E.; Beverstock, G.; Danen, E.H.; Jager, M.J. Establishment and Characterization of an Uveal-Melanoma Cell Line. *Int. J. Cancer* **1995**, *62*, 155–161. [CrossRef] [PubMed]
69. Jager, M.J.; Magner, J.A.; Ksander, B.R.; Dubovy, S.R. Uveal Melanoma Cell Lines: Where do they come from? (An American Ophthalmological Society Thesis). *Trans. Am. Ophthalmol. Soc.* **2016**, *114*, T5.
70. Schindelin, J.; Arganda-Carreras, I.; Frise, E.; Kaynig, V.; Longair, M.; Pietzsch, T.; Preibisch, S.; Rueden, C.; Saalfeld, S.; Schmid, B.; et al. Fiji: An Open-Source Platform for Biological-Image Analysis. *Nat. Methods* **2012**, *9*, 676–682. [CrossRef]

International Journal of
Molecular Sciences

MDPI

Article

Endothelial Mitochondria Transfer to Melanoma Induces M2-Type Macrophage Polarization and Promotes Tumor Growth by the Nrf2/HO-1-Mediated Pathway

Fu-Chen Kuo [1,2], Hsin-Yi Tsai [3,4], Bi-Ling Cheng [5], Kuen-Jang Tsai [6], Ping-Chen Chen [5], Yaw-Bin Huang [4], Chung-Jung Liu [7,8], Deng-Chyang Wu [7,8], Meng-Chieh Wu [8,9], Bin Huang [5,7,10,11,*] and Ming-Wei Lin [3,7,12,*]

1 School of Medicine, College of Medicine, I-Shou University, Kaohsiung 82445, Taiwan; ed100418@edah.org.tw
2 Department of Obstetrics & Gynecology, E-Da Hospital, I-Shou University, Kaohsiung 82445, Taiwan
3 Department of Medical Research, E-Da Hospital and E-Da Cancer Hospital, I-Shou University, Kaohsiung 82445, Taiwan; y7952pipi@gmail.com
4 School of Pharmacy, Kaohsiung Medical University, Kaohsiung 80708, Taiwan; yabihu@kmu.edu.tw
5 Department of Biological Sciences, National Sun Yat-sen University, Kaohsiung 80424, Taiwan; biling128@gmail.com (B.-L.C.); lajajaf@gmail.com (P.-C.C.)
6 Department of General Surgery, E-Da Cancer Hospital, I-Shou University, Kaohsiung 82445, Taiwan; ed108937@edah.org.tw
7 Regenerative Medicine and Cell Therapy Research Center, Kaohsiung Medical University, Kaohsiung 80708, Taiwan; pinkporkkimo@yahoo.com.tw (C.-J.L.); dechwu555@gmail.com (D.-C.W.)
8 Department of Internal Medicine, Kaohsiung Medical University Hospital, Kaohsiung 80708, Taiwan; 930293@mail.kmuh.org.tw
9 Department of Internal Medicine, Kaohsiung Municipal Ta-Tung Hospital, Kaohsiung 80145, Taiwan
10 Department of Biomedical Science and Environmental Biology, College of Life Science, Kaohsiung Medical University, Kaohsiung 80708, Taiwan
11 Department of Medical Research, Kaohsiung Medical University Hospital, Kaohsiung 80708, Taiwan
12 Department of Nursing, College of Medicine, I-Shou University, Kaohsiung 82445, Taiwan
* Correspondence: huangpin2@yahoo.com.tw (B.H.); ta990074@gmail.com (M.-W.L.); Tel.: +886-7-3121101 (ext. 2704) (B.H.); +886-7-6151100 (ext. 5413) (M.-W.L.)

Abstract: Gynecologic tract melanoma is a malignant tumor with poor prognosis. Because of the low survival rate and the lack of a standard treatment protocol related to this condition, the investigation of the mechanisms underlying melanoma progression is crucial to achieve advancements in the relevant gynecological surgery and treatment. Mitochondrial transfer between adjacent cells in the tumor microenvironment regulates tumor progression. This study investigated the effects of endothelial mitochondria on the growth of melanoma cells and the activation of specific signal transduction pathways following mitochondrial transplantation. Mitochondria were isolated from endothelial cells (ECs) and transplanted into B16F10 melanoma cells, resulting in the upregulation of proteins associated with tumor growth. Furthermore, enhanced antioxidation and mitochondrial homeostasis mediated by the Sirt1-PGC-1α-Nrf2-HO-1 pathway were observed, along with the inhibition of apoptotic protein caspase-3. Finally, the transplantation of endothelial mitochondria into B16F10 cells promoted tumor growth and increased M2-type macrophages through Nrf2/HO-1-mediated pathways in a xenograft animal model. In summary, the introduction of exogenous mitochondria from ECs into melanoma cells promoted tumor growth, indicating the role of mitochondrial transfer by stromal cells in modulating a tumor's phenotype. These results provide valuable insights into the role of mitochondrial transfer and provide potential targets for gynecological melanoma treatment.

Keywords: melanoma; endothelial cells; mitochondrial transplantation; Nrf2; tumor microenvironment; M2-type macrophage; tumor growth

1. Introduction

Melanoma, the most aggressive type of skin cancer, grows rapidly and can metastasize to other organs. In particular, gynecologic tract melanoma has a poor prognosis, with a 5-year survival rate lower than 25%. Because of the low survival rate and the lack of a standard treatment approach related to gynecologic tract melanoma [1–3], elucidation of the mechanisms underlying melanoma progression is crucial for achieving advancements in relevant gynecological surgery and treatment. Studies have indicated that extracellular signal-regulated kinase (ERK) and phosphoinositide 3-kinase/protein kinase B (AKT) pathways play major roles in the progression of melanoma [4–6]. In addition, genes implicated in cell cycle progression, including cyclin D1 and cyclin E, are commonly amplified in melanoma [7]. Furthermore, the progression of melanoma involves interactions with surrounding stromal cells in the tumor microenvironment (TME). Interactions between melanoma cells and endothelial cells (ECs) are crucial in tumor biology and enable tumor cells to undergo proliferation and metastasis [8]. In addition, such interactions—which occur through paracrine communication, direct contact, or gap junctions—facilitate the release of various signaling molecules—including growth factors, extracellular vesicles, and mitochondria—into the TME [8,9]. In the TME, M1-type antitumor macrophages expressing inducible nitric oxide synthase (iNOS) are polarized into M2-type macrophages expressing arginase 1 (Arg1), thereby promoting cancer cell proliferation and metastasis. Furthermore, cancer cells stimulate the differentiation of nonactivated macrophages into an M2-like tumor-associated macrophage (TAM) phenotype through the action of transforming growth factor β (TGF-β) [10–13].

Mitochondria, also regarded as endosymbiotic organelles, not only produce the majority of cellular energy, but also are involved in cellular exchanges, modulating the fate and function of cells [14,15]. Nuclear respiratory factor 2 (Nrf2) is a key modulator of peroxisome proliferator-activated receptor-gamma coactivator 1-α (PGC-1α)-mediated mitochondrial activity and protects against reactive oxygen species (ROS) generation and oxidative damage [16,17]. Mitochondrial transfer between adjacent cells occurs through tunneling nanotubes, microvesicles, gap junctional intercellular communication, and extrusion [9,15] the transfer of mitochondria from vascular smooth muscle cells to mesenchymal stem cells (MSCs) enhances cell proliferation [18]. In addition, the mitochondria from MSCs alleviate stress in patients with osteoarthritis [19]. Furthermore, the mitochondria obtained from bone-marrow-derived MSCs can rescue cardiomyocytes from ischemia-induced oxidative stress and cell death [20]. MSCs donate their healthy mitochondria to damaged cells, thereby enhancing the recipient cells' oxidative stress resistance, proliferation, and antiapoptotic capability [21]. In addition, such intercellular mitochondrial transfer is involved in the regulation of cancer progression [21–24]. Nevertheless, the mechanisms through which endothelial mitochondria affect melanoma progression, and subsequently regulate TAMs to promote tumor growth after their transfer, remain to be elucidated.

In recent years, mitochondrial transplants have emerged as a method for examining the functions of recipient cancer cells after their uptake of mitochondria from donor cells in the TME [25,26]. A common approach to mitochondrial transplants involves co-culturing recipient cells with isolated mitochondria from donor cells [27,28]. In the present study, we transplanted mitochondria from ECs into melanoma cells and used signaling pathways and tumor xenograft animal models to investigate the role of mitochondrial transfer in melanoma progression.

2. Results

2.1. *Transplanted Endothelial Mitochondria Upregulated Mitochondrial Biogenesis with Mediation by the Redox-Sensitive Transcription Factor Nrf2*

Silent mating-type information regulation 2 homolog (Sirt1), an NAD^+-dependent class III histone deacetylase, plays a key role in both mitochondrial biogenesis and cellular redox homeostasis through the PGC-1α and Nrf2 pathways [29]. Nrf2, a redox-sensitive transcription factor, subsequently induces heme oxygenase-1 (HO-1) expression. Upregulation of HO-1 is vital for protecting cancer cells against oxidative stress [30]. To investigate the intracellular effects of endothelial mitochondrial transplantation, mitochondria isolated from human umbilical vein ECs (HUVECs; 5×10^6 cells) were incubated with 5×10^6 B16F10 melanoma cells. After 24 or 48 h of coincubation, we examined the expression levels of Nrf2, HO-1, PGC-1α, Sirt1, and autophagic biomarker LC3B. The results indicated time-dependent increases in the levels of Nrf2, HO-1, PGC-1α, and Sirt1 proteins and a reduction in the level of LC3B (Figure 1).

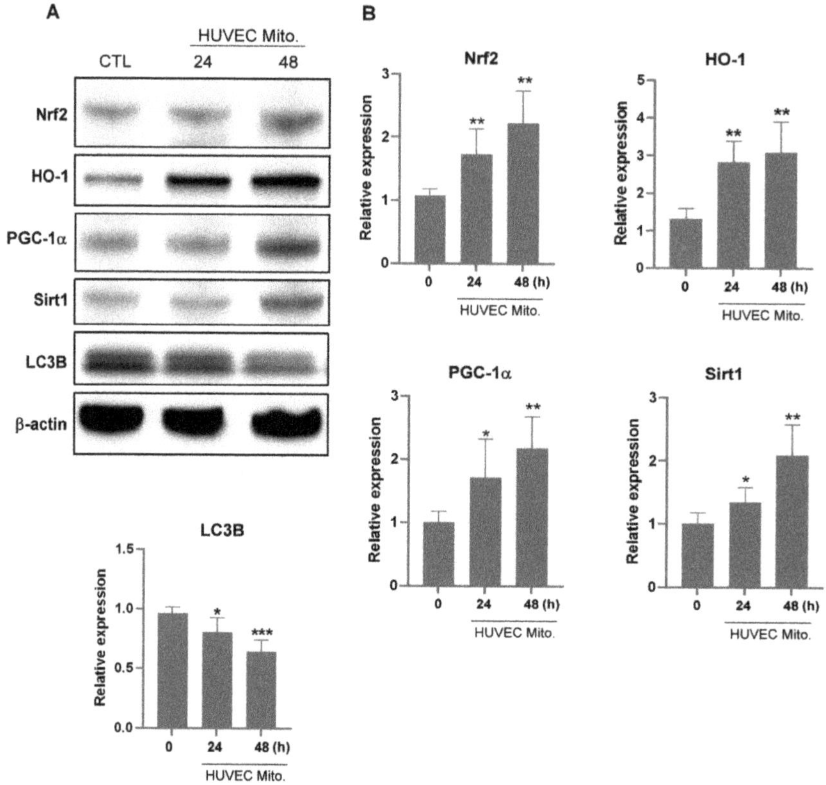

Figure 1. Transplanted HUVEC mitochondria upregulated the expression of antioxidant and mitochondria biogenesis proteins in B16F10 cells. (**A**) Western blot analysis demonstrating the protein expression levels of Nrf2, HO-1, PGC-1α, Sirt1, and LC3B in B16F10 cells with or without HUVEC mitochondrial transplantation at 24 and 48 h. (**B**) Quantitative analysis of Nrf2, HO-1, PGC-1α, Sirt1, and LC3B expression levels in B16F10 cells after the transplantation of HUVEC mitochondria, as determined through Western blotting at 24 and 48 h. Data are presented as the mean ± standard error after ≥3 independent experiments. Statistical significance was assessed using Student's *t* test: * $p < 0.05$, ** $p < 0.01$, *** $p < 0.005$.

2.2. *Transplanted Endothelial Mitochondria Enhanced Melanoma Cells' Viability through Activation of ERK and AKT Signaling and Suppression of Apoptosis*

After confirming that HUVEC mitochondria can be transplanted into B16F10 cells, a process that affects both mitochondrial biogenesis and cellular redox homeostasis, we identified the proteins involved in cancer cell proliferation and apoptosis. The results revealed that the transplantation of HUVEC endothelial mitochondria significantly enhanced the phosphorylation capabilities of ERK and AKT in a time-dependent manner (Figure 2A,B). The expression of cyclin D1 and cyclin E, which regulate cell proliferation, is deregulated in many cancers, including melanoma [31]. We observed upregulated expression of both cyclin D1 and cyclin E (Figure 2C,D). Moreover, the transplantation of endothelial mitochondria enhanced the viability of B16F10 cells (Figure 2E). The cleaved caspase-3 was increased at 24 h and then reduced the level of apoptotic protein cleaved caspase-3 at 48 h (Figure 2F,G).

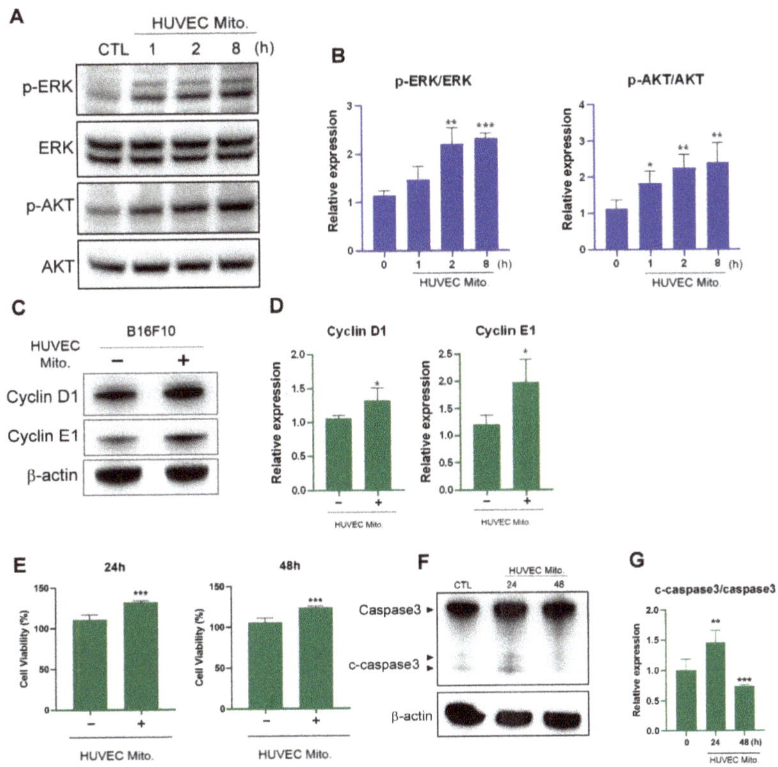

Figure 2. Transplanted HUVEC mitochondria-activated proliferative signaling and inhibited apoptosis in B16F10 cells. (**A**) Western blot analysis demonstrating the activation of the ERK and AKT signaling pathways at 1, 2, and 8 h following HUVEC mitochondrial transplantation. (**B**) Quantitative analysis of the phosphorylation ratios of ERK and AKT after treatment with HUVEC mitochondria, as determined through Western blotting. (**C**) Expression levels of cyclin D1 and cyclin E in B16F10 cells treated with HUVEC mitochondria for 48 h, as determined through Western blotting. (**D**) Quantitative analysis of cyclin D1 expression and cyclin E expression. (**E**) Viability of B16F10 cells at 24 and 48 h after treatment, as evaluated using the CCK8 assay. (**F**) Caspase-3 and cleaved caspase-3 levels in B16F10 cells, analyzed through Western blotting at 24 and 48 h after treatment with HUVEC mitochondria. (**G**) Quantification of the cleaved caspase-3-caspase-3 expression ratio. Data are presented as the mean $\pm$ standard error of the mean after $\geq$3 independent experiments. Statistical significance was assessed using a two-tailed Student's *t*-test: * $p < 0.05$, ** $p < 0.01$, *** $p < 0.005$.

2.3. *Transplanted Endothelial Mitochondria-Suppressed AKT, Oxidative Stress and Apoptosis of Melanoma Cells through Activation of Nrf2-Mediated Signaling*

To determine whether Nrf2 plays a pivotal role in AKT or ERK signaling, oxidative stress adaption, or apoptosis in melanoma cells after the uptake of endothelial mitochondria, we used brusatol, an Nrf2 inhibitor, and AI-1, an Nrf2 activator, to evaluate the activities of AKT, ERK, ROS, and apoptotic protein caspase-3. As shown in Figure 3, treatment with brusatol (40 nM) for 48 h revealed that the suppression of Nrf2 inhibited AKT signaling, increased ROS, and promoted apoptosis. By contrast, AI-1-activated AKT signaling reduced ROS and inhibited apoptosis, specifically AI-1- or brusatol-regulated AKT phosphorylation but not ERK (Figure 3).

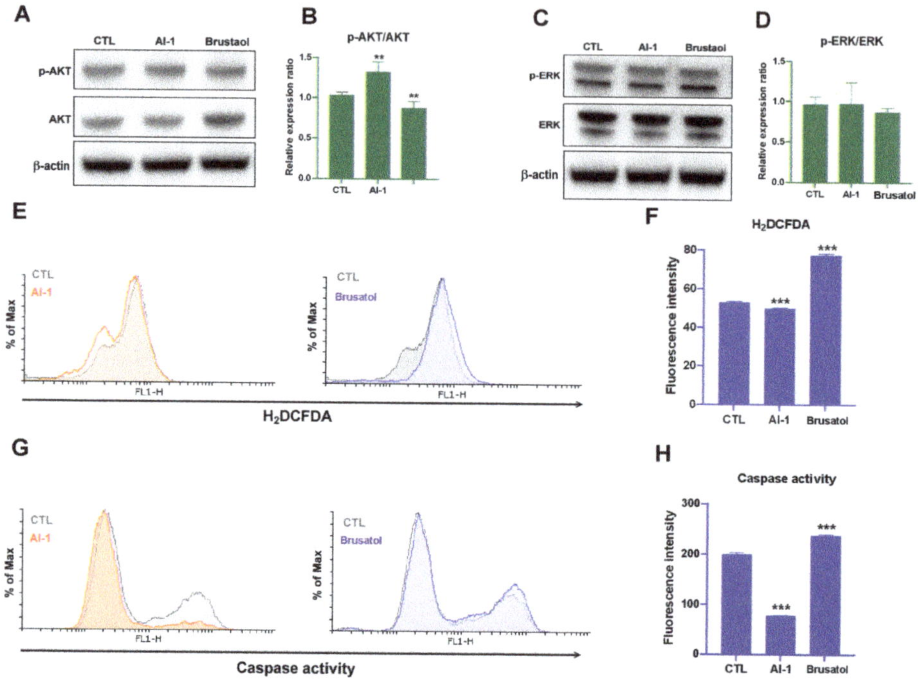

Figure 3. Effects of AI-1 and brusatol on B16F10 Cells. (**A**) Western blot analysis comparing the ratio of p-AKT/AKT in B16F10 cells treated with AI-1 (10 μ) and brusatol (40 nM) at 48 h. (**B**) Quantitative analysis of the p-AKT/AKT ratio after treatment with AI-1 and brusatol, as determined through Western blotting at 48 h. (**C**) Western blot analysis comparing the ratio of p-ERK/ERK in B16F10 cells treated with AI-1 (10 μ) and brusatol (40 nM) at 48 h. (**D**) Quantitative analysis of the p-ERK/ERK ratio after treatment with AI-1 and brusatol, as measured through Western blotting at 48 h. (**E**) Cellular ROS levels of B16F10 cells treated with AI-1 (10 μ) and brusatol (40 nM) at 48 h, as determined through flow cytometry. (**F**) Quantification of ROS levels in B16F10 cells treated with AI-1 (10 μM) and brusatol (40 nM) at 48 h, as determined through flow cytometry. (**G**) Evaluation of caspase activity in B16F10 cells treated with AI-1 (10 μM) and brusatol (40 nM) at 48 h, as determined through flow cytometry. (**H**) Quantitative analysis of caspase activity in B16F10 cells treated with AI-1 (10 μ) and brusatol (40 nM) at 48 h, as determined through flow cytometry. Data are presented as the mean ± standard error of the mean after ≥3 independent experiments. Statistical significance was assessed using a two-tailed Student's *t*-test: ** $p < 0.01$, *** $p < 0.005$.

2.4. *Transplantation of Endothelial Mitochondria-Promoted Melanoma Tumor Growth through Nrf2-Mediated Pathway in a Tumor Xenograft Animal Model*

Mice were inoculated with B16F10 cells containing HUVEC mitochondria. After 10 days, the tumors in these mice were larger than those in the mice injected with B16F10 cells without HUVEC mitochondria (Figure 4A,B). Protein expression in the tumors in these mice was similar to that observed in melanoma cells after the uptake of endothelial mitochondria (Figure 4C–F). These results indicate that the uptake of endothelial mitochondria by melanoma cells promotes tumor growth through AKT/ERK and Nrf2-mediated pathways.

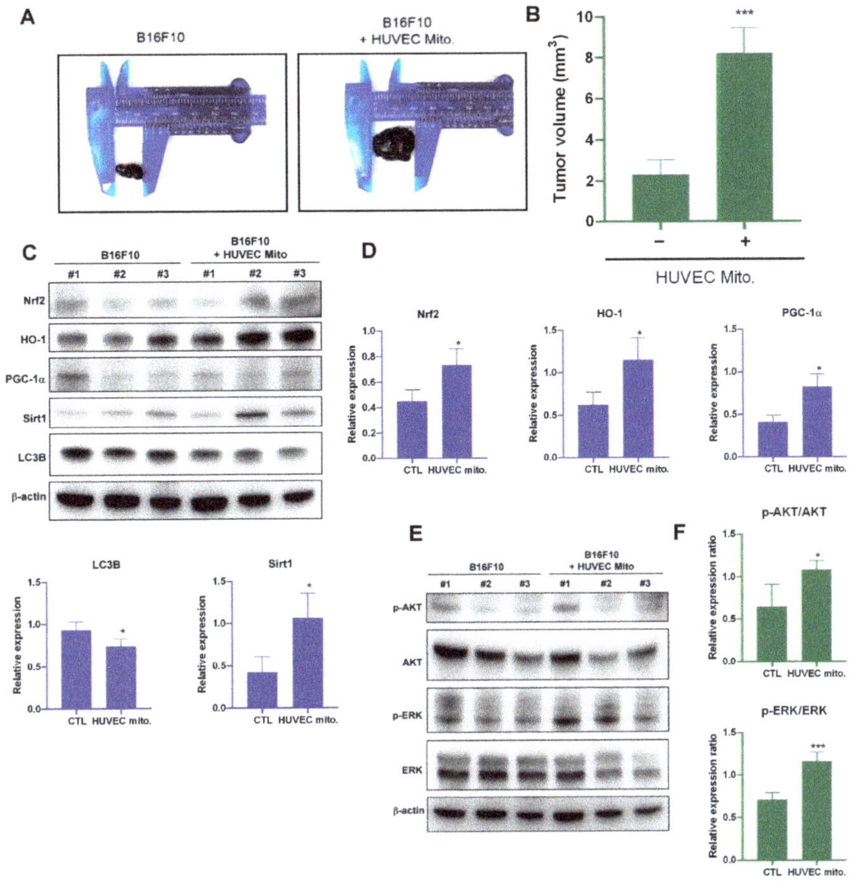

Figure 4. Xenograft analysis of melanoma tumor growth. (**A**) Mice were inoculated with B16F10 cells that underwent HUVEC mitochondrial transplantation and were monitored for 10 days. (**B**) Tumor size analysis in six mice. (**C**) Western blot analysis comparing the protein expression levels of Nrf2, HO-1, PGC-1α, Sirt1, and LC3B in B16F10 tumors with or without HUVEC mitochondrial transplantation at 10 days. (**D**) Quantification of the protein expression levels of Nrf2, HO-1, PGC-1α, Sirt1, and LC3B in B16F10 tumors with or without HUVEC mitochondrial transplantation at 10 days. (**E**) Western blot analysis of AKT or ERK signaling in B16F10 tumors with or without HUVEC mitochondrial transplantation at 10 days. (**F**) Quantitative analysis of p-AKT/AKT and p-ERK/ERK ratios in B16F10 tumors with or without HUVEC mitochondrial transplantation at 10 days. Data are presented as the mean ± standard error of the mean after ≥3 independent experiments. Statistical significance was assessed using a two-tailed Student's *t*-test: * $p < 0.05$, *** $p < 0.005$.

2.5. Transplant of Endothelial Mitochondria to Melanoma Upregulated Matrix Metallopeptidase 9, TGF-β1 and Induced M2-Type TAM in a Tumor Xenograft Animal Model

Nrf2 activates several oncogenes, including matrix metallopeptidase 9 (MMP9). MMP9 is the main enzyme able to remodel the extracellular matrix by favoring the tumor invasive processes [32,33]. Protein expression in the tumors and melanoma cells revealed the upregulation of MMP-9 and TGF-β1 after the transplantation of endothelial mitochondria (Figure 5A–D). The TGF-β signaling pathway plays a role in melanoma metastasis and macrophage polarization. TGF-β induces macrophage polarization into M2-like TAMs. These cells expressed the enzyme Arg1 display tumorigenic functions with increased metastatic potential and tumor cell proliferation [10–13,34]. TGF-β induces macrophages to express the M2-type marker Arg1 and downregulates the expression of the M1-type marker iNOS. In the mitochondrial transplantation groups, Arg1 was upregulated not only in a tumor xenograft animal model, but also in a B16F10 melanoma cell model. However, iNOS was downregulated in the mitochondrial transplant groups but not in the control groups (Figure 5E,F). Finally, TGF-β-induced macrophage Arg1 expression was confirmed in TGF-β1-treated RAW264.7 macrophage cells (Figure 5G,H).

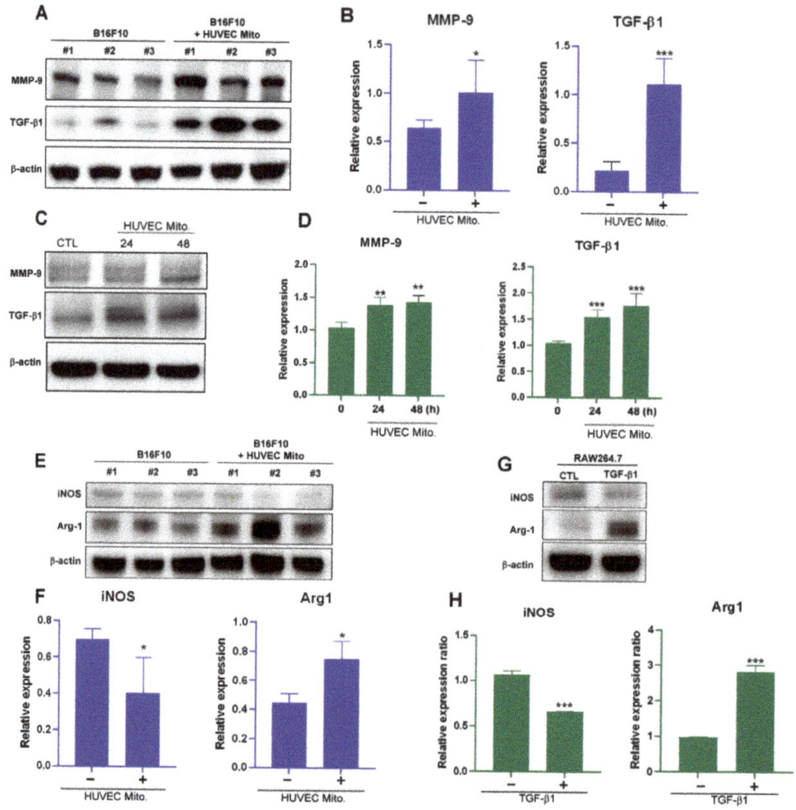

Figure 5. Xenograft analysis of melanoma tumor growth. (**A**) Western blot analysis comparing the protein expression levels of MMP-9 and TGF-β1 in B16F10 tumors with or without HUVEC mitochondrial transplantation at 10 days. (**B**) Quantitative analysis of MMP-9 and TGF-β1 protein expression levels in B16F10 tumors with or without HUVEC mitochondrial transplantation at 10 days. (**C**) Western blot analysis comparing the protein expression levels of MMP-9 and TGF-β1 in B16F10 cells with and without HUVEC mitochondrial transplantation at 24 or 48 h. (**D**) Quantification of MMP-9 and TGF-β1 expression after treatment with HUVEC mitochondria, as measured through Western blotting at 24 or 48 h. (**E**) Western blot analysis comparing iNOS and Arg1 protein levels in B16F10 tumors with or without HUVEC mitochondrial transplantation at 10 days. (**F**) Quantitative analysis of iNOS and MMP-9 protein levels in B16F10 tumors with or without HUVEC mitochondrial transplantation at 10 days. (**G**) Western blot analysis comparing iNOS and Arg1 protein expression levels in RAW264.7 cells treated with or without TGF-β1 (20 ng/mL) at 48 h. (**H**) Quantification of iNOS and MMP-9 protein levels in RAW264.7 cells treated with or without TGF-β1 (20 ng/mL) at 48 h. Data are presented as the mean ± standard error of the mean after ≥3 independent experiments. Statistical significance was assessed using a two-tailed Student's *t*-test: * $p < 0.05$, ** $p < 0.01$, *** $p < 0.005$.

2.6. *Transplant of Endothelial Mitochondria into Melanoma Cells Upregulated TGF-β Expression through the Nrf2-Mediated Pathway*

To determine whether Nrf2 also plays a role in TGF-β expression, we used SB431540, a TGF-β inhibitor, and brusatol to evaluate the expression of TGF-β in B16F10 cells containing HUVEC mitochondria. SB431540 inhibited TGF-β1 expression but did not affect Nrf2 expression (Figure 6A,B). By contrast, brusatol inhibited the expression of both Nrf2 and TGF-β1 (Figure 6C,D), indicating that Nrf2 plays a role in TGF-β expression in melanoma containing endothelial mitochondria.

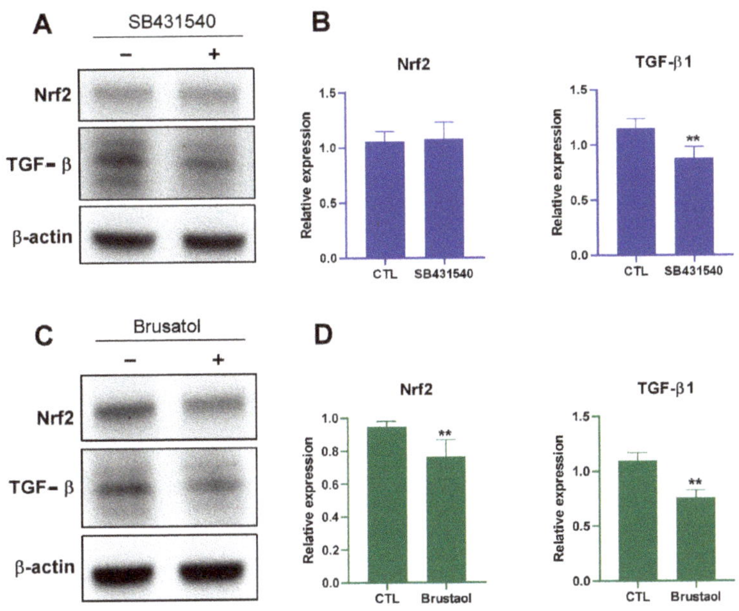

Figure 6. Effects of SB431540 and brusatol on B16F10 Cells. (**A**) Western blot analysis comparing Nrf2 and TGF-β1 protein levels in B16F10 cells with or without SB431540 (10 μM) treatment at 48 h. (**B**) Quantification of Nrf2 and TGF-β1 expression levels after treatment with or without SB431540, measured through Western blotting at 48 h. (**C**) Western blot analysis comparing Nrf2 and TGF-β1 in B16F10 cells treated with or without brusatol (40 nM) at 48 h. (**D**) Quantification of Nrf2 and TGF-β1 expression levels at 48 h after treatment with or without brusatol, as determined through Western blotting. Data are presented as the mean ± standard error of the mean after ≥3 independent experiments. Statistical significance was assessed using a two-tailed Student's *t*-test: ** $p < 0.01$.

3. Discussion

The TME plays a vital role in cancer development. Melanoma cells rely on their interactions with various other cells in their TME because such interactions are crucial for acquiring the characteristics typical of solid cancers. ECs are among the key interacting cell types in the gynecologic melanoma microenvironment. Studies have highlighted that although several mechanisms facilitate crosstalk between cancer and stromal cells, mitochondrial transfer supports cancer progression [22,35]. Thus, other studies have extensively investigated the effects of mitochondrial transfer on cell survival and antiapoptotic processes [24,35]. Cancer-associated fibroblasts (CAFs), which are predominant in the stromal compartment of many solid cancers, contribute to both tumor initiation and tumor progression. In particular, CAFs promote prostate cancer malignancy through mitochondrial transfer and metabolic reprogramming [36]. However, the role of endothelial mitochondria in melanoma progression remains unclear. Multiple methods for delivering exogenous mitochondria to recipient cells have been developed. Mitochondrial transplantation is one such method used to specifically examine the functional changes in recipient cancer cells after the uptake of mitochondria from donor cells in the TME. Various approaches—including coculturing, direct injection, and intracoronary vascular infusion in animal models—can be employed for mitochondrial transplantation [28]. Coculturing is the simplest approach for investigating the effects of mitochondrial uptake on the function of recipient cells. In addition, exogenous mitochondria can be introduced into cells through cell fusion, actin-dependent endocytosis, or micropinocytosis [37]. The present study investigated the effects of endothelial mitochondrial transplantation on melanoma progression.

Specifically, this study demonstrated that transplanting exogenous heterologous mitochondria from HUVECs into B16F10 melanoma cells resulted in the successful uptake of these mitochondria, thereby promoting the survival and proliferation of melanoma cells. However, the intricate mechanisms underlying this process remain unclear. Melanoma cells exhibit a high proliferative capacity mainly because of the constitutive activation of the ERK and AKT pathways, which results in rapid cell growth through the upregulation of cyclin D1 and cyclin E [38–40]. The increased expression of cyclin D1 in both primary and metastatic melanoma [41] indicates its crucial role in tumor progression. Although the caspase-3 increased and then decreased at 48 h, in the present study, after the transplantation of HUVEC mitochondria, B16F10 cells exhibited enhanced ERK and AKT signaling and increased cyclin D1 and cyclin E expression, suggesting that the transfer of endothelial mitochondria from the TME supports the growth of melanoma, a finding corroborated by relevant studies. Mitochondrial transfer between ECs and cancer cells causes phenotypic changes and induces chemoresistance in cancer cells [22]. In addition, one study demonstrated that stem cells donate their mitochondria to neighboring cells, aiding oxidative stress resistance and improving metabolic conditions, and thus promoting cell proliferation and enhancing antiapoptotic capability [42]. For instance, the introduction of healthy mitochondria into human prostate cancer PC-3 cells promoted cell proliferation and rescued cells from cisplatin-induced death [23]. Moreover, the engulfment of foreign somatic-derived mitochondria by MSCs increased the expression of the cytoprotective enzyme HO-1 and stimulated mitochondrial biogenesis [42].

HO-1 is a downstream protein of Nrf2 [30]. In this study, after the transplantation of HUVEC mitochondria, we observed increases in Nrf2, HO-1, PGC-1α, and Sirt1 levels. Sirt1 plays a key role in metabolic control and regulates the proliferation and viability of melanoma cancer cells [43]. It also contributes to mitochondrial biogenesis and maintains cellular redox homeostasis by increasing PGC-1α expression [44] and promoting Nrf2 activation [45]. Nrf2 activation promotes the transcription of cytoprotective genes and antioxidant enzymes, thereby protecting against oxidative stress in melanoma [46]. Our findings revealed that the autophagic marker LC3B was downregulated in melanoma cells and in a xenograft tumor animal model. Autophagy modulation occurs through an ROS-dependent mechanism. Inhibition of the antioxidant protein HO-1 induced autophagy in cancer cells [47]. As depicted in Figure 3E, the ROS level was reduced by the Nrf2 inhibitor. These results suggest that autophagy is inhibited through Nrf2/HO-1-mediated ROS elimination in melanoma cells containing endothelial mitochondria. In addition, AKT phosphorylation activates Nrf2-dependent mitochondrial biogenesis [48]. In the present study, the Nrf2 inhibitor suppressed AKT signaling (Figure 3C), suggesting that Nrf2 regulates AKT activity in melanoma cells through a positive feedback loop after the uptake of endothelial mitochondria. TGF-β promotes MMP-9-mediated tumor invasion [49]. In addition, TGF-β1not only promotes cancer cell invasion and metastasis, but also induces M2-type TAM polarization. Macrophages in primary malignant melanoma may contain the melanin pigment [50]. M2-type TAMs are recognized as a predictor of poor prognosis in patients with cutaneous malignant melanoma [51]. Finally, brusatol suppressed TGF-β (Figure 6C), indicating that Nrf2 may play a role in TGF-β1-induced M2-type TAM polarization after the uptake of mitochondria from ECs in the TME of melanoma cells.

The present study observed a time-dependent increase in AKT phosphorylation following mitochondrial transplantation, suggesting that endothelial mitochondrial transplantation contributes to melanoma proliferation by enabling AKT-mediated PGC-1α–Nrf2-dependent mitochondrial biogenesis and cellular redox homeostasis, which in turn promotes cell proliferation and inhibit apoptosis. Nrf2 was involved in endothelial mitochondria transfer-mediated melanoma growth (Figure S1). Moreover, Nrf2 plays a role in TGF-β1-induced M2-type TAM polarization after the uptake of mitochondria from ECs in the TME of melanoma cells. Xenograft experiments revealed that tumors in the experimental group were significantly larger than those in the control group. These results indicated that melanoma cells became more proliferative following the incorporation of exogenous mitochondria into their mitochondrial network (Figure 7). This finding further supports the role of the endothelium in tumor development in the TME.

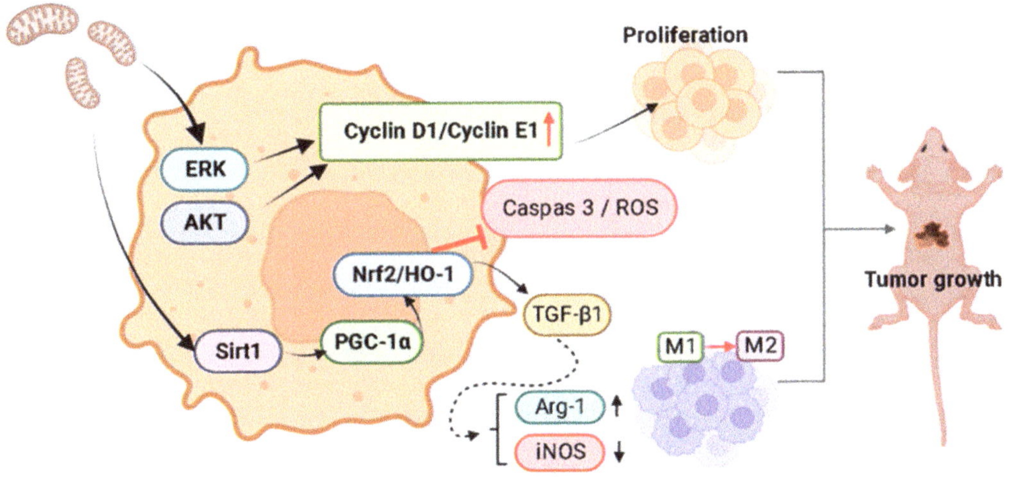

Figure 7. Schematic depicting how exogenous mitochondria from ECs can regulate melanoma tumor growth by activating proliferative signaling pathways, upregulating antioxidant molecules, and subsequently inhibiting apoptosis. Exogenous endothelial mitochondria activate the ERK/AKT and Sirt1/PGC-1a/Nrf2/HO-1 signaling pathways in melanoma cancer cells. The activated ERK/AKT signaling induces cyclin D1/cyclin E1-mediated cell proliferation. Upregulation of Sirt1/PGC-1a/Nrf2/HO-1 signaling inhibits ROS and caspase-3 activation and induces M2 macrophage polarization (by Arg-1 upregulation and iNOS downregulation) by Nrf-2/TGF-β signaling, thereby promoting tumor growth.

4. Materials and Methods

4.1. Cell Culture and Reagents

B16F10 melanoma cells, purchased from Merck (Darmstadt, Germany), were cultured in Dulbecco's Modified Eagle's Medium (DMEM) (Gibco, Waltham, MA, USA) supplemented with 10% FBS. Human umbilical vein ECs (HUVECs), purchased from Thermo Fisher Scientific (Waltham, MA, USA), were cultured in the M199 medium supplemented with 20% fetal bovine serum (FBS). Mouse monocyte macrophage RAW264.7, purchased from ATCC (Manassas, VA, USA), were cultured in DMEM (Gibco, Waltham, MA, USA) supplemented with 10% FBS. These cells were incubated at 37 °C in a growth chamber containing CO_2 (5%). Brusatol (MedChemExpress, NJ, USA), AI-1 (Focus biomolecules, Plymouth Meeting, PA, USA), and SB431542 (Sigma-Aldrich, St. Louis, MO, USA) in dimethyl sulfoxide (DMSO) (Sigma-Aldrich, St. Louis, MO, USA) were prepared and dissolved in a culture medium before treatment. Recombinant Human TGF-β1 (Cell Guidance Systems; GFH39-5, Cambridge, UK) was prepared and dissolved in a culture medium.

4.2. Isolation of Mitochondria and Mitochondrial Transplantation

Mitochondria were isolated following the protocol provided by Abcam. The cells were subjected to trypsinization and then collected through centrifugation. Lysis was performed using 500 μL of cytosol extraction buffer followed by moderate shaking for 20 min. The mixture was then centrifuged at 700× g for 20 min, after which the supernatant was transferred to a new tube. Additional centrifugation at 10,000× g was performed to precipitate the mitochondria. The mitochondria isolated from 5×10^6 HUVECs were co-incubated with B16F10 cells for a specified duration.

4.3. Cell Viability Analysis

B16F10 melanoma cells were seeded in 96-well dishes in quadruplicate at 6000 cells/well and cultured for 24 h before mitochondrial transplantation. Cell viability was analyzed using Cell Counting Kit-8 (Sigma–Aldrich, St. Louis, MO, USA) and absorbance was measured at 450 nm by using a microplate reader.

4.4. Cellular ROS Assay

The cells were harvested and washed with phosphate-buffered saline (PBS) and stained with 2',7'-dichlorodihydrofluorescein diacetate (H_2DCFDA; Med Chem Express, Monmouth Junction, NJ, USA) for 15 min. The cells were then washed twice with cold PBS, and analyzed through flow cytometry.

4.5. Caspase Activity Analysis

The cells were harvested, washed with PBS, and stained with a Cleaved Caspase-3 Staining Kit (Abcam, Cambridge, UK). The stained cells were then analyzed through flow cytometry.

4.6. Western Blot

Total proteins from the B16F10 cells into which HUVEC mitochondria were transplanted were extracted using a lysis buffer composed of HEPES (50 mM, pH 7.7), EDTA (1 mM), neocuproine (0.1 mM), and CHAPS (0.4%, w/v). Forty micrograms of proteins were mixed with a sample buffer containing Tris-HCl (62.5 mM, pH 6.8), SDS (3%, w/v), 2-mercaptoethanol (5%, v/v), and glycerol (10%, v/v). The proteins were then separated through SDS–polyacrylamide gel electrophoresis and transferred to a PVDF membrane (Millipore, Billerica, MA, USA). The membrane was incubated with primary antibodies against Nrf2 (1:1000; ABclonal, Woburn, MA, USA), PGC-1α (1:1000; NOVUS, CO, USA), sirt1 (1:1000; ABclonal, Woburn, MA, USA), HO-1 (1:1000; Cell Signaling, Danvers, MA, USA), LC3B (1:1000; Cell Signaling, Danvers, MA, USA), AKT (1:1000; Cell Signaling, Danvers, MA, USA), p-AKT (1:1000; Cell Signaling, Danvers, MA, USA), ERK (1:1000; Cell Signaling, Danvers, MA, USA), p-ERK (1:1000; Cell Signaling, Danvers, MA, USA), cyclin D1 (1:1000; Cell Signaling, Danvers, MA, USA), Cyclin E (1:1000; Cell Signaling, Danvers, MA, USA), caspase-3 (1:1000; Cell Signaling, Danvers, MA, USA), cleaved caspase-3 (c-caspase-3) (1:1000; Cell Signaling, Danvers, MA, USA), MMP9 (1:1000; arigo Biolaboratories, Hsinchu City, Taiwan), TGF-β1 (1:1000; Abcam, Cambridge, UK), iNOS (1:1000; ABclonal, Woburn, MA, USA), Arg-1 (1:1000; Proteintech, Planegg-Martinsried, Germany), or β-actin (1:1000; Cell Signaling, Danvers, MA, USA) at 4 °C. Subsequently, the membranes were incubated with secondary antibodies at room temperature for 1 h and analyzed using an electrochemiluminescence detection system.

4.7. Xenograft Tumor Experiments

After the HUVEC endothelial mitochondria had been transplanted into the B16F10 cells, these cells were then harvested and subcutaneously inoculated (5×10^6 cells/0.1 mL in PBS) into 6-week-old BALB/c nude mice (BioLASCO, Taipei City, Taiwan). The tumor volume was calculated using the formula $V = L \times W^2/2$ (L, length; W, width) and the tumors were harvested after 10 days.

4.8. Statistical Analysis

All data were analyzed using GraphPad Prism version 8 (GraphPad Software, San Diego, CA, USA). Results are presented as the mean ± standard error of the mean. Statistical significance was determined using Student's *t*-test, with the significance threshold set at $p < 0.05$.

5. Conclusions

The present study demonstrates that exogenous mitochondria from ECs can regulate the growth of melanoma tumors. This regulatory effect is achieved through the activation of proliferative signaling pathways, the upregulation of antioxidant molecules, and the subsequent inhibition of apoptosis. These results provide valuable insights into the role of mitochondrial transfer from ECs to melanoma cells in the regulation of the TME, and highlight potential targets for the treatment of gynecologic tract melanoma.

Supplementary Materials: The following supporting information can be downloaded at: https://www.mdpi.com/article/10.3390/ijms25031857/s1.

Author Contributions: Conceptualization, writing F.-C.K., B.H. and M.-W.L.; methodology, B.H. and M.-W.L.; validation, H.-Y.T., B.-L.C., P.-C.C. and K.-J.T.; investigation, H.-Y.T., B.-L.C., P.-C.C., K.-J.T. and C.-J.L.; resources, D.-C.W.; data curation, H.-Y.T., B.-L.C., P.-C.C., K.-J.T., C.-J.L. and M.-C.W.; writing—original draft preparation, F.-C.K., B.H. and M.-W.L.; writing—review and editing, B.H. and M.-W.L.; visualization, M.-C.W.; supervision, D.-C.W. and Y.-B.H.; project administration, H.-Y.T.; funding acquisition, B.H., M.-C.W. and D.-C.W. All authors have read and agreed to the published version of the manuscript.

Funding: This work was supported by Kaohsiung Medical University (KMU-TC112A02, 105-P032, 106-P009, kmtth 106-031, kmtth 107-030, kmtth 108-012) and the National Science and Technology Council of Taiwan (former Ministry of Science and Technology MOST 109-2314-B-037-118, MOST 110-2314-B-037-140, 111-2314-B-037-008).

Institutional Review Board Statement: The studies involving animal participants were reviewed and approved by the Affidavit of Approval of the Animal Use Protocol IACUC of E-Da Hospital (approval code: 112015).

Data Availability Statement: All data sets generated or analyzed in this study are included in the published article. Detailed data sets supporting the current study are available from the co-responding author upon request. This study did not generate new codes.

Conflicts of Interest: The authors declare no conflict of interest.

References

1. Mitra, D.; Farr, M.; Nagarajan, P.; Ho, J.; Bishop, A.J.; Jhingran, A.; Farooqi, A.S.; Frumovitz, M.; Amaria, R.N.; McQuade, J.L.; et al. Gynecologic tract melanoma in the contemporary therapeutic era: High rates of local and distant disease progression. *Gynecol. Oncol.* **2022**, *167*, 483–489. [CrossRef] [PubMed]
2. Bai, S.; Wu, Q.; Song, L.; Wu, W. Treatment of primary vaginal malignant melanoma and review of previous literature: A case report. *Medicine* **2023**, *102*, e36128.
3. Khayyat, A.; Pour, M.A.E.; Mousavi, S.; Khalili-Toosi, A.-R.; Amin, A. Primary Malignant Melanoma of the Genitourinary System: A Systemic Review and Report of Eight Cases. *Cureus* **2022**, *14*, e30444. [CrossRef]
4. Yajima, I.; Kumasaka, M.Y.; Thang, N.D.; Goto, Y.; Takeda, K.; Yamanoshita, O.; Iida, M.; Ohgami, N.; Tamura, H.; Kawamoto, Y.; et al. RAS/RAF/MEK/ERK and PI3K/PTEN/AKT Signaling in Malignant Melanoma Progression and Therapy. *Dermatol. Res. Pract.* **2011**, *2011*, 354191. [CrossRef]
5. Davies, M.A. The Role of the PI3K-AKT Pathway in Melanoma. *Cancer J.* **2012**, *18*, 142–147. [CrossRef]
6. Savoia, P.; Fava, P.; Casoni, F.; Cremona, O. Targeting the ERK Signaling Pathway in Melanoma. *Int. J. Mol. Sci.* **2019**, *20*, 1483. [CrossRef]
7. Ramirez, J.A.; Guitart, J.; Rao, M.S.; Diaz, L.K. Cyclin D1 expression in melanocytic lesions of the skin. *Ann. Diagn. Pathol.* **2005**, *9*, 185–188. [CrossRef]
8. Villanueva, J.; Herlyn, M. Melanoma and the tumor microenvironment. *Curr. Oncol. Rep.* **2008**, *10*, 439–446. [CrossRef]
9. Lou, E. A Ticket to Ride: The Implications of Direct Intercellular Communication via Tunneling Nanotubes in Peritoneal and Other Invasive Malignancies. *Front. Oncol.* **2020**, *10*, 559548. [CrossRef] [PubMed]

10. Boutilier, A.J.; Elsawa, S.F. Macrophage Polarization States in the Tumor Microenvironment. *Int. J. Mol. Sci.* **2021**, *22*, 6995. [CrossRef] [PubMed]
11. Wu, K.; Lin, K.; Li, X.; Yuan, X.; Xu, P.; Ni, P.; Xu, D. Redefining Tumor-Associated Macrophage Subpopulations and Functions in the Tumor Microenvironment. *Front. Immunol.* **2020**, *11*, 1731. [CrossRef]
12. Arlauckas, S.P.; Garren, S.B.; Garris, C.S.; Kohler, R.H.; Oh, J.; Pittet, M.J.; Weissleder, R. Arg1 expression defines immunosuppressive subsets of tumor-associated macrophages. *Theranostics* **2018**, *8*, 5842–5854. [CrossRef]
13. Zhang, F.; Wang, H.; Wang, X.; Jiang, G.; Liu, H.; Zhang, G.; Wang, H.; Fang, R.; Bu, X.; Cai, S.; et al. TGF-β induces M2-like macrophage polarization via SNAIL-mediated suppression of a pro-inflammatory phenotype. *Oncotarget* **2016**, *7*, 52294–52306. [CrossRef] [PubMed]
14. Al Amir Dache, Z.; Thierry, A.R. Mitochondria-derived cell-to-cell communication. *Cell Rep.* **2023**, *42*, 112728. [CrossRef] [PubMed]
15. Eugenin, E.; Camporesi, E.; Peracchia, C. Direct Cell-Cell Communication via Membrane Pores, Gap Junction Channels, and Tunneling Nanotubes: Medical Relevance of Mitochondrial Exchange. *Int. J. Mol. Sci.* **2022**, *23*, 6133. [CrossRef]
16. Spiegelman, B.M. Transcriptional control of mitochondrial energy metabolism through the PGC1 coactivators. *Novartis Found Symp.* **2007**, *287*, 60–63.
17. Wu, Z.; Puigserver, P.; Andersson, U.; Zhang, C.; Adelmant, G.; Mootha, V.; Troy, A.; Cinti, S.; Lowell, B.; Scarpulla, R.C.; et al. Mechanisms Controlling Mitochondrial Biogenesis and Respiration through the Thermogenic Coactivator PGC-1. *Cell* **1999**, *98*, 115–124. [CrossRef] [PubMed]
18. Vallabhaneni, K.C.; Haller, H.; Dumler, I. Vascular Smooth Muscle Cells Initiate Proliferation of Mesenchymal Stem Cells by Mitochondrial Transfer via Tunneling Nanotubes. *Stem Cells Dev.* **2012**, *21*, 3104–3113. [CrossRef] [PubMed]
19. Fahey, M.; Bennett, M.; Thomas, M.; Montney, K.; Vivancos-Koopman, I.; Pugliese, B.; Browning, L.; Bonassar, L.J.; Delco, M. Mesenchymal stromal cells donate mitochondria to articular chondrocytes exposed to mitochondrial, environmental, and mechanical stress. *Sci. Rep.* **2022**, *12*, 21525. [CrossRef] [PubMed]
20. Han, H.; Hu, J.; Yan, Q.; Zhu, J.; Zhu, Z.; Chen, Y.; Sun, J.; Zhang, R. Bone marrow-derived mesenchymal stem cells rescue injured H9c2 cells via transferring intact mitochondria through tunneling nanotubes in an in vitro simulated ischemia/reperfusion model. *Mol. Med. Rep.* **2016**, *13*, 1517–1524. [CrossRef] [PubMed]
21. Yang, X.; Ning, K.; Wang, D.-E.; Xu, H. Progress of Bone Marrow Mesenchymal Stem Cell Mitochondrial Transfer in Organ Injury Repair. *Stem Cells Dev.* **2023**, *32*, 379–386. [CrossRef]
22. Pasquier, J.; Guerrouahen, B.S.; Al Thawadi, H.; Ghiabi, P.; Maleki, M.; Abu-Kaoud, N.; Jacob, A.; Mirshahi, M.; Galas, L.; Rafii, S.; et al. Preferential transfer of mitochondria from endothelial to cancer cells through tunneling nanotubes modulates chemoresistance. *J. Transl. Med.* **2013**, *11*, 94. [CrossRef]
23. Nikoo, A.; Roudkenar, M.H.; Sato, T.; Kuwahara, Y.; Tomita, K.; Pourmohammadi-Bejarpasi, Z.; Najafi-Ghalehlou, N.; Roushandeh, A.M. Mitochondrial transfer in PC-3 cells fingerprinted in ferroptosis sensitivity: A brand new approach targeting cancer metabolism. *Hum. Cell* **2023**, *36*, 1441–1450. [CrossRef]
24. Nakhle, J.; Khattar, K.; Özkan, T.; Boughlita, A.; Moussa, D.A.; Darlix, A.; Lorcy, F.; Rigau, V.; Bauchet, L.; Gerbal-Chaloin, S.; et al. Mitochondria Transfer from Mesenchymal Stem Cells Confers Chemoresistance to Glioblastoma Stem Cells through Metabolic Rewiring. *Cancer Res. Commun.* **2023**, *3*, 1041–1056. [CrossRef]
25. Caicedo, A.; Fritz, V.; Brondello, J.-M.; Ayala, M.; Dennemont, I.; Abdellaoui, N.; de Fraipont, F.; Moisan, A.; Prouteau, C.A.; Boukhaddaoui, H.; et al. MitoCeption as a new tool to assess the effects of mesenchymal stem/stromal cell mitochondria on cancer cell metabolism and function. *Sci. Rep.* **2015**, *5*, 9073. [CrossRef]
26. Clemente-Suárez, V.J.; Martín-Rodríguez, A.; Yáñez-Sepúlveda, R.; Tornero-Aguilera, J.F. Mitochondrial Transfer as a Novel Therapeutic Approach in Disease Diagnosis and Treatment. *Int. J. Mol. Sci.* **2023**, *24*, 8848. [CrossRef] [PubMed]
27. Liu, Q.; Liu, M.; Yang, T.; Wang, X.; Cheng, P.; Zhou, H. What can we do to optimize mitochondrial transplantation therapy for myocardial ischemia-reperfusion injury? *Mitochondrion* **2023**, *72*, 72–83. [CrossRef] [PubMed]
28. Liu, Z.; Sun, Y.; Qi, Z.; Cao, L.; Ding, S. Mitochondrial transfer/transplantation: An emerging therapeutic approach for multiple diseases. *Cell Biosci.* **2022**, *12*, 66. [CrossRef] [PubMed]
29. Wang, Z.; Yuan, S.; Li, Y.; Zhang, Z.; Xiao, W.; Tang, D.; Ye, K.; Liu, Z.; Wang, C.; Zheng, Y.; et al. Regulation on SIRT1-PGC-1α/Nrf2 pathway together with selective inhibition of aldose reductase makes compound hr5F a potential agent for the treatment of diabetic complications. *Biochem. Pharmacol.* **2018**, *150*, 54–63. [CrossRef] [PubMed]
30. Nitti, M.; Piras, S.; Marinari, U.M.; Moretta, L.; Pronzato, M.A.; Furfaro, A.L. HO-1 Induction in Cancer Progression: A Matter of Cell Adaptation. *Antioxidants* **2017**, *6*, 29. [CrossRef]
31. Bales, E.S.; Dietrich, C.; Bandyopadhyay, D.; Schwahn, D.J.; Xu, W.; Didenko, V.; Leiss, P.; Conrad, N.; Pereira-Smith, O.; Orengo, I.; et al. High Levels of Expression of p27KIP1 and Cyclin E in Invasive Primary Malignant Melanomas. *J. Investig. Dermatol.* **1999**, *113*, 1039–1046. [CrossRef] [PubMed]
32. Napoli, S.; Scuderi, C.; Gattuso, G.; Bella, V.D.; Candido, S.; Basile, M.S.; Libra, M.; Falzone, L. Functional Roles of Matrix Metalloproteinases and Their Inhibitors in Melanoma. *Cells* **2020**, *9*, 1151. [CrossRef] [PubMed]
33. Zimta, A.-A.; Cenariu, D.; Irimie, A.; Magdo, L.; Nabavi, S.M.; Atanasov, A.G.; Berindan-Neagoe, I. The Role of Nrf2 Activity in Cancer Development and Progression. *Cancers* **2019**, *11*, 1755. [CrossRef] [PubMed]

34. Sumitomo, R.; Menju, T.; Shimazu, Y.; Toyazaki, T.; Chiba, N.; Miyamoto, H.; Hirayama, Y.; Nishikawa, S.; Tanaka, S.; Yutaka, Y.; et al. M2-like tumor-associated macrophages promote epithelial-mesenchymal transition through the transforming growth factor β/Smad/zinc finger e-box binding homeobox pathway with increased metastatic potential and tumor cell proliferation in lung squamous cell carcinoma. *Cancer Sci.* **2023**, *114*, 4521–4534. [PubMed]
35. Borcherding, N.; Brestoff, J.R. The power and potential of mitochondria transfer. *Nature* **2023**, *623*, 283–291. [CrossRef]
36. Goliwas, K.F.; Libring, S.; Berestesky, E.; Gholizadeh, S.; Schwager, S.C.; Frost, A.R.; Gaborski, T.R.; Zhang, J.; Reinhart-King, C.A. Mitochondrial transfer from cancer-associated fibroblasts increases migration in aggressive breast cancer. *J. Cell Sci.* **2023**, *136*, jcs260419. [CrossRef] [PubMed]
37. Patel, D.; Rorbach, J.; Downes, K.; Szukszto, M.J.; Pekalski, M.L.; Minczuk, M. Macropinocytic entry of isolated mitochondria in epidermal growth factor-activated human osteosarcoma cells. *Sci. Rep.* **2017**, *7*, 12886. [CrossRef]
38. Jiang, L.; Campagne, C.; Sundström, E.; Sousa, P.; Imran, S.; Seltenhammer, M.; Pielberg, G.; Olsson, M.J.; Egidy, G.; Andersson, L.; et al. Constitutive activation of the ERK pathway in melanoma and skin melanocytes in Grey horses. *BMC Cancer* **2014**, *14*, 857. [CrossRef]
39. Dhawan, P.; Singh, A.B.; Ellis, D.L.; Richmond, A. Constitutive activation of Akt/protein kinase B in melanoma leads to up-regulation of nuclear factor-kappaB and tumor progression. *Cancer Res.* **2002**, *62*, 7335–7342. [PubMed]
40. Ciołczyk-Wierzbicka, D.; Gil, D.; Laidler, P. Treatment of melanoma with selected inhibitors of signaling kinases effectively reduces proliferation and induces expression of cell cycle inhibitors. *Med. Oncol.* **2017**, *35*, 7. [CrossRef]
41. Gammon, B.; Ali, L.; Guitart, J.; Gerami, P. Homogeneous Staining Regions for Cyclin D1, a Marker of Poor Prognosis in Malignant Melanoma. *Am. J. Dermatopathol.* **2012**, *34*, 487–490. [CrossRef]
42. Mahrouf-Yorgov, M.; Augeul, L.; Da Silva, C.C.; Jourdan, M.; Rigolet, M.; Manin, S.; Ferrera, R.; Ovize, M.; Henry, A.; Guguin, A.; et al. Mesenchymal stem cells sense mitochondria released from damaged cells as danger signals to activate their rescue properties. *Cell Death Differ.* **2017**, *24*, 1224–1238. [CrossRef]
43. Ohanna, M.; Bonet, C.; Bille, K.; Allegra, M.; Davidson, I.; Bahadoran, P.; Lacour, J.P.; Ballotti, R.; Bertolotto, C. SIRT1 promotes proliferation and inhibits the senescence-like phenotype in human melanoma cells. *Oncotarget* **2014**, *5*, 2085–2095. [CrossRef] [PubMed]
44. Scarpulla, R.C. Metabolic control of mitochondrial biogenesis through the PGC-1 family regulatory network. *Biochim. Biophys. Acta* **2011**, *1813*, 1269–1278. [CrossRef] [PubMed]
45. Aquilano, K.; Baldelli, S.; Pagliei, B.; Cannata, S.M.; Rotilio, G.; Ciriolo, M.R. p53 Orchestrates the PGC-1α-Mediated Antioxidant Response Upon Mild Redox and Metabolic Imbalance. *Antioxidants Redox Signal.* **2013**, *18*, 386–399. [CrossRef] [PubMed]
46. Carpenter, E.L.; Becker, A.L.; Indra, A.K. NRF2 and Key Transcriptional Targets in Melanoma Redox Manipulation. *Cancers* **2022**, *14*, 1531. [CrossRef] [PubMed]
47. Ahmad, I.M.; Dafferner, A.J.; Salloom, R.J.; Abdalla, M.Y. Heme Oxygenase-1 Inhibition Modulates Autophagy and Augments Arsenic Trioxide Cytotoxicity in Pancreatic Cancer Cells. *Biomedicines* **2023**, *11*, 2580. [CrossRef] [PubMed]
48. Gureev, A.P.; Shaforostova, E.A.; Popov, V.N. Regulation of Mitochondrial Biogenesis as a Way for Active Longevity: Interaction Between the Nrf2 and PGC-1α Signaling Pathways. *Front. Genet.* **2019**, *10*, 435. [CrossRef]
49. Festuccia, C.; Angelucci, A.; Gravina, G.L.; Villanova, I.; Teti, A.; Albini, A.; Bologna, M.; Abini, A. Osteoblast-derived TGF-beta1 modulates matrix degrading protease expression and activity in prostate cancer cells. *Int. J. Cancer* **2000**, *85*, 407–415. [CrossRef]
50. Khalbuss, W.E.; Hossain, M.; Elhosseiny, A. Primary malignant melanoma of the urinary bladder diagnosed by urine cytology: A case report. *Acta Cytol.* **2001**, *45*, 631–635. [CrossRef]
51. Asai, Y.; Yanagawa, N.; Osakabe, M.; Yamada, N.; Sugimoto, R.; Sato, A.; Ito, K.; Koike, Y.; Tanji, T.; Sakuraba, M.; et al. The clinicopathological impact of tumor-associated macrophages in patients with cutaneous malignant melanoma. *J. Surg. Oncol.* **2024**, *129*, 381–391. [CrossRef] [PubMed]

International Journal of
Molecular Sciences

MDPI

Article

Kinase Suppressor of RAS 1 (KSR1) Maintains the Transformed Phenotype of BRAFV600E Mutant Human Melanoma Cells

Zhi Liu [1], Aleksandar Krstic [1], Ashish Neve [1], Cristina Casalou [2], Nora Rauch [1], Kieran Wynne [1], Hilary Cassidy [1,3], Amanda McCann [4,5], Emma Kavanagh [4], Brendan McCann [1], Alfonso Blanco [5], Jens Rauch [1,3,*] and Walter Kolch [1,4,*]

1 Systems Biology Ireland (SBI), School of Medicine, University College Dublin, D04 V1W8 Dublin, Ireland; 09liuzhi@sina.com (Z.L.); aleksandar.krstic@ucd.ie (A.K.); ashish.neve@ucd.ie (A.N.); nora.rauch@ucd.ie (N.R.); kieran.wynne1@ucd.ie (K.W.); hilary.cassidy@ucd.ie (H.C.); brendan.mccann@cantab.net (B.M.)

2 Charles Institute of Dermatology, School of Medicine, University College Dublin, D04 V1W8 Dublin, Ireland; cristina.casalou@ucd.ie

3 School of Biomolecular & Biomedical Science, University College Dublin, D04 V1W8 Dublin, Ireland

4 School of Medicine, University College Dublin, D04 V1W8 Dublin, Ireland; amanda.mccann@ucd.ie (A.M.); emma.kavanagh@ucdconnect.ie (E.K.)

5 Conway Institute, University College Dublin, D04 V1W8 Dublin, Ireland; alfonso.blanco@ucd.ie

* Correspondence: jens.rauch@ucd.ie (J.R.); walter.kolch@ucd.ie (W.K.); Tel.: +353-1-716-6337 (J.R.); +353-1-716-6303 (W.K.)

Abstract: Kinase Suppressor of RAS 1 (KSR1) is a scaffolding protein for the RAS-RAF-MEK-ERK pathway, which is one of the most frequently altered pathways in human cancers. Previous results have shown that KSR1 has a critical role in mutant RAS-mediated transformation. Here, we examined the role of KSR1 in mutant BRAF transformation. We used CRISPR/Cas9 to knock out KSR1 in a BRAFV600E-transformed melanoma cell line. KSR1 loss produced a complex phenotype characterised by impaired proliferation, cell cycle defects, decreased transformation, decreased invasive migration, increased cellular senescence, and increased apoptosis. To decipher this phenotype, we used a combination of proteomic ERK substrate profiling, global protein expression profiling, and biochemical validation assays. The results suggest that KSR1 directs ERK to phosphorylate substrates that have a critical role in ensuring cell survival. The results further indicate that KSR1 loss induces the activation of p38 Mitogen-Activated Protein Kinase (MAPK) and subsequent cell cycle aberrations and senescence. In summary, KSR1 function plays a key role in oncogenic BRAF transformation.

Keywords: melanoma; KSR1; apoptosis; senescence; proliferation

1. Introduction

The RAS-RAF-MEK-ERK pathway (hereafter called the ERK pathway) is a central signalling pathway in the cell. It is mutationally altered in 30–40% of all human cancers and may be hyperactivated in the majority of cancers due to crosstalk with other pathways [1]. The ERK pathway has a bewildering array of functions [2], and this versatility is tightly coordinated by activation dynamics and scaffolding proteins [3,4]. The scaffold protein Kinase Suppressor of RAS 1 (KSR1) has emerged as a major facilitator of normal and oncogenic RAS signalling by binding all three kinases in the pathway, i.e., RAF, MEK, and ERK. Originally, KSR1 was considered a platform that facilitates RAF phosphorylation of MEK and MEK phosphorylation of ERK by bringing the kinases into physical proximity. However, a more nuanced view of KSR1 functions is emerging [5]. KSR1 not only binds to these kinases but also regulates their activation. For instance, MEK binding to KSR1 stimulates its binding to BRAF, resulting in the allosteric activation of BRAF's kinase activity towards MEK [6]. Similarly, KSR1 preferentially binds to ERK dimers and directs them to cytosolic substrates [7].

Perhaps the most intriguing finding is that KSR1 knockout mice are healthy, but resistant to oncogenic RAS tumorigenesis [8]. While this protection may not be complete in all cancer types [9], it has sparked substantial interest in finding out more about KSR1 functions in oncogenic transformation. As a result, we now know that KSR1 regulates several aspects of oncogenic RAS and RAF transformation, including cell proliferation [10], apoptosis [11], senescence [12,13], and the epithelial–mesenchymal transition (EMT) [14]. Most of these KSR1 functions facilitate RAS transformation, and KSR1 has become a plausible drug target for combating RAS-driven cancers [15].

However, how KSR1 may contribute to transformation by mutant, oncogenic BRAF is not well understood. Therefore, KSR1 was knocked out in BRAFV600E-driven melanoma cells. The knockout resulted in a complex phenotype with features of cell cycle aberration, senescence, invasion, and enhanced apoptosis. Analysis of the molecular mechanisms suggests a multi-layered mechanism that includes KSR1 control of ERK substrate specificity.

2. Results

2.1. Knocking Out KSR1 in BRAFV600E-Mutated SK-MEL-239 Cells Does Not Impact Bulk RAF-ERK Signalling

To knock out KSR1 gene expression in SK-MEL-239 cells, we used the CRISPR/Cas9-OFP system with three crRNAs [16] that target exon 5 of KSR1 (Figures 1A and S1A). This exon is common to different KSR1 splice variants and located close to the start of the coding sequence. Its disruption is expected to result in a complete loss of KSR1 protein expression. After isolating successfully transfected, i.e., OFP-expressing, cells, KSR1 knockout clones were identified by Genomic Cleavage Detection (GCD) assays and Sanger sequencing (Figure S1B). We selected three clones with homozygous indels in KSR1 exon 5 that cause a complete loss of KSR1 protein expression, as detectable by Western blotting (Figure 1B). There was no compensatory upregulation of KSR2 expression, and the KSR1 knockout did not affect the protein levels of BRAF, CRAF, MEK, or ERK. Interestingly, we only observed a slightly increased activation of MEK and ERK, suggesting that KSR1 function is not required to sustain MEK-ERK activity in these cells. To ensure the lineage fidelity, we genotyped the parental and KSR1 knockout cells and found that they all retained the same genotype (Table S2).

2.2. The Biological Phenotype of KSR1 Loss

In order to test the biological consequences of the KSR1 knockout, we assayed different biological traits. KSR1 knockout cells proliferated significantly slower than the parental cells (Figure 2A). Cell cycle analysis showed that KSR1 loss did not prevent cells from exiting interphase (G0/G1) but retarded their progression through late S (by 4–10%) and G2/M phases (by 7–16%) (Figures 2B and S2), suggesting that KSR1 function is needed to complete the cell cycle after DNA replication.

We noticed that KSR1$^{-/-}$ cultures contained large, flat cells that resembled the phenotype of senescent cells. Performing a stain for acidic β-galactosidase confirmed an increase in the number of senescent cells in KSR1 KO1-3 clones (Figure 3A,B). The expression of the proliferation marker Ki67 was attenuated in the phenotypically senescent cells (Figure 3C). Interestingly, most of the non-proliferative, acidic β-galactosidase-positive cells were multinucleated, further supporting the interpretation of the cell cycle data that KSR1$^{-/-}$ cells can replicate DNA but are unable to complete mitosis and cell fission. Cells that arrest in mitosis for a prolonged time typically die by apoptosis or exit mitosis without dividing, causing a multinucleated phenotype [17]. Indeed, all KSR1 KO clones showed increased rates of apoptosis (Figure 3D) and DNA damage, as indicated by increased phosphorylation of pCHK1 (Figure 3E). Taken together, these data suggest that the decrease in cell proliferation is caused by a combined increase in senescence and apoptosis.

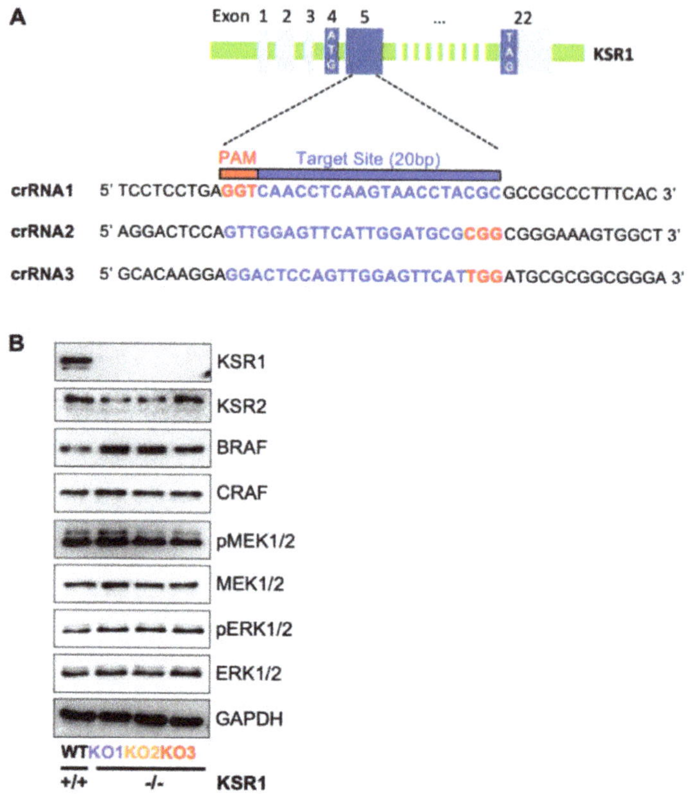

Figure 1. Knockout of KSR1 in BRAFV600E-mediated SK-MEL-239 cells does not impact bulk RAF-ERK signalling. (**A**) Schematic of KSR1 exon 1–5 structure and sequence of sgRNAs targeting exon 5. Untranslated exons are shown in light blue, and translated exons are in dark blue. Translation start (ATG) and stop (TAG) codons are indicated. Genomic target sites of the three crRNAs and corresponding PAM sites are shown in blue and red, respectively. (**B**) KSR1/2 and RAF-MEK-ERK pathway proteins were detected by Western blotting in wildtype (WT) cells and three KSR1 knockout clones (KO1-3). MEK and ERK activation was assessed using phosphospecific antibodies (pMEK and pERK).

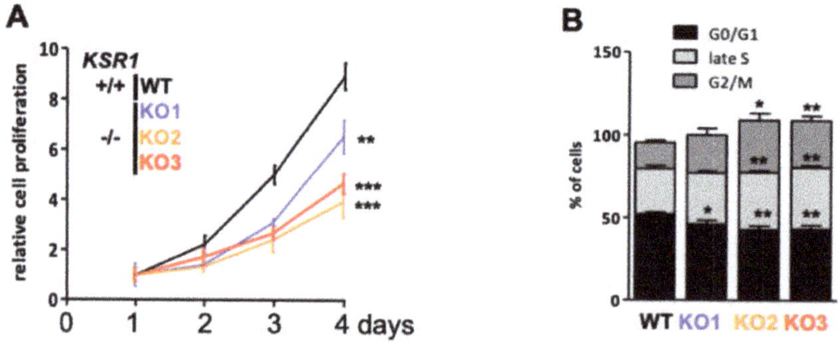

Figure 2. KSR1 loss decreases proliferation by retarding cell cycle progression through late S and G2/M phases. (**A**) Cell proliferation. (**B**) Cell cycle analysis. * $p < 0.05$, ** $p < 0.01$, *** $p < 0.001$ (Student's t-test).

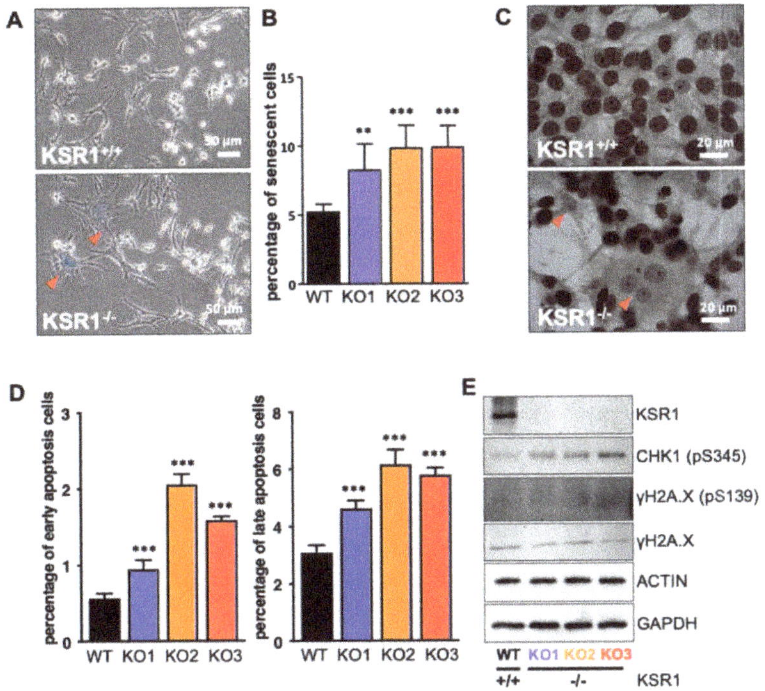

Figure 3. KSR1 loss increases senescence, apoptosis, and DNA damage. (**A**) Increased expression of the senescence marker acidic β-galactosidase in KSR1$^{-/-}$ cells. Shown are representative acidic β-galactosidase stains; red arrowheads indicate β-galactosidase-positive cells. (**B**) Quantification of relative β-galactosidase activity. (**C**) Ki-67 stain indicating proliferative cells. Red arrowheads indicate multinucleated cells with senescent morphology. (**D**) Percentage of early- and late-stage apoptotic cells measured by the YO-PRO™-1 Iodide assay. (**E**) Western blot validation of key protein expression changes involved in DNA damage. ** $p < 0.01$, *** $p < 0.001$ (Student's *t*-test).

These results indicate that KSR1 may have a role in sustaining the transformed phenotype of melanoma cells. Therefore, we tested the effects of KSR1 knockout on the ability of cells to grow in 3D soft agar cultures, which is a reliable in vitro indicator of tumorigenicity in vivo [18]. KSR1$^{-/-}$ cells failed to grow in soft agar, whereas parental cells formed readily visible colonies (Figure 4A). Similarly, KSR1 knockout severely compromised the ability of SK-MEL-239 cells to migrate through a Transwell membrane (Figure 4B,C). In addition, 3D tumour spheroid invasion was assessed by plating cells into Ultra Low Attachment (ULA) 96-well round-bottom plates (Figure 4D,E) or agarose-coated 96-well round-bottom plates (Figure S3). Spheroids were embedded into growth-factor-reduced Matrigel, allowing melanoma cells to invade and spread out of the spheroid. While a clear and homogeneous invasive cell front was only visible in parental SK-MEL-239 cells, loss of KSR1 resulted in non-homogeneous fronts of invasion. The quantification of 3D spheroid invasion clearly indicates a significant impairment of the invasion capacity in all KSR1$^{-/-}$ clones (Figures 4E and S3B). In conclusion, KSR1 loss interferes not only with cell proliferation and cell cycle progression but also with several traits of oncogenic transformation, including the ability to undergo anchorage-independent growth in soft agar and invasive migration.

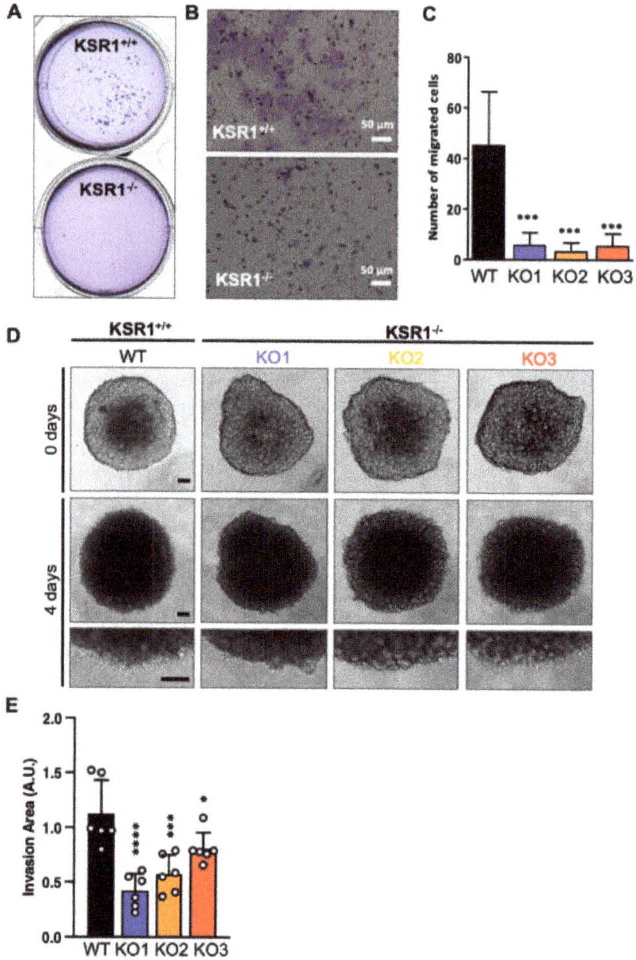

Figure 4. KSR1 loss inhibits growth in soft agar, migration, and 3D invasion. (**A**) A representative assay showing that KSR1$^{-/-}$ cells fail to form colonies in soft agar. (**B**) Transwell migration assay. Cells were stained with Giemsa, and cells able to migrate through the membrane were counted. Shown are representative images. (**C**) Quantification of cells that have migrated through the membrane. (**D**) Three-dimensional spheroid formation. SK-MEL-239 cells and KSR1$^{-/-}$ cells were grown in 96-well ultra-low-attachment surface plates and embedded in Matrigel, and invasion distance was monitored over a 4-day period of incubation. Representative images showing spheroid formation (0 days) and invasion after 4 days (upper panel). Expanded regions of invasion areas (lower panel). Scale bar 100 µm. (**E**) Three-dimensional spheroid formation was quantified by subtracting the cell-covered area from the spheroid core area (fold change). The graph shows the relative representation of the invasion areas in each condition ± SD; n = 6; ordinary one-way ANOVA test was used to test significance. * $p < 0.05$; *** $p < 0.001$; **** $p < 0.0001$.

2.3. ERK Substrateomics

The above results suggest that KSR1 plays an important role in maintaining the transformed state of BRAF mutant melanoma cells. As ERK activation is considered a main effector of mutant BRAF signalling, we re-examined the role of ERK in more depth. Given the lack of impact of KSR1 loss on global ERK activity (Figure 1B), we hypothesised that KSR1 may direct ERK to specific substrates rather than being required for general ERK activation. ERK fulfils its pleiotropic biological functions via almost 500 bona fide substrates [19], whose phosphorylation plausibly needs to be selective in order to achieve specific biological outcomes. Therefore, we assessed the impact of KSR1 loss on the phosphorylation of ERK substrates.

For this, we enriched ERK substrates using an antibody that recognises sites phosphorylated by ERK (P-X-pS-P and pS-X-R/K) and identified and quantified the immunoprecipitated ERK substrates by mass spectrometry (MS) (Figure 5A). Consistent with the observation that KSR1 knockout did not impact global MEK and ERK activation, the pattern of ERK-phosphorylated proteins resolved by gel electrophoresis was highly similar between WT and KSR1 KO cells (Figure 5B). However, MS analysis revealed a small number of ERK substrates that were differentially phosphorylated (Figure 5C,D; Table S3). Of 399 proteins specially immunoprecipitated (i.e., enriched >2-fold over a control immunoprecipitation with an isotype-matched IgG) in KSR1 KO1-3 cells, 85 were known ERK substrates [20]. Analysing differences between parental and KSR1$^{-/-}$ cells using a fold change of >2 and p-value of <0.05 as the cut-off for differential phosphorylation, we identified 29–34 substrates showing enhanced and 28–33 substrates showing decreased phosphorylation in the KSR1 KO1-3 clones versus parental cells. This finding supports our hypothesis that KSR1 may direct ERK to specific substrates. Interestingly, only six up- and four downregulated substrate phosphorylations were shared between all three KSR1 knockout clones, suggesting that cells can adapt to KSR1 loss *via* different mechanisms that share common core processes (Figure 5C,D).

These core adaptations include a very significant increase in the phosphorylation of caspase 3, BAG3 (Bcl-2-associated athanogene 3), VAPA (VAMP-Associated Protein A), VPS26A (Vacuolar Protein Sorting-Associated Protein 26A), CEP41 (Centrosomal Protein 41), and PRPS2 (Phosphoribosyl Pyrophosphate Synthetase 2). Caspase 3 integrates both extrinsic and intrinsic apoptosis pathways and is a key effector of apoptosis [21]. Caspase 3 has an ERK docking site, and ERK can activate caspase 3 [22], which could help explain the enhanced apoptosis in KSR1$^{-/-}$ cells. BAG3 is a multifunctional protein that is involved in protein folding, autophagy, and apoptosis [23]. Interestingly, ERK phosphorylation neutralises its protective function against oxidative-stress-induced apoptosis [24], suggesting that the enhanced BAG3 phosphorylation common to KSR$^{-/-}$ cells can contribute to their increased apoptosis rates. VAPA and VPS26A function in vesicle transport [25,26]. CEP41 is a centrosomal protein that regulates the function of cilia [27]. PRPS2 functions in the deoxynucleotide synthesis pathway, and its overexpression stimulates the proliferation and metastatic capacity of melanoma cells [28]. Proteins whose phosphorylation at ERK target sites was significantly downregulated in all KSR1$^{-/-}$ clones include PPP2R1A (Protein Phosphatase 2 Regulatory Subunit A α), PTMA (Prothymosin α), NEDD4L (NEDD4 Like E3 Ubiquitin Protein Ligase), and BOLA1 (BolA Family Member 1). PPP2R1A is a subunit of the serine/threonine phosphatase PP2, which directs PP2 to specific substrates and functions as a tumour suppressor in endometrial cancer [29]. PTMA is an immunomodulatory protein that can enhance T-cell responses to tumours [30]. On the other hand, PTMA expression in melanoma cells enhances their growth and aggressiveness in a preclinical mouse model [31]. These different actions could conceivably be dependent on posttranslational modifications, such as phosphorylation. NEDD4L is an E3 ubiquitin ligase, which can be overexpressed in melanoma and promote tumour growth [32]. ERK can phosphorylate NEDD4L on S448, and this phosphorylation is reduced in melanoma cells that are resistant to the RAF inhibitor PLX4720 [33]. Phosphorylation of this site disrupts substrate binding and is an effective inhibitor of NEDD4L function [34]. BOLA1 helps maintain the mitochondrial redox balance by counteracting the effects of glutathione depletion [35].

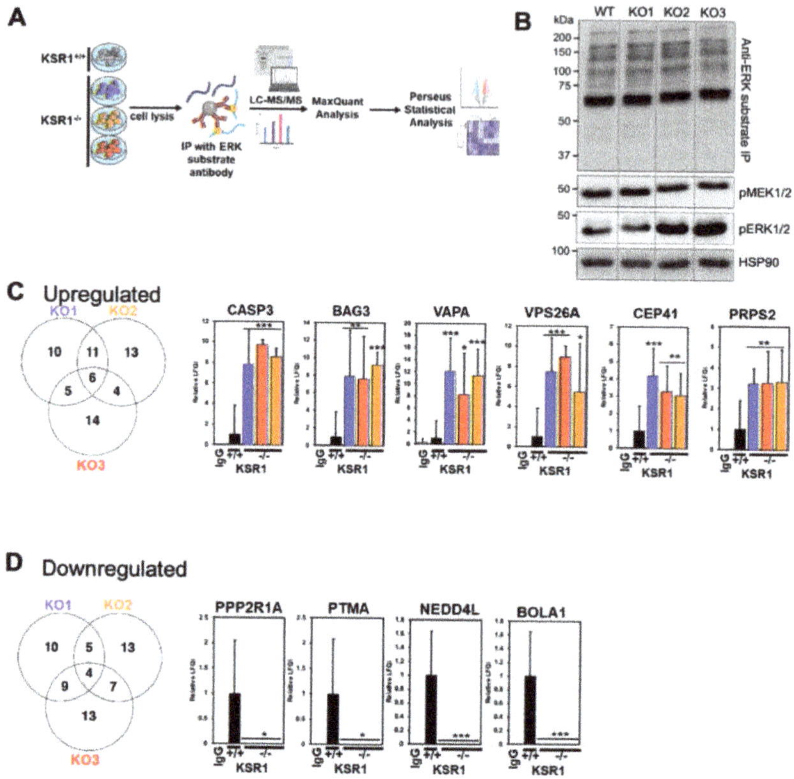

Figure 5. ERK substrateomics. (**A**) Workflow. (**B**) Western blot of ERK substrate immunoprecipitation (IP) stained with ERK substrate antibody. Lysates were blotted for activated MEK (pMEK) and ERK (pERK). HSP90 served as loading control. (**C**,**D**) Proteins whose phosphorylation was up- or downregulated in KSR1$^{-/-}$ cells. The changes shared by KSR1 KO1-3 clones are shown as bar graphs from 3 biological replicates.* $p < 0.05$; ** $p < 0.01$; *** $p < 0.001$ (Student's *t*-test).

Of these 10 proteins, only two are listed in the "Compendium of ERK targets" [20], specifically, BAG3 and NEDD4L. In both cases, ERK phosphorylation inhibits their function. The effects are consistent with the phosphorylation changes observed in KSR$^{-/-}$ cells, i.e., the increase in BAG3 phosphorylation, reducing cell survival, and the decrease in NEDD4L phosphorylation, blocking invasive cell migration. The distinct phosphorylation changes in ERK substrates in KSR1 knockout cells require further investigation in dedicated functional studies. They, however, support our hypothesis that KSR1 can direct ERK substrate phosphorylation.

2.4. *KSR1-Dependent Global Changes in Protein Expression*

The specific changes in ERK substrate phosphorylation caused by KSR1 knockout prompted us to investigate whether KSR1 knockout also alters protein expression. We used label-free quantitative proteomics to profile global protein expression in parental SK-MEL-239 cells and the three KSR1$^{-/-}$ clones (Figure 6A). The expression of several proteins was differentially regulated between parental and KSR1$^{-/-}$ SK-MEL-239 cells (Figures 6B and S4, Table S4). The expression of 36/21 proteins was up/downregulated, respectively. The proteins downregulated in KSR1$^{-/-}$ cells are involved in tetrahydrofolate and pyrimidine (deoxythymidine) synthesis (Figure 6C), which may contribute to the S-phase delay in KSR1$^{-/-}$ cells (Figures 2B and S2). The upregulated proteins mapped onto signalling pathways for apoptosis, senescence, autophagy, and the p53 network, among the top hits (Figure 6C). These mappings correspond well to the observed phenotype of the KSR1$^{-/-}$ cells. While ERK substrateomics provided plausible explanations for the apoptosis and migration phenotype, the senescence and cell cycle phenotypes remained elusive.

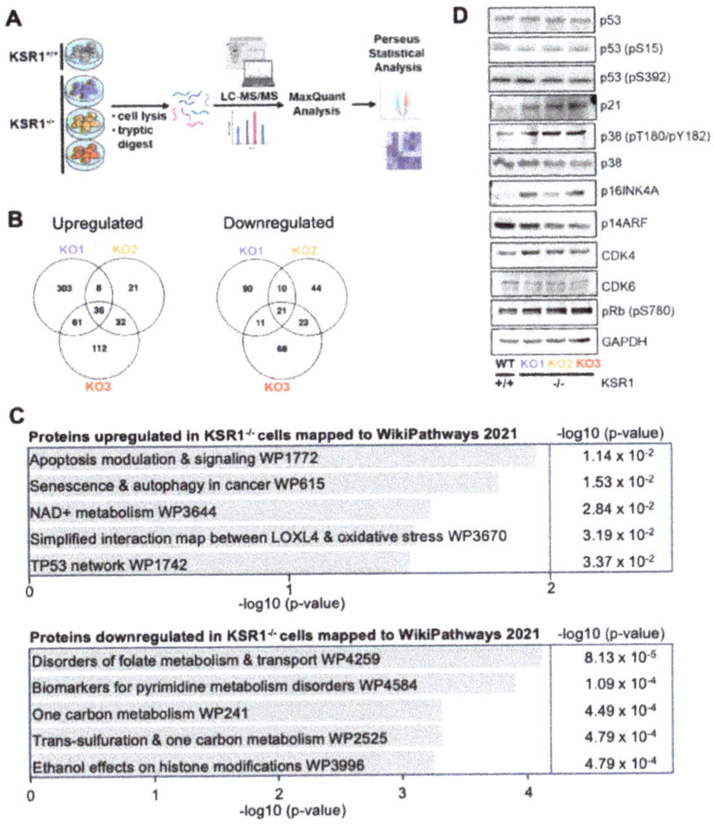

Figure 6. Global proteomic expression profiling. (**A**) Workflow. (**B**) Venn diagram of proteins differentially regulated in the KSR1 KO1-3 clones vs. parental SK-MEL-239 cells. (**C**) ENRICHR analysis of the differentially expressed proteins. The combined score is the log *p*-value multiplied by the Z-score of the deviation from the expected rank. (**D**) Western blot validation of key protein expression changes found by MS-based proteomic expression profiling.

Given that the global expression proteomics highlighted senescence and p53, and that p53 is a major player in both senescence and cell cycle regulation [36], we examined the status of the p53 pathway in the KSR1$^{-/-}$ cells in more detail using the Western blot analysis of key proteins (Figure 6D). These proteins were chosen based on existing knowledge of pathways that connect cell cycle, senescence, and p53. Surprisingly, Western blot analysis showed no changes in p53 abundance or the phosphorylation of sites that regulate p53 activity. However, the protein expression of the cell cycle inhibitor p21, a classic transcriptional p53 target gene, was upregulated. The p38 kinase can stabilise the p21 mRNA and thereby enhance p21 protein expression independently of p53 [37], and p38 is also implicated in senescence [38]. Indeed, p38 was activated in the KSR1$^{-/-}$ cells. The many roles of p38 in senescence induction include the activation of p16INK induction [39]. The p16INK protein is encoded by the *CDKN2A* gene, which also encodes the p14ARF tumour suppressor protein. MS analysis showed that p16INK was upregulated in KSR1$^{-/-}$ cells, and this result was confirmed by the Western blot analysis. The p14ARF protein, which regulates p53 protein stability, was downregulated in the KSR1$^{-/-}$ cells. This is consistent with the observation that p53 levels did not change in the KSR1$^{-/-}$ cells. The p16INK protein binds to and inhibits the cell cycle kinases CDK4 and CDK6, which promote cell cycle entry by phosphorylating and inactivating the retinoblastoma protein RB1. The expression levels of CDK4 and CDK6 were similar in parental and KSR1$^{-/-}$ cells, suggesting that the KSR1 knockout affects their regulation rather than their expression. Interestingly, phosphorylation of the RB1 protein at S780 was enhanced in the KSR1$^{-/-}$ cells. This phosphorylation is critical for the inactivation of RB1 and the progression of cells into the S phase [40]. While the enhanced inactivation of RB1 in KSR1$^{-/-}$ cells seems counterintuitive, it fits the observed phenotype. KSR1$^{-/-}$ cells can still synthesise DNA and enter the S phase, before being slowed down in the late S and G2 phases (Figures 2B and 3B). S780 can be phosphorylated by CDK4/6 and several other kinases, including p38, in the context of proapoptotic signalling [41]. Alternatively, at low concentrations, p21 serves as a scaffold that promotes the assembly of CDK4/6 complexes with cyclin D, enhancing CDK4/6 activity before it inhibits it at high p21 concentrations [42]. These possibilities are not mutually exclusive and will be interesting to dissect in future studies.

In addition to these effects on the cell cycle, apoptosis, and senescence, we also found protein expression changes that suggest a role for KSR1 in cell differentiation and adhesion (Figure S4). The expression of the tumour suppressor protein PDCD4 (Programmed Cell Death 4) correlates with a good prognosis in melanoma [43] and is upregulated in KSR1$^{-/-}$ cells. Likewise, CAV1 (Caveolin) is slightly overexpressed in KSR1$^{-/-}$ cells. It functions as tumour suppressor in melanoma and restricts cell growth and motility [44]. In mouse embryo fibroblasts, CAV1 associates with KSR1 and enhances KSR1 functions [13]. Similarly, MITF (Melanocyte-Inducing Transcription Factor) is upregulated in KSR1$^{-/-}$ cells. MITF is a transcription factor that initiates and maintains the melanocyte lineage [45]. By contrast, TYRP1 (Tyrosinase-Related Protein 1) protein expression is severely downregulated in KSR1$^{-/-}$ cells. TYRP1 functions in melanin synthesis, although high expression is associated with a poor prognosis due to sequestration of the tumour suppressor miRNA-16 [46]. Likewise, β-catenin expression is strongly suppressed in KSR1$^{-/-}$ cells. β-Catenin is part of the classic WNT signalling pathway and increases tumorigenicity, metastasis, and drug resistance in melanoma [47]. Interestingly, enhanced WNT signalling in melanoma cells also inhibits T-cell infiltration and response to immunotherapies [48]. These molecular changes are largely consistent with the observed phenotypical changes in response to KSR1 knockout. However, further investigations are required to determine the exact roles of these multiple changes in the KSR1$^{-/-}$ phenotype.

In order to corroborate the observed key changes in RAF-ERK signalling and senescence upon KSR1 depletion in other melanoma cell lines, BRAFV600E-driven melanoma cell lines SK-MEL-28 and A375 were transfected with KSR1 siRNA, and adaptations were analysed by Western blotting (Figure S5). The results confirm that the reduced expression of KSR1 in these cells does not impact RAF-ERK signalling and activation. Furthermore, KSR1 knockdown resulted in the increased expression of PDCD4, MITF, and p16INK4a, while p14ARF expression was downregulated. Thus, knocking down KSR1 by siRNA in two other BRAFV600E-driven melanoma cell lines results in the same key adaptations as observed in the KSR1$^{-/-}$ SK-MEL-239 cells. Importantly, these results suggest that the adaptive changes are KSR1-specific rather than cell-line-specific.

3. Discussion

Our study confirms the emerging intricacy of KSR1 functions [5]. Knocking out KSR1 in the BRAFV600E-driven melanoma cell line SK-MEL-239 resulted in a complex phenotype that shows features of aberrant cell cycle regulation, enhanced senescence, and increased apoptosis. Interestingly, KSR1 seems to support BRAFV600E-driven transformation through different functions, which are not fully explainable by known mechanisms. The decrease in proliferation caused by KSR1 knockout is mainly due to a slowing down of S-phase exit and G2-phase completion. Examining the activity of cell cycle checkpoints showed an upregulation of p21 and p16INK4A in KSR1$^{-/-}$ cells. These proteins are classic inhibitors of S-phase entry and should decrease the phosphorylation and inactivation of RB1, which controls G1/S progression. Our results show that RB1 phosphorylation increased in the KSR1$^{-/-}$ cells. This is consistent with the cells being able to replicate DNA but does not explain why they have difficulties progressing through the late S and G2 phases. We did not find any changes in the expression of mitotic CDK inhibitors, such as p27, but a recent report suggests that p21 can also control later stages of the cell cycle [49]. An alternative and non-mutually exclusive explanation could be that the p38 MAPK, which is activated in KSR1$^{-/-}$ cells, can phosphorylate and inactivate RB1 independently of CDKs [41]. Moreover, the decrease in the expression of proteins involved in pyrimidine synthesis (Figure 6C) may decelerate the late S phase by causing cells to run out of nucleotides for DNA synthesis.

The increase in senescence caused by KSR1 knockout is also unorthodox. KSR1$^{-/-}$ cells showed a clear increase in cells with the classic senescent morphology and expression of the classic senescence marker acidic β-galactosidase, as well as an increase in the expression of p21 and p16INK. However, they did not show other hallmark features of senescence, such as the upregulation of p53, p27, and proteins typical of the senescence-associated secretory phenotype (SASP). As DNA replication occurred in KSR1$^{-/-}$ cells, with multinucleated cells appearing that mainly also had a senescent appearance, it is possible that senescence is triggered by endoreplication [50]. Nevertheless, it is an unorthodox senescence phenotype, as judged by the usual criteria [51].

The clearest explanation can be provided for the increase in apoptosis and DNA damage. KSR1$^{-/-}$ cells exhibited an increase in the inactivation of BAG3 and presumably the activation of Caspase 3 phosphorylation. This would remove a protective mechanism and activate an apoptosis executioner molecule, which could plausibly account for the increase in apoptosis and DNA damage in KSR1$^{-/-}$ cells.

How does this all fit together? Within the limitations that more detailed studies of each aspect will be required to fully disentangle the molecular mechanisms underpinning the KSR1 knockout phenotype, we propose the following model (Figure 7). Our results suggest that KSR1 regulates the ERK substrate choice. When KSR1 is lost, ERK activates the executioner Caspase 3 and inactivates the apoptosis antagonist BAG3 to promote apoptosis in our BRAFV600E-driven melanoma models. In the p53 and RB1 networks, the increase in p21 and p16INK could be due to the direct effects of the p38 MAPK, which can increase the expression of both proteins [39,41]. Thus, our results indicate that KSR1 might have a multi-layered role in facilitating transformation by oncogenic BRAF mutants and that some of these traits could lend themselves to therapeutic interference in the future.

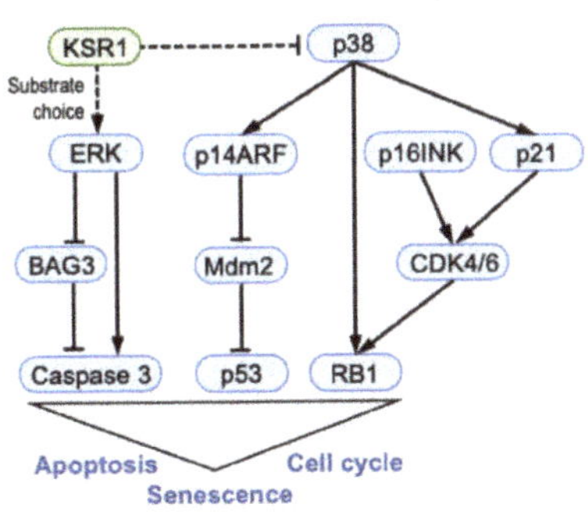

Figure 7. Summary model of KSR1 functions in BRAF mutant melanoma cells. See text for details. Arrows indicate activation; blunt lines indicate inhibition; broken lines indicate that the regulatory mechanism is not entirely clear.

4. Materials and Methods

Cells. SK-MEL-28 and A375 were obtained from ATCC. SK-MEL-239 cells (RRID:CVCL_6122) were obtained from Dr Poulikos Poulikakos, Memorial Sloan-Kettering Cancer Center, New York, NY, USA. All cells were cultured in RPMI-1640 complete medium (Gibco™, Thermo Fisher Scientific, Waltham, MA, USA, Cat# 21875034) containing 10% FBS and 2 mM L-Glutamine (Gibco, Cat# 25030081). Cells were authenticated using the AmpFlSTR® Identifiler® Plus PCR Amplification Kit (Thermo Fisher Scientific, Waltham, MA, USA, Cat# A26182; Figure S1).

CRISPR/Cas9 knockout. Three crRNAs (Table S1) that target exon 5 of KSR1 (Ensembl transcript ID ENST00000509603.6) were designed using GeneArt (https://www.thermofisher.com/ie/en/home/life-science/genome-editing/geneart-crispr/geneart-crispr-search-and-design-tool.html; accessed on 1 September 2015) and cloned into the GeneArt™ CRISPR Nuclease Vector with OFP (orange fluorescent protein) Reporter (Thermo Fisher Scientific, Waltham, MA, USA, Cat# A21174). Twenty-four hours after transfection, 288 single cells expressing OFP were sorted for each crRNA using a FACSAria III instrument (BD Biosciences, San Jose, CA, USA). Twenty-four surviving single-cell clones for each crRNA were tested for indels using the GeneArt™ Genomic Cleavage Detection Kit (Thermo Fisher Scientific, Waltham, MA, USA, Cat# A24372). Positive clones were Sanger-sequenced, and the sequence containing mixed base calls from different KSR1 alleles was decomposed by using the Synthego webtool (https://ice.synthego.com/#/; accessed on 1 March 2019) (Figure S1).

Cell proliferation was measured using the Cell Counting Kit-8 (Sigma-Aldrich, Burlington, MA, USA, Cat# 96992-500) according to the manufacturer's instructions.

Cell senescence was measured using the Senescence β-Galactosidase Staining Kit (Cell Signaling Technologies, Danvers, MA, USA, Cat# 9860). Senescent (β-Galactosidase positive) cells were counted manually from three randomly taken fields.

Anchorage-independent growth was measured using soft agar assays as previously described [52]. Colonies were stained with 0.005% crystal violet solution for two hours and manually enumerated.

Cell cycle analysis. Cells at 80% confluence were collected and resuspended in 1 mL of phosphate-buffered saline (PBS) containing 10 μM BrdU (BD Biosciences, San Jose, CA, USA, Cat# 556028) for 1 h. Cells were then fixed in 70% ethanol for 30 min and labelled with 10 μg/mL propidium-iodide (Sigma, Burlington, MA, USA, Cat# P4864) for 30 min prior to cell cycle analysis using a BD Accuri C6 Flow Cytometer® (BD Biosciences).

Cell apoptosis. When the cells reached 70–80% confluence, they were gently washed with PBS and resuspended in PBS containing 0.1 μM YO-PRO-1 (Thermo Fisher Scientific, Waltham, MA, USA, Cat# Y3603) and 1 μM propidium-iodide (Sigma, Burlington, MA, USA, Cat# P4864) for 20 min prior to analysis on a BD Accuri C6 Flow Cytometer®.

Transwell cell migration was measured using Corning® Transwell® 8 μm pore polycarbonate membrane cell culture inserts (Corning Inc., Corning, NY, USA, Cat# CLS3422). A total of 1×10^6 cells in serum-free RPMI medium were added to the inserts with RPMI containing 10% FBS serving as a chemoattractant in the bottom chamber. After 24 h, cells migrating through the membrane were fixed with 70% ethanol, stained with Giemsa, and counted.

Three-dimensional (3D) invasion assay. SK-MEL-239 and KSR1$^{-/-}$ cells were used to generate spheroids (2000 cells/sphere) using two distinct approaches. Briefly, the distinct cells were distributed in 96-well low-attachment surface plates (Nunclon sphera 96-well plates; Thermo Fisher Scientific, Waltham, MA, USA) or in 1.5% agarose-coated 96-well round bottom plates and cultured in standard culture conditions, and spheroids were allowed to form for 5 days. Every other day, 75 mL of medium was carefully replaced, and after 48 h, this change of media was made with the supplement of 3 μg/mL rat tail collagen I (Gibco™ Thermo Fisher Scientific, Waltham, MA, USA; Cat# A10483-01) to promote spheroid formation. For the 3D invasion assay, each spheroid was embedded in 4.2 mg/mL Matrigel (Corning Inc., Corning, NY, USA, Cat#3542380), and plates were incubated for 30 min under standard culture conditions for Matrigel solidification. Spheroids were overlaid with 100 μL of complete culture media, and invasion was followed for a total period of 5 days. For each of the 2 independent experiments, 3–6 spheroids were generated by each cell line, and spheroid invasion was registered using brightfield images with an Olympus CKX41 microscope equipped with a Leica DFC295 camera. Invasion areas were quantified by image analysis using ImageJ/FijI software (v. 2.14.0). To calculate invasion areas, digital images (300 pixels/inch) were converted to 8 bits, and the total area of invaded cells leaving the core spheroid was measured [53,54]. Data were further analysed using GraphPad Prism.

Immunocytochemistry. Cells were fixed with ice-cold methanol (Sigma-Aldrich, Cat# 24229) and stained with Ki67 antibody (Thermo Fisher Scientific, Waltham, MA, USA, Cat# MA5-15690, RRID:AB_10979995, 1:1000 dilution) using the Novolink Polymer Detection kit (Leica Biosystems, Wetzlar, Germany, Cat# RE7140-CE). Cells were counterstained with haematoxylin (Reagecon Diagnostics, Ltd., Shannon, Ireland, Cat# RBA-4201-00A).

Western blotting. Proteins were separated by SDS-polyacrylamide gel electrophoresis and transferred to a polyvinylidene difluoride membrane using the XCell SureLock® Mini-Cell chamber wet transfer system according to the manufacturer's instructions (Thermo Fisher Scientific, Waltham, MA, USA). Membranes were blocked with 5% non-fat dry milk in TBST (20 mM TrisHCl, pH 7.4; 150 mM NaCl, 0.1% Tween 20) for 30 min and washed 3 × 5 min in TBST buffer. Then, membranes were incubated overnight with primary antibody in TBST with 4% bovine serum albumin, washed 3 × 5 min in TBST buffer, and incubated with secondary antibody (horse radish peroxidase-conjugated) in TBST with 5% non-fat dry milk for 1 h. After three 5-min washes, the membrane was briefly rinsed with water and developed with Pierce-ECL (enhanced chemiluminescence) reagent (Thermo Fisher Scientific, Waltham, MA, USA, Cat# 32109). Bands were visualised using the ChemiImager (Advanced Molecular Vision, London, UK, accompanied with Chemostar software v. 0.3.23) or iBright™ CL750 Imaging System (Invitrogen™ Thermo Fisher Scientific, Waltham, MA, USA). To re-use membranes, antibodies were removed by incubation in stripping buffer for 15 min (0.2 M glycine, pH 2.5, 1% SDS).

Antibodies used for Western blotting were from the following vendors: Cell Signaling Technologies, Danvers, MA, USA: KSR1 (Cat# 4640, RRID:AB_10544539), pMEK1/2 (Cat# 9121, RRID:AB_331648), MEK1/2 (Cat# 9122, RRID:AB_823567), GAPDH (Cat# 2118, RRID:AB_561053), HSP90 (Cat# 4877, RRID:AB_2233307), p-p38 (Cat# 9211, RRID:AB_331641), p38 (Cat# 9212, RRID:AB_330713), p53 and p53 phospho-forms pS15 and pS392 (Phospho-p53 Antibody Sampler Kit #9919, RRID:AB_330019), Rb1 pS780 (Cat# 9307, RRID:AB_330015), E-Cadherin (Cat# 3195, RRID:AB_2291471), MITF (Cat# 97800S, RRID:AB_2800289), p14ARF (Cat# 74560S, RRID:AB_2923025), PDCD4 (Cat# 9535, RRID:AB_2162318), phospho-CHK1 (Ser345) (Cat# 2348, RRID:AB_331212), Histone H2A.X (Cat#7631, RRID: AB_10860771), phospho-Histone H2A.X (Ser139) (Cat#9718, RRID: AB_2118009), horse radish peroxidase-linked anti-mouse IgG (Cat#7076, RRID:AB_330924), horse radish peroxidase-linked anti-rabbit IgG (Cat#7074, RRID:AB_2099233); Santa Cruz (Dallas, TX, USA): KSR2 (Cat# sc-100421, RRID:AB_1124518), BRAF (Cat# sc-5284, RRID:AB_626760), CRAF (Cat# sc-133, RRID:AB_632305), p21 (Cat# Sc-6246, RRID:AB_628073), CDK4 (Cat# sc-23896, RRID:AB_627239), CDK6 (Cat# sc-7961, RRID:AB_627242), Caveolin 1 (Cat# sc-894, RRID:AB_2072042); Sigma-Aldrich (Burlington, MA, USA): pERK1/2 (Cat# M8159, RRID:AB_477245), ERK1/2 (Cat# M5670, RRID:AB_477245); BD Biosciences (San Jose, CA, USA), p16INK4A (Cat# 550834, RRID:AB_2078446); Abcam (Cambridge, UK): TYRP1 (Cat# Ab235447, RRID:AB_2923026).

Immunoprecipitation. Cells were lysed in 20 mM Tris-HCl (pH 7.5), 150 mM NaCl, 0.5% NP-40, 1 mM EDTA, and 1 mM EGTA containing protease inhibitor cocktail (cOmplete™ Mini Protease Inhibitor Cocktail, Roche Diagnostics (Rotkreuz, Switzerland, Cat# 11836170001) and phosphatase inhibitor cocktail (PhosSTOP, Roche Diagnostics, Rotkreuz, Switzerland, Cat# 4906837001). Cell lysates were cleared by centrifugation at 15,000× g at 4 °C for 10 min. The protein concentration of the lysates was determined by Pierce® BCA Protein Assay (Thermo Fisher Scientific, Waltham, MA, USA, Cat# 23225). Potential ERK substrates were immunoprecipitated using Phospho-MAPK/CDK Substrates sepharose beads (Cell Signaling, Danvers, MA, USA, Cat# 5501) from cell lysates at 4 °C for 6 h. The immunoprecipitates were washed 3× with lysis buffer and processed for mass spectrometry as described previously [19].

Mass spectrometry analysis of immunoprecipitates was performed as previously reported [55]. Total protein expression profiling was performed as previously reported [56] and a detailed description has been submitted to PRIDE (PXD036265). The raw data were analysed by MaxQuant and Perseus [57].

Lysate-based proteomics. Cells were resuspended in 100 μL of 8 M urea, 50 mM Tris-HCl pH 8.0, supplemented with cOmplete™ Mini Protease Inhibitor Cocktail (Roche Diagnostics, Rotkreuz, Switzerland, Cat# 11836170001), and phosphatase inhibitor cocktail (PhosSTOP, Roche Diagnostics, Rotkreuz, Switzerland, Cat# 4906837001). Samples were sonicated for 2 × 9 seconds at a power setting of 15% to disrupt cell pellets (Syclon Ultrasonic Homogeniser). Samples were reduced by adding 8 mM dithiothreitol (DTT) for 60 min and subsequently carboxylated using 20 mM iodoacetamide for 30 min in the dark while mixing (Thermomixer 1200 rpm, 30 °C). The solution was diluted with 50 mM Tris-HCl pH 8.0 to a final urea concentration of 2 M. Sequencing Grade Modified Trypsin (Promega, Madison, WI, USA, Cat# V5111) was resuspended in 50 mM Tris-HCL at a concentration of 0.5 ug/μl and added at a 1:100 enzyme-to-protein ratio. Samples were digested overnight with gentle shaking (thermomixer 850 rpm, 37 °C). The tryptic digest was terminated by adding formic acid to 1% final concentration, and samples were desalted using C18 HyperSep™ SpinTips (Thermo Fisher Scientific, Waltham, MA, USA, Cat# 60109-412).

Geneset Enrichment analysis (GSEA) was performed using EnrichR [58].

Statistics. Two-tailed, paired, or unpaired Student's T-Test was performed to analyse the significance of differences between two groups. Ordinary one-way ANOVA test was used to analyse the significance in 3D invasion assays. GraphPad Prism version 5.01 (RRID:SCR_002798) was used to create graphs. Error bars represent standard error of the mean (SEM) or standard deviation (SD) as indicated; 1–4 asterisks indicate significance at the 0.05, 0.01, 0.001, and 0.0001 probability levels, respectively; *n.s.* indicates non-significant. As the work focuses on the molecular mechanistic analysis of KSR1 loss in cell lines, blinding, power analysis, randomisation, and considerations regarding differences between males and females were not required for the study.

Supplementary Materials: The supporting information can be downloaded at: https://www.mdpi.com/article/10.3390/ijms241411821/s1.

Author Contributions: Conceptualization, W.K., J.R. and Z.L.; methodology, Z.L, A.K., A.N., C.C., N.R., K.W., A.M., E.K., B.M., A.B. and J.R.; software, Z.L., A.N., A.K., C.C., K.W., A.B. and J.R.; validation, Z.L, A.N., N.R., C.C. and J.R.; formal analysis, Z.L, A.K., A.N., C.C., N.R., K.W., H.C., E.K., B.M., A.B. and J.R.; investigation, Z.L, A.K., A.N., C.C., N.R. and J.R.; resources, B.M., K.W. and A.B.; data curation, J.R., Z.L., K.W., A.K. and A.N.; writing—original draft preparation, W.K., J.R. and Z.L.; writing—review and editing, J.R., A.N., A.K., Z.L., C.C. and N.R.; visualization, Z.L., J.R., W.K. and C.C.; supervision, J.R., W.K. and A.M.; project administration, W.K. and J.R.; funding acquisition, W.K. and J.R. All authors have read and agreed to the published version of the manuscript.

Funding: Financial support was provided by Science Foundation Ireland (SFI) and National Children's Research Centre/Children's Health Foundation through the Precision Oncology Ireland grant 18/SPP/3522 (WK, AK), the SFI investigator grant 14/IA/2395 (WK, JR), the Comprehensive Molecular Analytical Platform (CMAP) under the SFI Research Infrastructure Programme, 18/RI/5702 (WK), the UCD-Chinese Scholarship Council (CSC) Scholarship Scheme 2015 (ZL), and the Irish Research Council postgraduate scholarship GOIPG/2018/1910 (AN, JR).

Data Availability Statement: The proteomics data supporting the findings of this study were submitted to the EMBL Proteomics Identification Database PRIDE (https://www.ebi.ac.uk/pride/ accessed on 1 July 2023): PXD036265 (full lysate proteomics analysis) and PXD036261 (ERK substrateome analysis).

Acknowledgments: We thank the Conway Institute Core Technologies, UCD for expert assistance with proteomics and flow cytometry. Similarly, we thank the Charles Institute for Dermatology, UCD, for expert assistance with cell invasion assays and Philip Cotter for help with data upload to PRIDE.

Conflicts of Interest: The authors declare no potential conflicts of interest.

References

1. Lee, S.; Rauch, J.; Kolch, W. Targeting MAPK Signaling in Cancer: Mechanisms of Drug Resistance and Sensitivity. *Int. J. Mol. Sci.* **2020**, *21*, 1102. [CrossRef]
2. Roskoski, R. Targeting ERK1/2 protein-serine/threonine kinases in human cancers. *Pharmacol. Res.* **2019**, *14*, 151–168. [CrossRef] [PubMed]
3. Kolch, W.; Halasz, M.; Granovskaya, M.; Kholodenko, B.N. The dynamic control of signal transduction networks in cancer cells. *Nat. Rev. Cancer* **2015**, *15*, 515–527. [CrossRef] [PubMed]
4. Kolch, W. Coordinating ERK/MAPK signalling through scaffolds and inhibitors. *Nat. Rev. Mol. Cell Biol.* **2005**, *6*, 827–837. [CrossRef] [PubMed]
5. Frodyma, D.; Neilsen, B.; Costanzo-Garvey, D.; Fisher, K.; Lewis, R. Coordinating ERK signaling via the molecular scaffold Kinase Suppressor of Ras. *F1000Research* **2017**, *6*, 1621. [CrossRef]
6. Lavoie, H.; Sahmi, M.; Maisonneuve, P.; Marullo, S.A.; Thevakumaran, N.; Jin, T.; Kurinov, I.; Sicheri, F.; Therrien, M. MEK drives BRAF activation through allosteric control of KSR proteins. *Nature* **2018**, *554*, 549–553. [CrossRef]
7. Casar, B.; Arozarena, I.; Sanz-Moreno, V.; Pinto, A.; Agudo-Ibáñez, L.; Marais, R.; Lewis, R.E.; Berciano, M.T.; Crespo, P. Ras subcellular localization defines extracellular signal-regulated kinase 1 and 2 substrate specificity through distinct utilization of scaffold proteins. *Mol. Cell. Biol.* **2009**, *29*, 1338–1353. [CrossRef] [PubMed]
8. Lozano, J.; Xing, R.; Cai, Z.; Jensen, H.L.; Trempus, C.; Mark, W.; Cannon, R.; Kolesnick, R. Deficiency of kinase suppressor of Ras1 prevents oncogenic ras signaling in mice. *Cancer Res.* **2003**, *63*, 4232–4238.
9. Germino, E.A.; Miller, J.P.; Diehl, L.; Swanson, C.J.; Durinck, S.; Modrusan, Z.; Miner, J.H.; Shaw, A.S. Homozygous KSR1 deletion attenuates morbidity but does not prevent tumor development in a mouse model of RAS-driven pancreatic cancer. *PLoS ONE* **2018**, *13*, e0194998. [CrossRef]
10. Kortum, R.L.; Lewis, R.E. The molecular scaffold KSR1 regulates the proliferative and oncogenic potential of cells. *Mol. Cell. Biol.* **2004**, *24*, 4407–4416. [CrossRef]
11. Yan, F.; John, S.K.; Wilson, G.; Jones, D.S.; Washington, M.K.; Polk, D.B. Kinase suppressor of Ras-1 protects intestinal epithelium from cytokine-mediated apoptosis during inflammation. *J. Clin. Investig.* **2004**, *114*, 1272–1280. [CrossRef] [PubMed]
12. Kortum, R.L.; Johnson, H.J.; Costanzo, D.L.; Volle, D.J.; Razidlo, G.L.; Fusello, A.M.; Shaw, A.S.; Lewis, R.E. The molecular scaffold kinase suppressor of Ras 1 is a modifier of RasV12-induced and replicative senescence. *Mol. Cell. Biol.* **2006**, *26*, 2202–2214. [CrossRef] [PubMed]
13. Kortum, R.L.; Fernandez, M.R.; Costanzo-Garvey, D.L.; Johnson, H.J.; Fisher, K.W.; Volle, D.J.; Lewis, R.E. Caveolin-1 is required for kinase suppressor of Ras 1 (KSR1)-mediated extracellular signal-regulated kinase 1/2 activation, H-RasV12-induced senescence, and transformation. *Mol. Cell. Biol.* **2014**, *34*, 3461–3472. [CrossRef] [PubMed]
14. Rao, C.; Frodyma, D.E.; Southekal, S.; Svoboda, R.A.; Black, A.R.; Guda, C.; Mizutani, T.; Clevers, H.; Johnson, K.R.; Fisher, K.W.; et al. KSR1- and ERK-dependent translational regulation of the epithelial-to-mesenchymal transition. *eLife* **2021**, *10*, e66608. [CrossRef] [PubMed]
15. Neilsen, B.K.; Frodyma, D.E.; Lewis, R.E.; Fisher, K.W. KSR as a therapeutic target for Ras-dependent cancers. *Expert Opin. Ther. Targets* **2017**, *21*, 499–509. [CrossRef] [PubMed]
16. Liang, X.; Potter, J.; Kumar, S.; Zou, Y.; Quintanilla, R.; Sridharan, M.; Carte, J.; Chen, W.; Roark, N.; Ranganathan, S.; et al. Rapid and highly efficient mammalian cell engineering via Cas9 protein transfection. *J. Biotechnol.* **2015**, *208*, 44–53. [CrossRef]
17. Topham, C.H.; Taylor, S.S. Mitosis and apoptosis: How is the balance set? *Curr. Opin. Cell Biol.* **2013**, *25*, 780–785. [CrossRef]
18. Lemmens, M.; Fischer, B.; Zogg, M.; Rodrigues, L.; Kerr, G.; Del Rio-Espinola, A.; Schaeffer, F.; Maddalo, D.; Dubost, V.; Piaia, A.; et al. Evaluation of two in vitro assays for tumorigenicity assessment of CRISPR-Cas9 genome-edited cells. *Mol. Ther. Methods Clin. Dev.* **2021**, *23*, 241–253. [CrossRef]
19. Yang, L.; Zheng, L.; Chng, W.J.; Ding, J.L. Comprehensive Analysis of ERK1/2 Substrates for Potential Combination Immunotherapies. *Trends Pharmacol. Sci.* **2019**, *40*, 897–910. [CrossRef]
20. Ünal, E.B.; Uhlitz, F.; Blüthgen, N. A compendium of ERK targets. *FEBS Lett.* **2017**, *591*, 2607–2615. [CrossRef]
21. Nagata, S. Apoptosis and Clearance of Apoptotic Cells. *Annu. Rev. Immunol.* **2018**, *36*, 489–517. [CrossRef]
22. Zhuang, S.; Yan, Y.; Daubert, R.A.; Han, J.; Schnellmann, R.G. ERK promotes hydrogen peroxide-induced apoptosis through caspase-3 activation and inhibition of Akt in renal epithelial cells. *Am. J. Physiol. Ren. Physiol* **2007**, *292*, F440–F447. [CrossRef] [PubMed]
23. Sturner, E.; Behl, C. The Role of the Multifunctional BAG3 Protein in Cellular Protein Quality Control and in Disease. *Front. Mol. Neurosci.* **2017**, *10*, 177. [CrossRef] [PubMed]
24. Kim, H.Y.; Kim, Y.S.; Yun, H.H.; Im, C.N.; Ko, J.H.; Lee, J.H. ERK-mediated phosphorylation of BIS regulates nuclear translocation of HSF1 under oxidative stress. *Exp. Mol. Med.* **2016**, *48*, e260. [CrossRef]

25. Wang, S.; Bellen, H.J. The retromer complex in development and disease. *Development* **2015**, *142*, 2392–2396. [CrossRef]
26. Weir, M.L.; Xie, H.; Klip, A.; Trimble, W.S. VAP-A binds promiscuously to both v- and tSNAREs. *Biochem. Biophys. Res. Commun.* **2001**, *286*, 616–621. [CrossRef]
27. Lee, J.E.; Silhavy, J.L.; Zaki, M.S.; Schroth, J.; Bielas, S.L.; Marsh, S.E.; Olvera, J.; Brancati, F.; Iannicelli, M.; Ikegami, K.; et al. CEP41 is mutated in Joubert syndrome and is required for tubulin glutamylation at the cilium. *Nat. Genet.* **2012**, *44*, 193–199. [CrossRef]
28. Mannava, S.; Grachtchouk, V.; Wheeler, L.J.; Im, M.; Zhuang, D.; Slavina, E.G.; Mathews, C.K.; Shewach, D.S.; Nikiforov, M.A. Direct role of nucleotide metabolism in C-MYC-dependent proliferation of melanoma cells. *Cell Cycle* **2008**, *7*, 2392–2400. [CrossRef] [PubMed]
29. Remmerie, M.; Janssens, V. PP2A: A Promising Biomarker and Therapeutic Target in Endometrial Cancer. *Front. Oncol.* **2019**, *9*, 462. [CrossRef] [PubMed]
30. Birmpilis, A.I.; Karachaliou, C.E.; Samara, P.; Ioannou, K.; Selemenakis, P.; Kostopoulos, I.V.; Kavrochorianou, N.; Kalbacher, H.; Livaniou, E.; Haralambous, S.; et al. Antitumor Reactive T-Cell Responses Are Enhanced In Vivo by DAMP Prothymosin Alpha and Its C-Terminal Decapeptide. *Cancers* **2019**, *11*, 1764. [CrossRef]
31. Fortis, S.P.; Anastasopoulou, E.A.; Voutsas, I.F.; Baxevanis, C.N.; Perez, S.A.; Mahaira, L.G. Potential Prognostic Molecular Signatures in a Preclinical Model of Melanoma. *Anticancer. Res.* **2017**, *37*, 143–148. [CrossRef] [PubMed]
32. Kito, Y.; Bai, J.; Goto, N.; Okubo, H.; Adachi, Y.; Nagayama, T.; Takeuchi, T. Pathobiological properties of the ubiquitin ligase Nedd4L in melanoma. *Int. J. Exp. Pathol.* **2014**, *95*, 24–28. [CrossRef] [PubMed]
33. Parker, R.; Vella, L.J.; Xavier, D.; Amirkhani, A.; Parker, J.; Cebon, J.; Molloy, M.P. Phosphoproteomic Analysis of Cell-Based Resistance to BRAF Inhibitor Therapy in Melanoma. *Front. Oncol.* **2015**, *5*, 95. [CrossRef] [PubMed]
34. Kim, J.E.; Lee, D.S.; Kim, M.J.; Kang, T.C. PLPP/CIN-mediated NEDD4-2 S448 dephosphorylation regulates neuronal excitability via GluA1 ubiquitination. *Cell Death Dis.* **2019**, *10*, 545. [CrossRef]
35. Willems, P.; Wanschers, B.F.; Esseling, J.; Szklarczyk, R.; Kudla, U.; Duarte, I.; Forkink, M.; Nooteboom, M.; Swarts, H.; Gloerich, J.; et al. BOLA1 is an aerobic protein that prevents mitochondrial morphology changes induced by glutathione depletion. *Antioxid. Redox Signal.* **2013**, *18*, 129–138. [CrossRef]
36. Rufini, A.; Tucci, P.; Celardo, I.; Melino, G. Senescence and aging: The critical roles of p53. *Oncogene* **2013**, *32*, 5129. [CrossRef]
37. Lafarga, V.; Cuadrado, A.; Lopez de Silanes, I.; Bengoechea, R.; Fernandez-Capetillo, O.; Nebreda, A.R. p38 Mitogen-activated protein kinase- and HuR-dependent stabilization of p21(Cip1) mRNA mediates the G(1)/S checkpoint. *Mol. Cell. Biol.* **2009**, *29*, 4341–4351. [CrossRef]
38. Iwasa, H.; Han, J.; Ishikawa, F. Mitogen-activated protein kinase p38 defines the common senescence-signalling pathway. *Genes Cells* **2003**, *8*, 131–144. [CrossRef]
39. Spallarossa, P.; Altieri, P.; Barisione, C.; Passalacqua, M.; Aloi, C.; Fugazza, G.; Frassoni, F.; Podestà, M.; Canepa, M.; Ghigliotti, G.; et al. p38 MAPK and JNK antagonistically control senescence and cytoplasmic p16INK4A expression in doxorubicin-treated endothelial progenitor cells. *PLoS ONE* **2010**, *5*, e15583. [CrossRef]
40. Chew, Y.P.; Ellis, M.; Wilkie, S.; Mittnacht, S. pRB phosphorylation mutants reveal role of pRB in regulating S phase completion by a mechanism independent of E2F. *Oncogene* **1998**, *17*, 2177–2186. [CrossRef]
41. Cho, H.J.; Park, S.M.; Hwang, E.M.; Baek, K.E.; Kim, I.K.; Nam, I.K.; Im, M.J.; Park, S.H.; Bae, S.; Park, J.Y.; et al. Gadd45b mediates Fas-induced apoptosis by enhancing the interaction between p38 and retinoblastoma tumor suppressor. *J. Biol. Chem.* **2010**, *285*, 25500–25505. [CrossRef] [PubMed]
42. LaBaer, J.; Garrett, M.D.; Stevenson, L.F.; Slingerland, J.M.; Sandhu, C.; Chou, H.S.; Fattaey, A.; Harlow, E. New functional activities for the p21 family of CDK inhibitors. *Genes Dev.* **1997**, *11*, 847–862. [CrossRef]
43. Tran, T.T.; Rane, C.K.; Zito, C.R.; Weiss, S.A.; Jessel, S.; Lucca, L.; Lu, B.Y.; Oria, V.O.; Adeniran, A.; Chiang, V.L.; et al. Clinical Significance of PDCD4 in Melanoma by Subcellular Expression and in Tumor-Associated Immune Cells. *Cancers* **2021**, *13*, 1049. [CrossRef]
44. Nakashima, H.; Hamamura, K.; Houjou, T.; Taguchi, R.; Yamamoto, N.; Mitsudo, K.; Tohnai, I.; Ueda, M.; Urano, T.; Furukawa, K.; et al. Overexpression of caveolin-1 in a human melanoma cell line results in dispersion of ganglioside GD3 from lipid rafts and alteration of leading edges, leading to attenuation of malignant properties. *Cancer Sci.* **2007**, *98*, 512–520. [CrossRef]
45. Goding, C.R.; Arnheiter, H. MITF—The first 25 years. *Genes Dev.* **2019**, *33*, 983–1007. [CrossRef] [PubMed]
46. Gautron, A.; Migault, M.; Bachelot, L.; Corre, S.; Galibert, M.D.; Gilot, D. Human TYRP1: Two functions for a single gene? *Pigment. Cell Melanoma Res.* **2021**, *34*, 836–852. [CrossRef] [PubMed]
47. Sinnberg, T.; Menzel, M.; Ewerth, D.; Sauer, B.; Schwarz, M.; Schaller, M.; Garbe, C.; Schittek, B. β-Catenin signaling increases during melanoma progression and promotes tumor cell survival and chemoresistance. *PLoS ONE* **2011**, *6*, e23429. [CrossRef]
48. Spranger, S.; Bao, R.; Gajewski, T.F. Melanoma-intrinsic β-catenin signalling prevents anti-tumour immunity. *Nature* **2015**, *523*, 231–235. [CrossRef]
49. Koyano, T.; Namba, M.; Kobayashi, T.; Nakakuni, K.; Nakano, D.; Fukushima, M.; Nishiyama, A.; Matsuyama, M. The p21 dependent G2 arrest of the cell cycle in epithelial tubular cells links to the early stage of renal fibrosis. *Sci. Rep.* **2019**, *9*, 12059. [CrossRef]
50. Lee, H.O.; Davidson, J.M.; Duronio, R.J. Endoreplication: Polyploidy with purpose. *Genes Dev.* **2009**, *23*, 2461–2477. [CrossRef]

51. Hernandez-Segura, A.; Nehme, J.; Demaria, M. Hallmarks of cellular senescence. *Trends Cell Biol.* **2018**, *28*, 436–453. [CrossRef] [PubMed]
52. Dhillon, A.S.; Meikle, S.; Peyssonnaux, C.; Grindlay, J.; Kaiser, C.; Steen, H.; Shaw, P.E.; Mischak, H.; Eychène, A.; Kolch, W. A Raf-1 mutant that dissociates MEK/extracellular signal-regulated kinase activation from malignant transformation and differentiation but not proliferation. *Mol. Cell. Biol.* **2003**, *23*, 1983–1993. [CrossRef] [PubMed]
53. Berens, E.B.; Holy, J.M.; Riegel, A.T.; Wellstein, A. A Cancer Cell Spheroid Assay to Assess Invasion in a 3D Setting. *J. Vis. Exp.* **2015**, *105*, e53409. [CrossRef]
54. De Wever, O.; Hendrix, A.; De Boeck, A.; Westbroek, W.; Braems, G.; Emami, S.; Sabbah, M.; Gespach, C.; Bracke, M. Modeling and quantification of cancer cell invasion through collagen type I matrices. *Int. J. Dev. Biol.* **2010**, *54*, 887–896. [CrossRef] [PubMed]
55. Turriziani, B.; Garcia-Munoz, A.; Pilkington, R.; Raso, C.; Kolch, W.; von Kriegsheim, A. On-beads digestion in conjunction with data-dependent mass spectrometry: A shortcut to quantitative and dynamic interaction proteomics. *Biology* **2014**, *3*, 320–332. [CrossRef]
56. Howard, J.; Wynne, K.; Moldenhauer, E.; Clarke, P.; Maguire, C.; Bollard, S.; Yin, X.; Brennan, L.; Mooney, L.; Fitzsimons, S.; et al. A comparative analysis of extracellular vesicles (EVs) from human and feline plasma. *Sci. Rep.* **2022**, *12*, 10851. [CrossRef]
57. Tyanova, S.; Temu, T.; Sinitcyn, P.; Carlson, A.; Hein, M.Y.; Geiger, T.; Mann, M.; Cox, J. The Perseus computational platform for comprehensive analysis of (prote)omics data. *Nat. Methods* **2016**, *13*, 731–740. [CrossRef]
58. Chen, E.Y.; Tan, C.M.; Kou, Y.; Duan, Q.; Wang, Z.; Meirelles, G.V.; Clark, N.R.; Ma'ayan, A. Enrichr: Interactive and collaborative HTML5 gene list enrichment analysis tool. *BMC Bioinform.* **2013**, *14*, 128. [CrossRef]

International Journal of
Molecular Sciences

MDPI

Review

Immune Checkpoint Inhibitor Therapy for Metastatic Melanoma: What Should We Focus on to Improve the Clinical Outcomes?

Sultana Mehbuba Hossain †, Kevin Ly †, Yih Jian Sung, Antony Braithwaite and Kunyu Li *

Department of Pathology, Dunedin School of Medicine, University of Otago, Dunedin 9016, New Zealand; mehbuba.hossain@otago.ac.nz (S.M.H.); kevin.ly@otago.ac.nz (K.L.); yihjian.sung@otago.ac.nz (Y.J.S.); antony.braithwaite@otago.ac.nz (A.B.)

* Correspondence: kunyu.li@otago.ac.nz

† These authors contributed equally to this work.

Abstract: Immune checkpoint inhibitors (ICIs) have transformed cancer treatment by enhancing anti-tumour immune responses, demonstrating significant efficacy in various malignancies, including melanoma. However, over 50% of patients experience limited or no response to ICI therapy. Resistance to ICIs is influenced by a complex interplay of tumour intrinsic and extrinsic factors. This review summarizes current ICIs for melanoma and the factors involved in resistance to the treatment. We also discuss emerging evidence that the microbiota can impact ICI treatment outcomes by modulating tumour biology and anti-tumour immune function. Furthermore, microbiota profiles may offer a non-invasive method for predicting ICI response. Therefore, future research into microbiota manipulation could provide cost-effective strategies to enhance ICI efficacy and improve outcomes for melanoma patients.

Keywords: ICI; melanoma; treatment resistance; epigenetic regulation; microbiota; anti-tumour immune response; predicting treatment outcomes

1. Introduction

Immune checkpoint molecules (ICMs), such as CTLA-4 and PD-1, are key immune checkpoint regulators involving T cell exhaustion and tolerance to prevent excess immune response and pathology [1]. However, tumours often hijack these regulatory mechanisms to evade immune detection [2]. ICIs are monoclonal antibodies designed to block these signalling pathways, thereby countering T cell exhaustion and tolerance, leading to a prolonged anti-tumour immune response [3]. ICIs have significantly transformed the treatment of advanced melanoma, leading to substantial improvements in long-term progression-free survival for many patients [4,5]. These therapies target immune checkpoint molecules (ICMs) such as cytotoxic T-lymphocyte-associated protein 4 (CTLA-4) and programmed cell death protein 1 (PD-1), which are involved in T cell exhaustion and tolerance. By inhibiting these checkpoints, ICIs restore the ability of T cells to attack tumour cells. Despite these advancements, over 50% of patients experience limited or no benefit from these therapies, highlighting a major challenge in current cancer treatment [6,7]. Recent research has emphasised the significant role of the gut microbiota in influencing cancer development and response to treatment [8]. Although the precise molecular mechanisms underlying these effects are not yet fully understood, emerging research suggests that the composition and function of the gut microbiota influence the anti-tumour immune responses and treatment outcomes of ICI [9,10]. This manuscript explores the complexities of resistance to ICI therapy in melanoma, with a focus on how the microbiota affects tumour biology and the anti-tumour immune response. By examining the impact of the microbiota on ICI efficacy and investigating potential mechanisms for incorporating microbiota-based approaches into clinical treatment, this study aims to provide new insights and identify future research avenues to enhance ICI immunotherapy through microbiota modulation.

2. Overview of ICI Therapy in Melanoma

Clinical research on ICI therapy is advancing (Table 1), starting with the most well-known ICMs CTLA-4 and PD-1, where blocking signalling through these molecules has been shown to promote T cell infiltration and expansion at the tumour site and to activate intratumoral natural killer (NK) cells [11–14]. Since 2011, the U.S. Food and Drug Administration (FDA) has approved several ICIs as first-line treatments for metastatic melanoma, including Ipilimumab, a monoclonal antibody against CTLA-4, and Nivolumab and Pembrolizumab, which block PD-1. These ICIs have become standard first-line treatments for advanced melanoma, demonstrating better response rates than other therapies such as IL-2 and interferons (IFN)-α immunotherapies. Dual targeting of CTLA-4 and PD-1 has been explored in both preclinical and clinical studies. A 2015 phase 3 trial of combined ICI therapy in 945 patients with unresectable stage III and IV melanomas found that those receiving both Ipilimumab and Nivolumab had longer median progression-free survival (11.5 months) compared to those receiving Ipilimumab (2.9 months) or Nivolumab (6.9 months) alone [15]. Another trial reported a higher 3-year overall survival (OS) rate in the combination therapy group (58%) compared to 52% and 34% in the Nivolumab and Ipilimumab groups, respectively [16]. Additionally, the FDA has approved Ipilimumab, Nivolumab, and Pembrolizumab for use as adjuvant therapy in high-risk melanoma, showing improved recurrence-free survival (RFS) and OS compared to high-dose IFN-α2b in resected high-risk melanoma [17]. However, combination therapy was associated with a higher incidence of treatment-related grade 3 or 4 adverse events (59%) compared to 16.3% and 27.3% in patients receiving only Nivolumab and Ipilimumab, respectively [16].

Lymphocyte activation gene 3 (LAG-3) is another checkpoint target that is expressed on activated T cells 3–4 days post-activation, where it suppresses T cell activation and prevents autoimmunity [18,19]. Blocking LAG-3 can restore T cell function and increase tumour infiltration. Research has demonstrated that anti-LAG-3 therapy can improve T cell proliferation, rejuvenate exhausted cytotoxic T lymphocytes, and increase tumour infiltration in murine cancer models [19]. Melanoma patients who responded to the combination therapy of anti-LAG-3 and anti-PD-1 were found to have higher NK cell levels in the tumours and greater transcriptional changes associated with IFN-γ responses, cytotoxicity, and degranulation [20]. Several anti-LAG-3 antibodies (e.g., Relatlimab) are now in clinical trials, both as monotherapies and in combination with other ICI therapies. A clinical study of Relatlimab/Nivolumab combination therapy (Opdualag) reported a significant improvement in progression-free survival (PFS) to 10.2 months versus 4.6 months with Nivolumab alone [21]. At 12 months, PFS was 48.0% for the combination therapy versus 36.9% for Nivolumab monotherapy [21]. Based on these results, the FDA approved this combination therapy in 2022, making LAG-3 the third checkpoint inhibitor approved for cancer treatment [22]. Post-treatment analysis of biospecimens from patients with advanced melanoma demonstrated that dual blockade of LAG-3 and PD-1 leads to enhanced capacity for $CD8^+$ T cell receptor signalling and cytotoxicity, despite the retention of an exhaustion profile [23]. However, the increased anti-tumour immune response with combined anti-LAG-3 and anti-PD-1 therapies comes with the cost of higher immune-related adverse events (irAEs), with 21.1% of patients on combination therapy experiencing grade 3 or 4 events compared to 11.1% with anti-PD-1 monotherapy [21]. Thus, optimizing dosages to balance survival benefits and treatment safety remains an active area of research on combined ICI therapies [24,25].

T cell immunoglobulin and mucin domain-containing protein 3 (TIM-3) is a type I transmembrane protein that is upregulated on exhausted NK cells, monocytes, and exhausted CD8 T cells, and its expression was found to be associated with poorer prognoses in melanoma patients [26]. While no anti-TIM-3 antibodies are currently FDA-approved, clinical and pre-clinical trials are underway to evaluate their efficacy in combination with other immune checkpoint inhibitors [27]. Treatment with a soluble TIM-3 blocking antibody has been shown to reverse the exhausted phenotype of NK cells isolated from melanoma patients [26]. Additionally, using a mouse glioma model, dual treatments with anti-TIM-3 antibody and either stereotactic radiosurgery (SRS) or anti-PD-1 were shown to improve survival of the tumour-bearing animals compared with anti-TIM-3 alone; triple therapy also resulted in a significant survival improvement compared to either dual therapy [28]. These results suggest that anti-TIM-3 is most effective as part of a combination therapy aimed at alleviating T cell and NK cell exhaustion.

Moreover, research is also investigating the co-administration of autologous natural killer cells and oncolytic viral adjuvants like TILT-123 or MEM-288 (which is a monoclonal antibody that targets TIM-3) to enhance immune cell activity and improve the anti-tumour response. Clinical studies are also exploring the combination of ICIs with small molecule inhibitors such as Dabrafenib and Trametinib, which target the BRAF-MEK pathway in BRAF-mutated tumours. Furthermore, novel ICI targets are under investigation, including anti-TIGIT (T cell immunoreceptor with Ig and ITIM domains) and anti-ILT4 (Inhibitory Ligand Tool 4) antibodies, which address immune evasion, and anti-CD40 and anti-CD27 antibodies, which aim to stimulate T-cell activation and proliferation. The dual-action ICI M7824, a bifunctional fusion protein targeting both Programmed Death-Ligand 1 (PD-L1) and Transforming Growth Factor-beta (TGF-β), is also being studied to inhibit immune suppression and enhance immune responses [29]. These innovative approaches are being tested across various cancers, including melanoma, with the goals of reducing treatment-related toxicity and improving objective response rates, progression-free survival, and OS. Overall, combination therapies often yield improved response rates but also increase the severity of irAEs, which can affect both OS and PFS [30]. Despite these advances, treatment resistance, which occurs in almost all anti-cancer therapies, remains a major challenge that limits the clinical outcomes of cancers.

Table 1. The development of ICI therapies over the last 2 decades.

Clinical Trial	Target	Stage of Melanoma/Study Phase	Key Findings
Ipilimumab (NCT00094653, 2004) [31]	anti-CTLA-4	phase 3 study in advanced melanoma.	Ipilimumab improved OS and provided durable responses in some patients
Nivolumab (NCT00730639, 2008) [32]	anti-PD-1	Phase 1 study in advanced melanoma	Nivolumab demonstrated an acceptable long-term safety profile and durable tumour regression
Pembrolizumab (KEYNOTE-001, NCT01295827, 2011) [33]	anti-PD-1	Phase 1 study in advanced melanoma that progressed after 2 doses of Ipilimumab therapy	Pembrolizumab was well tolerated and demonstrated significant anti-tumour effects in patients previously treated with Ipilimumab
Pembrolizumab (KEYNOTE-002, NCT01704287, 2012) [34]	anti-PD-1	Phase 2 study in advanced melanoma that progressed after Ipilimumab therapy	Pembrolizumab had a higher rate of progression-free survival compared standard-of-care chemotherapy
Nivolumab (CheckMate 037, NCT01721746, 2012) [35]	anti-PD-1	Phase 3 study in advanced melanoma that progressed after Ipilimumab therapy	Nivolumab demonstrated higher objective response rate compared to chemotherapy.
Pembrolizumab, Ipilimumab (KEYNOTE-006, NCT01866319, 2013) [36]	anti-PD-1, anti-CTLA-4	Phase 3 study in advanced melanoma with no more than one prior systemic therapy	Pembrolizumab improved progression-free survival and OS with lower rates of high-grade toxicity compared to Ipilimumab.
Nivolumab, Ipilimumab (CheckMate 064, NCT01783938, 2013) [37]	anti-PD-1, anti-CTLA-4	Phase 2 study in advanced melanoma, without prior treatment or with progression after prior systemic therapy	Sequential treatment with Nivolumab followed by Ipilimumab enhanced efficacy but higher frequency of adverse events, compared to the reverse order.
Nivolumab (CheckMate 066, NCT01721772, 2013) [38]	anti-PD-1	Phase 3 study in advanced melanoma without prior treatment	Nivolumab conferred a significant OS benefit compared to chemotherapy.

Table 1. *Cont.*

Clinical Trial	Target	Stage of Melanoma/Study Phase	Key Findings
Nivolumab, Ipilimumab (CheckMate 067, NCT01844505, 2013) [15].	anti-PD-1, anti-CTLA-4	Phase 3 study in untreated and unresectable advanced melanoma	Nivolumab, with or without Ipilimumab, showed longer progression-free survival and better objective response rates than Ipilimumab alone, especially in PD-L1-negative tumours.
Pembrolizumab, Ipilimumab (KEYNOTE-029, NCT02089685, 2014) [39]	anti-PD-1, anti-CTLA-4	Phases 1 & 2 study in advanced melanoma with no prior ICI therapy	standard-dose Pembrolizumab combined with reduced-dose Ipilimumab offers a manageable toxicity profile and robust anti-tumour activity
Nivolumab, Ipilimumab (CheckMate 238, NCT02388906, 2015) [40]	anti-PD-1, anti-CTLA-4	Phase 3 study as an adjuvant treatment in complete resection of stage IIIB, IIIC, or IV melanoma	Adjuvant Nivolumab significantly improved 12-month recurrence-free survival compared to Ipilimumab and was associated with fewer severe adverse events.
Pembrolizumab (KEYNOTE-054, NCT02362594, 2015) [41]	anti-PD-1	Phase 3 study as an adjuvant treatment in completely resected stage III melanoma with no other prior treatment	Adjuvant Pembrolizumab significantly improved recurrence-free survival compared to placebo, with a manageable safety profile
Ieramilimab, Spartalizumab (NCT02460224, 2015) [42]	anti-PD-1, anti-LAG-3	Phase I/II study in advanced melanoma that progressed after, or were unsuitable for, standard-of-care therapy	Ieramilimab, alone or with spartalizumab, was well tolerated, with modest anti-tumour activity and a safety profile similar to spartalizumab alone.
Pembrolizumab (KEYNOTE-151, NCT02821000, 2016) [43]	anti-PD-1	Phase 1 study in Chinese patients with advanced melanoma that progressed after first-line chemotherapy or targeted therapy	Pembrolizumab therapy was well tolerated in Chinese populations where acral or mucosal subtypes of melanoma are more prevalent and led to durable responses.
Nivolumab, Sotigalimab, Cabiralizumab (NCT03502330, 2018) [44]	anti-PD-1, anti-CD40L, anti-CSF-1R	Phase 1 study in advanced melanoma progressing after prior anti-PD-1/PD-L1 therapy	Combination of sotigalimab and cabiralizumab with or without Nivolumab is well tolerated in patients with anti-PD-1/PD-L1-resistant advanced melanoma.
Nivolumab, Relatlimab (RELATIVITY-047, NCT03470922, 2018) [45]	anti-PD-1, anti-LAG-3	Phases 2 & 3 studies in advanced melanoma with no prior anticancer treatment	Combination of Relatlimab and Nivolumab demonstrated longer progression-free survival than Nivolumab alone.
Nivolumab, Ipilimumab (CheckMate 238, NCT02388906, 2020) [46]	anti-PD-1, anti-CTLA-4	Phase 3 trial in resected stage IIIB-C or IV melanoma	Nivolumab showed a superior recurrence-free survival benefit compared to Ipilimumab, with similar OS rates and a more favourable safety profile
Nivolumab and Ipilimumab (CheckMate 238, 2023) [47]	anti-PD-1, anti-CTLA-4	Resected Stage III/IV Melanoma: 5-Year Efficacy	At 5 years, Nivolumab demonstrated superior recurrence-free survival and distant metastasis-free survival compared to Ipilimumab
Ieramilimab, spartalizumab, 2023 [48]	anti-PD-1, anti-LAG-3	phase 2 study in advanced solid tumours including melanoma, lung cancer, and TNBC with or without receiving prior anti-PD-1/L1 therapy	The combination therapy was well tolerated, showing durable responses, particularly those naive to anti-PD-1/L1 therapy.

3. Resistance to ICI Therapy in Melanoma

ICIs can be categorized into two subgroups: primary (innate) resistance and acquired resistance. Primary resistance occurs when patients never respond to treatment, typically due to a lack of tumour-reactive T cell infiltration, which is essential for the effectiveness of ICIs [49]. Acquired resistance, on the other hand, develops after an initial response and is often attributed to intratumoral heterogeneity and tumour diversification [49]. A preclinical study using combined genomic, transcriptomic, and high-dimensional flow cytometric profiling identified several distinct resistance programs involving both tumour-intrinsic and extrinsic factors, leading to multiple resistance mechanisms in melanoma [50].

3.1. The Involvement of Tumour-Intrinsic Factors

Several tumour-intrinsic factors are involved in treatment resistance to ICIs, including genetic mutations, altered antigen presentation, signalling pathways, tumour heterogeneity, and expression of other immunosuppressive molecules by the tumour cells. Key factors include mutations in the phosphatase and tensin homolog (PTEN), activation of the WNT/β-catenin signalling pathway, cytokine IFN-γ signalling, loss of heterozygosity in human leukocyte antigen (HLA) genes, and levels of neoantigen expression. PTEN loss or mutation is linked to reduced IFN-γ, granzyme B, and $CD8^+$ T cell infiltration [51], while β-catenin signalling activation can result in T cell exclusion in melanoma [52]. WNT/β-catenin signalling activation has also been found to correlate with poor T cell infiltration and a "cold tumour" phenotype. Other contributing factors include dendritic cells (DCs), interleukin-10 (IL-10), transforming growth factor-β (TGF-β), regulatory T cells (Tregs), and reduced $CD8^+$ T cell priming and infiltration, all leading to immune evasion and decreased cancer immunosurveillance [53,54]. Additionally, Hugo et al. (2017) identified a set of innate anti-PD-1 resistance signature (IPRES) genes involved in the mesenchymal transition, cell adhesion, extracellular matrix (ECM) remodelling, angiogenesis, and wound healing, which also control the MAPK signalling pathway and inhibit T cell function [55]. This study showed that prior anti-CTLA-4 treatment modifies genomic and transcriptomic features predictive of anti-PD-1 response, highlighting differences in baseline melanoma tumours across immunotherapy trials. Phenotypic switching in melanoma also plays a role in immune evasion, with non-responding tumours showing genes related to undifferentiated and neural crest-like states, while responding tumours display transitory and melanocytic gene signatures [56,57]. Furthermore, mutations in the tumour suppressor p53 (*TP53*) are associated with reduced efficacy of anti-CTLA-4 therapy, possibly due to downregulation of Fas transcription, decreasing susceptibility to CTL-induced apoptosis and reducing anti-CTLA-4 treatment effectiveness [58].

Epigenetic mechanisms, which involve DNA and RNA methylation as well as chromatin remodelling, are intrinsic cellular processes that regulate gene expression without altering the DNA sequence itself [59]. These mechanisms play a crucial role in cancer development and anti-tumour immune responses [60]. Changes in DNA methylation can affect the expression of immune checkpoint genes such as PD-1, PD-L1, PD-L2, and CTLA-4, leading to $CD8^+$ T cell exhaustion and altered immune cell recruitment [61]. In melanoma, global hypomethylation is linked to persistent PD-L1 expression and inhibitory cytokine production, contributing to immunosuppression and resistance to ICI therapy [62]. At the molecular level, DNA methyltransferase 3 (DNMT3) mediates new methylation during therapy, while PD-1 promoter demethylation can sustain $CD8^+$ T cell exhaustion [63]. DNMT and lysine methyltransferase 6A (KMT6A/EZH2) also suppress Th1-type chemokines like CXCL9 and CXCL10, crucial for T cell recruitment [64]. Global loss of methylation, especially in immunomodulatory genes related to Major Histocompatibility Complex (MHC) and cytokine interactions, correlates with chromosomal instability and reduced anti-tumour immune activity [65]. Chromosomal instability can impact tumour immune infiltration and inflammation via the activation of the cyclic guanosine monophosphate–adenosine monophosphate (GMP–AMP) synthase–stimulator of interferon genes (cGAS–STING) pathway [66], leading to suppression of anti-tumour immunity [67]. STING agonists, which stimulate both innate and adaptive immune responses, represent a novel class of cancer immunotherapy agents [68]. Notably, the expression of STING is epigenetically regulated by histone H3K4 lysine demethylases KDM5B and KDM5C and is activated by opposing H3K4 methyltransferases. Recent research has shown that inhibitors of KDM5 can induce STING expression, suggesting a potential new approach for cancer immunotherapy [68].

Epigenetic dysregulation of transposable elements (TEs) and human endogenous retroviruses (HERVs) can cause inappropriate immune gene activation. Research by Ye et al. highlights that TEs enriched in immune cells are vital for immune regulation [69]. Dysregulation affecting TE-derived enhancers can lead to the inappropriate activation of immune genes during disease progression. HERVs are typically cleared by endogenous immune responses [70], but their reactivation can stimulate immune responses and upregulate viral defence mechanisms, correlating with immune-infiltrating CD8$^+$ T cells [71,72]. Conversely, HERV-encoded oncogenes, such as Rec and NP9, can upregulate immunosuppressive pathways like β-catenin, inhibiting immune surveillance [73].

3.2. The Involvement of Tumour-Extrinsic Factors

Tumour-extrinsic mechanisms of immune evasion include the influence of immune cells, host microbiota, tumour stroma, and alterations in the local tumour microenvironment (TME), all of which contribute to resistance to ICIs [51,74]. The heterogeneity of immune cell composition in the TME of non-responders, particularly an increased presence of M2 macrophages, is associated with remodelling of the ECM and suppression of the immune system [75]. Even though CD8$^+$ T cells may be abundant during ICI therapy, they may lose their cytotoxic effectiveness due to mechanisms such as loss of tumour antigen recognition or tolerance to tumour-associated antigens (TAAs) [76]. Tumour-infiltrating macrophages also contribute to an immunosuppressive TME by secreting factors such as TGF-β, prostaglandins, and IL-10 [77]. These effectors promote the expansion of Treg populations and further recruit and polarize immunosuppressive tumour-associated macrophages (TAMs) [78]. Macrophages also facilitate melanoma progression, as evidenced by their increased density at the invasive front of melanoma lesions [79], and facilitate metastasis through the secretion of metalloproteinases like MMP-9, which remodel the ECM [78]. The ECM, a complex network of secreted molecules, defines tissue architecture and stiffness and influences cell behaviour by supporting cell adhesion, survival, and migration [80]. In melanoma, the ECM becomes highly heterogeneous and dysregulated, incorporating tumour cells, cancer-associated fibroblasts (CAFs), and newly formed blood vessels [80]. ECM molecules also promote TAM infiltration during tumorigenesis and regulate the spatial positioning of TAMs within the TME [81]

Cancer resistance arises from various factors that allow tumour cells to adapt to a changing environment. Therefore, a multifaceted approach may be necessary to address the diverse mechanisms of resistance in treating resistant cancers. Current clinical trials are tackling this issue by incorporating additional factors, such as patient ethnicities and delivery methods, to better evaluate treatment toxicity and efficacy. Moreover, recent studies in the microbiome have identified a significant role of gut or intratumoral microbiota in influencing cancer intrinsic factors, and anti-tumour immune responses, influencing the treatment efficacy and associated irAEs.

4. The Role of Microbiota in ICI Therapy

4.1. The Association between Microbiota and Cancer

The microbiota that inhabits the human body plays a crucial role in the well-being of its host [82]. Recent research has increasingly focused on its impact on health and disease, revealing that gut microbiota significantly modulates inflammation and immune defence [83,84]. Indeed, intratumoral microbiota can affect therapeutic outcomes by influencing both tumour-intrinsic and extrinsic factors, including genetic and epigenetic expression in tumour cells, signalling pathways like Wnt/β-catenin and NF-κB, metabolism of anti-cancer drugs, and immune cell infiltration and function [85]. Interactions between the host and gut microbes are mostly mediated by the gut metabolome. For example, a study of metabolomic profiles from patients with advanced colorectal adenomas, matched controls, and colorectal cancer (CRC) found that elevated levels of specific bioactive lipids could serve as early indicators of cancer development [86]. Additionally, analysis of the gut microbiome using 16S rRNA gene and shotgun metagenome sequencing revealed that higher microbial community richness and specific microbiome compositions were associated with longer PFS in melanoma patients undergoing immunotherapy [87]. These findings underscore the significant role of gut microbiome interactions in early cancer pathogenesis and therapeutic response.

4.2. The Effects of Microbiota on Tumour Genetic and Epigenetic Expression

Research indicates that intratumoral microbiota may contribute to carcinogenesis by releasing toxic byproducts that cause DNA damage, cell cycle arrest, and genomic instability [88]. Gut microbiota can also produce metabolites such as short-chain fatty acids (SCFAs) butyrate and propionate, to modulate host epigenetic machinery. These interactions influence the activity of epigenetic enzymes involved in gene regulation, ultimately affecting immune responses and cancer progression. A study on CRC utilized metagenomic and 16S rRNA gene sequencing to analyse microbiomes in faecal and tissue samples from CRC patients and healthy controls [89]. The study revealed significant differences in DNA methylation patterns between CRC tumours and adjacent normal tissues, with specific microbial-related pathways influencing these changes. Notably, microbial-associated DNA methylation was more evident in adjacent normal tissues but absent in tumours, indicating that gut microbiota and pathogenic bacteria play a crucial role in altering DNA methylation and contributing to CRC development. While the effects of microbiota and their byproducts on epigenetic modifications in melanoma need further investigation, these findings highlight the critical role of host–microbiome interactions in cancer progression.

4.3. The Effects of Microbiota in Anti-Tumour Immune Response

The mechanisms by which microbiota enhance anti-tumour immune responses include the upregulation of helper T cell (Th1) and DC functions and the downregulation of regulatory T cells (Tregs), thereby reducing immunosuppression and reinforcing immune activation against tumour cells [90]. By influencing the immune system, microbiota can also affect the efficacy of vaccines and cancer therapies, including ICIs [91,92]. For example, the MIND-DC phase III trial, which randomized 148 stage IIIB/C melanoma patients to receive either autologous DC therapy or a placebo, found that significant baseline differences in gut microbiota and metabolomic profiles affected treatment outcomes [93]. Specifically, the study observed baseline biases in gut microbial composition and metabolic profiles, such as lower levels of *F. prausnitzii* and perturbations in bile acids and acylcarnitines, which were correlated with prognosis and influenced the effectiveness of the dendritic cell therapy [93]. In addition, SCFAs pentanoate and butyrate from microbes can act as enhancers of anti-tumour immunity by modulating cytotoxic T lymphocytes and Chimeric Antigen Receptor (CAR) T cells through metabolic and epigenetic reprogramming, thus improving their efficacy in treating melanoma and pancreatic cancer [94]. The presence of polyclonal neoantigen-specific T cells is also a crucial determinant of effective anti-PD-1 therapy [95]. Interestingly, pre-resection antibiotics administration targeting anaerobic bacteria was found to substantially improve disease-free survival by 25.5% in patients with CRC [96]. Using a mouse CRC model, the authors found that antibiotic treatment generated microbial neoantigens that elicited anti-tumour $CD8^+$ T cell response [96]. Gut microbiota can also independently generate epitopes that resemble tumour neoantigens, which can enhance anti-tumour immune responses and contribute to more favourable long-term outcomes with immune checkpoint inhibitors [97].

Microbiota diversity is also a critical determinant of anti-tumour response. Differences in microbiome diversity and composition, along with enhanced systemic anti-tumour immune responses, were observed in melanoma patients who responded to anti-PD-1 ICI compared to non-responders [98]. In a melanoma animal model, the abundance of the commensal microbiota *Bifidobacterium* was associated with increased production of proinflammatory cytokines by DCs, leading to enhanced priming and recruitment of cytotoxic $CD8^+$ T cells into the TME [99]. Oral administration of *Bifidobacterium* alone improved tumour control to a degree comparable to that achieved with PD-L1-specific antibody therapy (checkpoint blockade), and combined treatment nearly abolished tumour outgrowth [99]. Similarly, in a preclinical melanoma model, *Lactobacillus reuteri*, found in the gastrointestinal (GI) tract of humans and animals, migrated to the tumour and released the dietary tryptophan catabolite indole-3-aldehyde (I3A). This promoted IFN-γ-producing $CD8^+$ T cells and enhanced ICI efficacy [100]. In addition, intratumoral microbiota, particularly the *Lachnoclostridium* genus, positively correlates with $CD8^+$ T cell infiltration and chemokine expression and influences survival in cutaneous melanoma [101]. The benefit of microbiota on ICI treatment efficacy is further supported by evidence that faecal microbiota transplantation (FMT) from cancer patients who responded to ICIs improved the anti-tumour effects of PD-1 blockade in germ-free and antibiotic-treated mice [102].

However, intratumoral microbiota can also promote cancer development by inducing genetic mutation, affecting epigenetic modifications, promoting inflammatory response, evading immune destruction, and activating invasion and metastasis. Abnormal gut microbiome composition, associated with dysbiosis, has also been linked to primary resistance to ICIs in patients with advanced cancer [103]. A clinical study analysed microbiomes from 1526 tumours across seven cancer types, including melanoma, and found that each type had a unique microbial profile [104]. Interestingly, intratumor bacteria, mostly intracellular within cancer and immune cells, correlated with tumour characteristics, smoking status, and immunotherapy responses [104]. The mechanisms by which intracellular bacteria within the tumour affect tumour biology and immune responses, and how they differ from extracellular bacteria within the tumour, are currently unknown and require further research. Nevertheless, these findings suggest that modulating the intratumoral microbiome could potentially enhance patient outcomes in immunotherapy.

It is fascinating how gut microbiota can influence anti-tumour immune responses at various sites in the body. Several pathways have been identified through which gut bacteria and their products can reach tumours in different organs. These pathways include passage through the intestinal mucosal barrier into the mesenteric lymph nodes, entry into the systemic circulation, or migration to distant organs due to increased intestinal wall permeability [105]. A recent study using a mouse model of subcutaneous melanoma has uncovered a novel mechanism by which gut microbiota translocation and modulation affect anti-tumour immune responses during ICI therapy [106]. The study demonstrated that ICI treatment induces DC activation, leading to the translocation of gut microbiota to the mesenteric lymph nodes (MLNs) and subsequent remodelling of these nodes. This remodelling facilitates the migration of gut bacteria to tumour-draining lymph nodes (TDLNs) and the subcutaneous primary tumour [106]. This process enhances the activation of effector $CD4^+$ and $CD8^+$ T cells in both the TDLNs and the tumour, as well as increases leukocyte infiltration and the proportion of IFN-γ and Granzyme B-producing $CD8^+$ T cells in the tumour. The presence of MLNs is crucial for the translocation of gut bacteria to extraintestinal tissues. Intestinal DCs are essential for transferring bacteria from the gut to the MLNs but are not required for the subsequent movement from MLNs to TDLNs and the tumour. These findings suggest a complex pathway for microbiota migration beyond the gut, with MLNs serving as a central hub and intestinal DCs acting as transporters to facilitate gut bacterial translocation under specific conditions.

5. Predicting Treatment Response to ICI Therapy

Predicting patient responses to ICIs remains a significant challenge in oncology. Several key biomarkers have been explored for this purpose. PD-1 expression on T cells and PD-L1 expression on tumour cells are well-established indicators for predicting responses to anti-PD-1 and anti-PD-L1 therapies. Higher baseline levels of PD-L1 expression generally correlate with improved responses to ICIs [107]. However, PD-L1 expression alone may not always accurately predict outcomes, as its levels can vary across different tumour regions or over time. Increased infiltration of $CD8^+$ T cells and other pro-inflammatory immune cells is generally associated with better responses to ICIs [108]. Conversely, high levels of myeloid-derived suppressor cells (MDSCs) correlate with resistance to therapy; reducing these cells enhanced anti-PD-1 therapy in a mouse model of melanoma [109]. Gene expression profiles related to T cell inflammation are also valuable for predicting treatment response. A gene profile associated with T cell inflammation has been connected to improved responses to anti-PD-1 therapy [110]. Variations in expression levels of specific genes, particularly those involved in immune signalling pathways, can help predict patient responses to treatment. Additionally, inflammation-related gene signatures (IRGS) in the TME can distinguish between "cold" and "hot" tumours and predict responses to immunotherapy [111]. Interestingly, High IRGS scores are associated with reduced $CD8^+$ T cell infiltration, increased M2 macrophage infiltration, more stroma-activated molecular subtypes, hypoxia, enriched myofibroblast-related signalling, and greater benefit from gemcitabine chemotherapy in prostate cancer [112].

Tumour mutational burden (TMB) is another important predictive factor [107]. The composition and density of immune cell populations within the TME can influence ICI efficacy. In patients with advanced melanoma, high TMB and high inflammatory gene expression scores were associated with longer survival; this was consistent across either Nivolumab and Ipilimumab alone, or in combination [113]. However, TMB alone is not always a reliable predictor of ICI response, as it has been less effective in predicting outcomes for ICIs in various other cancers [114,115]. For instance, ICI responders were found to have more frequent hypomethylation in specific genes, suggesting that methylation profiles could serve as potential predictors of ICI efficacy [116].

Additionally, Microbiota composition has been linked to treatment outcomes. A meta-analysis of four published shotgun metagenomic studies in metastatic melanoma patients identified a faecal microbiome signature associated with responders [117]. The authors found that specific microbial features, such as *Faecalibacterium* and *Barnesiella intestinihominis*, were associated with treatment response. Another meta-analysis study of anti-PD-1 ICI in melanoma patients identified two distinct microbial signatures that differentially affected treatment response [118]. Patients enriched for Actinobacteria and the *Lachnospiraceae/Ruminococcaceae* families of *Firmicutes* showed favourable clinical responses. In contrast, Gram-negative bacteria such as *Streptococcaceae spp* were associated with an inflammatory gene signature, increased blood neutrophil-to-lymphocyte ratio, and poor outcomes with distinct immune-related adverse effects [118]. Moreover, longitudinal microbiome profiling by Weersma et al. revealed several microbial species-level genome bins (SGBs) and pathways that could differentiate patients who achieved PFS of 12 months or longer from those with shorter PFS after ICI treatment [119].

Taken together, predicting responses to ICI therapy involves a multifaceted approach that includes tumour-intrinsic factors, immune cell infiltration, epigenetic profiles, and microbiota signatures. By leveraging these predictive biomarkers, clinicians can better tailor treatment strategies and improve outcomes for melanoma patients undergoing ICI therapy.

6. Summary and Future Perspective

In conclusion, the development of ICIs is advancing with a focus on identifying new targets and optimizing combination therapies tailored to individual patients. This progress involves balancing the therapeutic efficacy of ICIs with the management of irAEs [120]. Emerging research on the microbiome underscores its potential role in influencing cancer epigenetics, immune responses, and ICI outcomes (see Figure 1). The concept of a "symbiotic microecosystem" within tumours comprising intratumoral microbiota, tumour cells, and immune cells highlights a fundamental interplay in cancer development and treatment success [121]. Recent findings indicate that specific microbiota profiles can enhance responses to PD-1 inhibitors, suggesting promising interventions such as FMT, probiotics, and dietary adjustments [8,122]. These strategies could improve the presence of anti-tumour microbiota and, consequently, treatment outcomes. In addition, further research is needed to elucidate their role in tumour progression, identify strategies to promote anti-tumour microbiota infiltration into the tumours, and the molecular mechanisms behind these processes. Taken together, the field of anti-cancer therapy is evolving rapidly, with significant promise for both ICI and microbiome-based treatments. These approaches potentially offer more cost-effective and efficient strategies to improve cancer treatment outcomes in the future.

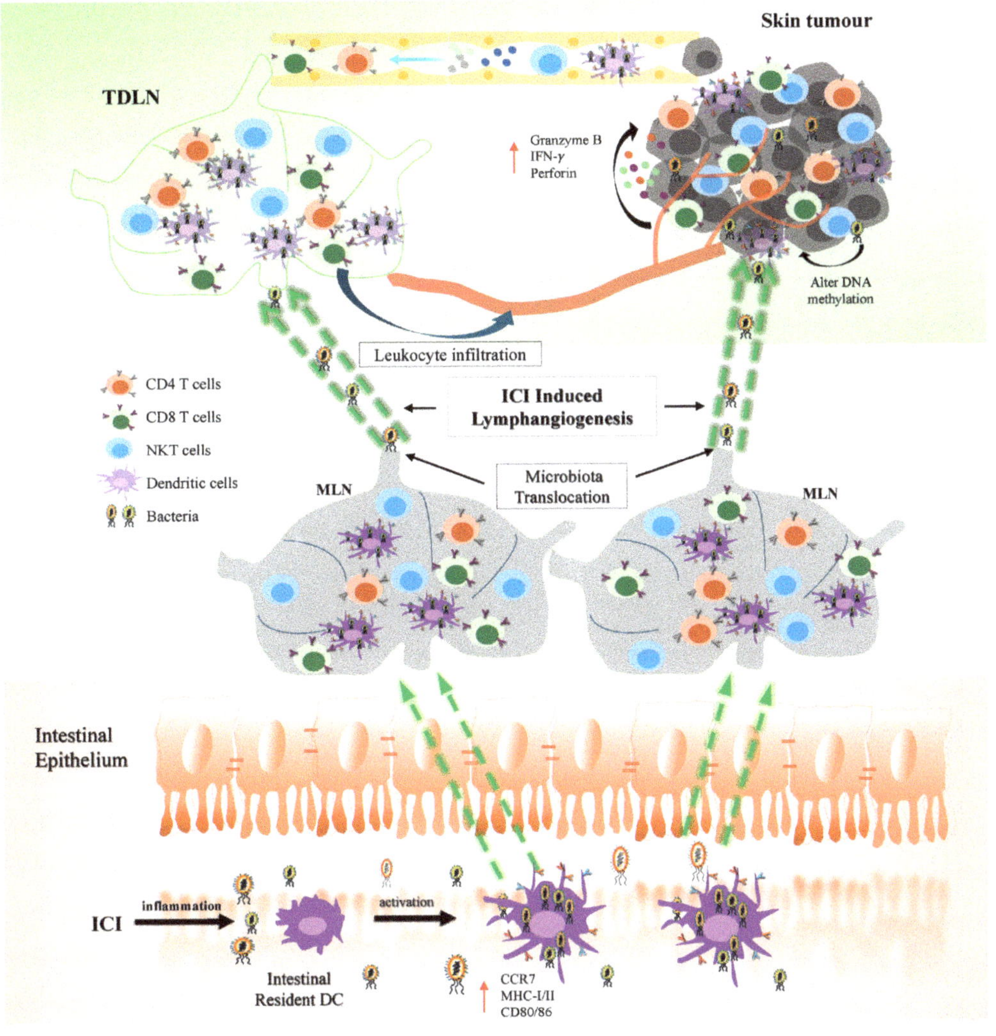

Figure 1. Synergistic response of ICI and gut microbiota. Inflammation-induced by ICI stimulates gut microbiota uptake by and activation of intestinal DCs, accompanied by the upregulation of MHC, CD86, and CCR7. This process facilitates the translocation of bacterial-retaining DCs into the MLNs, leading to bacterial translocation to the TDLNs and the tumour, where they alter epigenetic expression of the tumour cells, and upregulate the production of pro-inflammatory cytokines by effector immune cells, such as CD8 T cells and NKT cells. This procedure also results in increased leukocyte infiltration into the tumour and secretion of Granzyme B and perforin to initiate tumour elimination.

Author Contributions: S.M.H. collected all data related to anti-PD-1 therapy and genetic and epigenetic expression. Y.J.S. gathered data on anti-CTLA-4, TIM-3, and LAG-3 therapies. K.L. (Kevin Ly) compiled data on the microbiota and prepared the associated figures. A.B. reviewed the manuscript. K.L. (Kunyu Li) planned the manuscript structure, wrote the introduction and conclusion, and organized the overall content. All authors have read and agreed to the published version of the manuscript.

Funding: This research was funded by Otago Medical Research Foundation (AG-400). S.M.H. is supported by a Postdoctoral Fellowship from the New Zealand Institute for Cancer Research Trust. Kevin Ly is supported by New Zealand Cancer Society Postdoctoral Fellowship. A. Braithwaite is supported by New Zealand HRC programme grant (23/470). Y.J. Sung and Kunyu Li are supported by New Zealand HRC project grant (23/301).

Conflicts of Interest: All the authors declare that they have no conflicts of interest related to the publication of this manuscript.

References

1. Barnova, M.; Bobcakova, A.; Urdova, V.; Kosturiak, R.; Kapustova, L.; Dobrota, D.; Jesenak, M. Inhibitory immune checkpoint molecules and exhaustion of T cells in COVID-19. *Physiol. Res.* **2021**, *70*, S227–S247. [CrossRef] [PubMed]
2. Brunell, A.E.; Lahesmaa, R.; Autio, A.; Thotakura, A.K. Exhausted T cells hijacking the cancer-immunity cycle: Assets and liabilities. *Front. Immunol.* **2023**, *14*, 1151632. [CrossRef] [PubMed]
3. Disis, M.L. Mechanism of action of immunotherapy. *Semin. Oncol.* **2014**, *41* (Suppl. 5), S3–S13. [CrossRef]
4. Gong, J.; Chehrazi-Raffle, A.; Reddi, S.; Salgia, R. Development of PD-1 and PD-L1 inhibitors as a form of cancer immunotherapy: A comprehensive review of registration trials and future considerations. *J. Immunother. Cancer* **2018**, *6*, 8. [CrossRef]
5. Vaddepally, R.K.; Kharel, P.; Pandey, R.; Garje, R.; Chandra, A.B. Review of Indications of FDA-Approved Immune Checkpoint Inhibitors per NCCN Guidelines with the Level of Evidence. *Cancers* **2020**, *12*, 738. [CrossRef]
6. Bai, R.; Chen, N.; Li, L.; Du, N.; Bai, L.; Lv, Z.; Tian, H.; Cui, J. Mechanisms of Cancer Resistance to Immunotherapy. *Front. Oncol.* **2020**, *10*, 1290. [CrossRef]
7. Hossain, S.M.; Gimenez, G.; Stockwell, P.A.; Tsai, P.; Print, C.G.; Rys, J.; Cybulska-Stopa, B.; Ratajska, M.; Harazin-Lechowska, A.; Almomani, S.; et al. Innate immune checkpoint inhibitor resistance is associated with melanoma sub-types exhibiting invasive and de-differentiated gene expression signatures. *Front. Immunol.* **2022**, *13*, 955063. [CrossRef]
8. Wu, J.; Zhang, P.; Mei, W.; Zeng, C. Intratumoral microbiota: Implications for cancer onset, progression, and therapy. *Front. Immunol.* **2023**, *14*, 1301506. [CrossRef] [PubMed]
9. Jiang, H.; Zhang, Q. Gut microbiota influences the efficiency of immune checkpoint inhibitors by modulating the immune system (Review). *Oncol. Lett.* **2024**, *27*, 87. [CrossRef]
10. Aghamajidi, A.; Maleki Vareki, S. The Effect of the Gut Microbiota on Systemic and Anti-Tumor Immunity and Response to Systemic Therapy against Cancer. *Cancers* **2022**, *14*, 3563. [CrossRef]
11. Sanseviero, E.; O'Brien, E.M.; Karras, J.R.; Shabaneh, T.B.; Aksoy, B.A.; Xu, W.; Zheng, C.; Yin, X.; Xu, X.; Karakousis, G.C.; et al. Anti-CTLA-4 Activates Intratumoral NK Cells and Combined with IL15/IL15Rα Complexes Enhances Tumor Control. *Cancer Immunol. Res.* **2019**, *7*, 1371–1380. [CrossRef]
12. Friese, C.; Harbst, K.; Borch, T.H.; Westergaard, M.C.W.; Pedersen, M.; Kverneland, A.; Jönsson, G.; Donia, M.; Svane, I.M.; Met, Ö. CTLA-4 blockade boosts the expansion of tumor-reactive CD8(+) tumor-infiltrating lymphocytes in ovarian cancer. *Sci. Rep.* **2020**, *10*, 3914. [CrossRef]
13. Nagasaki, J.; Inozume, T.; Sax, N.; Ariyasu, R.; Ishikawa, M.; Yamashita, K.; Kawazu, M.; Ueno, T.; Irie, T.; Tanji, E.; et al. PD-1 blockade therapy promotes infiltration of tumor-attacking exhausted T cell clonotypes. *Cell Rep.* **2022**, *38*, 110331. [CrossRef]
14. Xiao, Z.; Yan, R.; Liu, H.; Huang, X.; Liang, Z.; An, G.; Ge, Y. Preventive Treatment with PD-1 Antibody Increases Tissue-resident Memory T Cells Infiltration and Delays Esophageal Carcinogenesis. *Cancer Prev. Res.* **2023**, *16*, 669–679. [CrossRef] [PubMed]
15. Larkin, J.; Chiarion-Sileni, V.; Gonzalez, R.; Grob, J.J.; Cowey, C.L.; Lao, C.D.; Schadendorf, D.; Dummer, R.; Smylie, M.; Rutkowski, P.; et al. Combined Nivolumab and Ipilimumab or Monotherapy in Untreated Melanoma. *N. Engl. J. Med.* **2015**, *373*, 23–34. [CrossRef] [PubMed]
16. Wolchok, J.D.; Chiarion-Sileni, V.; Gonzalez, R.; Rutkowski, P.; Grob, J.J.; Cowey, C.L.; Lao, C.D.; Wagstaff, J.; Schadendorf, D.; Ferrucci, P.F.; et al. Overall Survival with Combined Nivolumab and Ipilimumab in Advanced Melanoma. *N. Engl. J. Med.* **2017**, *377*, 1345–1356. [CrossRef] [PubMed]
17. Grossmann, K.F.; Othus, M.; Patel, S.P.; Tarhini, A.A.; Sondak, V.K.; Knopp, M.V.; Petrella, T.M.; Truong, T.G.; Khushalani, N.I.; Cohen, J.V.; et al. Adjuvant Pembrolizumab versus IFNα2b or Ipilimumab in Resected High-Risk Melanoma. *Cancer Discov.* **2022**, *12*, 644–653. [CrossRef]
18. Maruhashi, T.; Sugiura, D.; Okazaki, I.M.; Shimizu, K.; Maeda, T.K.; Ikubo, J.; Yoshikawa, H.; Maenaka, K.; Ishimaru, N.; Kosako, H.; et al. Binding of LAG-3 to stable peptide-MHC class II limits T cell function and suppresses autoimmunity and anti-cancer immunity. *Immunity* **2022**, *55*, 912–924.e918. [CrossRef]
19. Grosso, J.F.; Kelleher, C.C.; Harris, T.J.; Maris, C.H.; Hipkiss, E.L.; De Marzo, A.; Anders, R.; Netto, G.; Getnet, D.; Bruno, T.C.; et al. LAG-3 regulates CD8+ T cell accumulation and effector function in murine self- and tumor-tolerance systems. *J. Clin. Investig.* **2007**, *117*, 3383–3392. [CrossRef]
20. Huuhtanen, J.; Kasanen, H.; Peltola, K.; Lonnberg, T.; Glumoff, V.; Bruck, O.; Dufva, O.; Peltonen, K.; Vikkula, J.; Jokinen, E.; et al. Single-cell characterization of anti-LAG-3 and anti-PD-1 combination treatment in patients with melanoma. *J. Clin. Investig.* **2023**, *133*, e164809. [CrossRef]

21. Long, G.V.; Stephen Hodi, F.; Lipson, E.J.; Schadendorf, D.; Ascierto, P.A.; Matamala, L.; Salman, P.; Castillo Gutierrez, E.; Rutkowski, P.; Gogas, H.J.; et al. Overall Survival and Response with Nivolumab and Relatlimab in Advanced Melanoma. *NEJM Evid.* **2023**, *2*, EVIDoa2200239. [CrossRef] [PubMed]
22. Aggarwal, V.; Workman, C.J.; Vignali, D.A.A. LAG-3 as the third checkpoint inhibitor. *Nat. Immunol.* **2023**, *24*, 1415–1422. [CrossRef] [PubMed]
23. Cillo, A.R.; Cardello, C.; Shan, F.; Karapetyan, L.; Kunning, S.; Sander, C.; Rush, E.; Karunamurthy, A.; Massa, R.C.; Rohatgi, A.; et al. Blockade of LAG-3 and PD-1 leads to co-expression of cytotoxic and exhaustion gene modules in CD8(+) T cells to promote antitumor immunity. *Cell* **2024**, *187*, 4373–4388.e4315. [CrossRef] [PubMed]
24. Weber, J.S.; Schadendorf, D.; Del Vecchio, M.; Larkin, J.; Atkinson, V.; Schenker, M.; Pigozzo, J.; Gogas, H.; Dalle, S.; Meyer, N.; et al. Adjuvant Therapy of Nivolumab Combined With Ipilimumab Versus Nivolumab Alone in Patients With Resected Stage IIIB-D or Stage IV Melanoma (CheckMate 915). *J. Clin. Oncol.* **2023**, *41*, 517–527. [CrossRef] [PubMed]
25. Carlino, M.S.; Larkin, J.; Long, G.V. Immune checkpoint inhibitors in melanoma. *Lancet* **2021**, *398*, 1002–1014. [CrossRef]
26. da Silva, I.P.; Gallois, A.; Jimenez-Baranda, S.; Khan, S.; Anderson, A.C.; Kuchroo, V.K.; Osman, I.; Bhardwaj, N. Reversal of NK-cell exhaustion in advanced melanoma by Tim-3 blockade. *Cancer Immunol. Res.* **2014**, *2*, 410–422. [CrossRef]
27. Sauer, N.; Janicka, N.; Szlasa, W.; Skinderowicz, B.; Kołodzińska, K.; Dwernicka, W.; Oślizło, M.; Kulbacka, J.; Novickij, V.; Karłowicz-Bodalska, K. TIM-3 as a promising target for cancer immunotherapy in a wide range of tumors. *Cancer Immunol. Immunother.* **2023**, *72*, 3405–3425. [CrossRef]
28. Kim, J.E.; Patel, M.A.; Mangraviti, A.; Kim, E.S.; Theodros, D.; Velarde, E.; Liu, A.; Sankey, E.W.; Tam, A.; Xu, H.; et al. Combination Therapy with Anti-PD-1, Anti-TIM-3, and Focal Radiation Results in Regression of Murine Gliomas. *Clin. Cancer Res.* **2017**, *23*, 124–136. [CrossRef]
29. Karami, Z.; Mortezaee, K.; Majidpoor, J. Dual anti-PD-(L)1/TGF-β inhibitors in cancer immunotherapy—Updated. *Int. Immunopharmacol.* **2023**, *122*, 110648. [CrossRef]
30. Kuzmanovszki, D.; Kiss, N.; Tóth, B.; Kerner, T.; Tóth, V.; Szakonyi, J.; Lőrincz, K.; Hársing, J.; Imrédi, E.; Pfund, A.; et al. Anti-PD-1 Monotherapy in Advanced Melanoma-Real-World Data from a 77-Month-Long Retrospective Observational Study. *Biomedicines* **2022**, *10*, 1737. [CrossRef]
31. Hodi, F.S.; O'Day, S.J.; McDermott, D.F.; Weber, R.W.; Sosman, J.A.; Haanen, J.B.; Gonzalez, R.; Robert, C.; Schadendorf, D.; Hassel, J.C.; et al. Improved survival with ipilimumab in patients with metastatic melanoma. *N. Engl. J. Med.* **2010**, *363*, 711–723. [CrossRef] [PubMed]
32. Topalian, S.L.; Sznol, M.; McDermott, D.F.; Kluger, H.M.; Carvajal, R.D.; Sharfman, W.H.; Brahmer, J.R.; Lawrence, D.P.; Atkins, M.B.; Powderly, J.D.; et al. Survival, durable tumor remission, and long-term safety in patients with advanced melanoma receiving nivolumab. *J. Clin. Oncol.* **2014**, *32*, 1020–1030. [CrossRef] [PubMed]
33. Robert, C.; Ribas, A.; Wolchok, J.D.; Hodi, F.S.; Hamid, O.; Kefford, R.; Weber, J.S.; Joshua, A.M.; Hwu, W.J.; Gangadhar, T.C.; et al. Anti-programmed-death-receptor-1 treatment with pembrolizumab in ipilimumab-refractory advanced melanoma: A randomised dose-comparison cohort of a phase 1 trial. *Lancet* **2014**, *384*, 1109–1117. [CrossRef] [PubMed]
34. Ribas, A.; Puzanov, I.; Dummer, R.; Schadendorf, D.; Hamid, O.; Robert, C.; Hodi, F.S.; Schachter, J.; Pavlick, A.C.; Lewis, K.D.; et al. Pembrolizumab versus investigator-choice chemotherapy for ipilimumab-refractory melanoma (KEYNOTE-002): A randomised, controlled, phase 2 trial. *Lancet Oncol.* **2015**, *16*, 908–918. [CrossRef]
35. Weber, J.S.; D'Angelo, S.P.; Minor, D.; Hodi, F.S.; Gutzmer, R.; Neyns, B.; Hoeller, C.; Khushalani, N.I.; Miller, W.H., Jr.; Lao, C.D.; et al. Nivolumab versus chemotherapy in patients with advanced melanoma who progressed after anti-CTLA-4 treatment (CheckMate 037): A randomised, controlled, open-label, phase 3 trial. *Lancet Oncol.* **2015**, *16*, 375–384. [CrossRef]
36. Robert, C.; Schachter, J.; Long, G.V.; Arance, A.; Grob, J.J.; Mortier, L.; Daud, A.; Carlino, M.S.; McNeil, C.; Lotem, M.; et al. Pembrolizumab versus Ipilimumab in Advanced Melanoma. *N. Engl. J. Med.* **2015**, *372*, 2521–2532. [CrossRef] [PubMed]
37. Weber, J.S.; Gibney, G.; Sullivan, R.J.; Sosman, J.A.; Slingluff, C.L., Jr.; Lawrence, D.P.; Logan, T.F.; Schuchter, L.M.; Nair, S.; Fecher, L.; et al. Sequential administration of nivolumab and ipilimumab with a planned switch in patients with advanced melanoma (CheckMate 064): An open-label, randomised, phase 2 trial. *Lancet Oncol.* **2016**, *17*, 943–955. [CrossRef]
38. Robert, C.; Long, G.V.; Brady, B.; Dutriaux, C.; Maio, M.; Mortier, L.; Hassel, J.C.; Rutkowski, P.; McNeil, C.; Kalinka-Warzocha, E.; et al. Nivolumab in previously untreated melanoma without BRAF mutation. *N. Engl. J. Med.* **2015**, *372*, 320–330. [CrossRef]
39. Long, G.V.; Atkinson, V.; Cebon, J.S.; Jameson, M.B.; Fitzharris, B.M.; McNeil, C.M.; Hill, A.G.; Ribas, A.; Atkins, M.B.; Thompson, J.A.; et al. Standard-dose pembrolizumab in combination with reduced-dose ipilimumab for patients with advanced melanoma (KEYNOTE-029): An open-label, phase 1b trial. *Lancet Oncol.* **2017**, *18*, 1202–1210. [CrossRef]
40. Weber, J.; Mandala, M.; Del Vecchio, M.; Gogas, H.J.; Arance, A.M.; Cowey, C.L.; Dalle, S.; Schenker, M.; Chiarion-Sileni, V.; Marquez-Rodas, I.; et al. Adjuvant Nivolumab versus Ipilimumab in Resected Stage III or IV Melanoma. *N. Engl. J. Med.* **2017**, *377*, 1824–1835. [CrossRef]
41. Eggermont, A.M.M.; Blank, C.U.; Mandala, M.; Long, G.V.; Atkinson, V.; Dalle, S.; Haydon, A.; Lichinitser, M.; Khattak, A.; Carlino, M.S.; et al. Adjuvant Pembrolizumab versus Placebo in Resected Stage III Melanoma. *N. Engl. J. Med.* **2018**, *378*, 1789–1801. [CrossRef] [PubMed]
42. Schoffski, P.; Tan, D.S.W.; Martin, M.; Ochoa-de-Olza, M.; Sarantopoulos, J.; Carvajal, R.D.; Kyi, C.; Esaki, T.; Prawira, A.; Akerley, W.; et al. Phase I/II study of the LAG-3 inhibitor ieramilimab (LAG525) +/− anti-PD-1 spartalizumab (PDR001) in patients with advanced malignancies. *J. Immunother. Cancer* **2022**, *10*, e003776. [CrossRef]

43. Si, L.; Zhang, X.; Shu, Y.; Pan, H.; Wu, D.; Liu, J.; Lou, F.; Mao, L.; Wang, X.; Wen, X.; et al. A Phase Ib Study of Pembrolizumab as Second-Line Therapy for Chinese Patients With Advanced or Metastatic Melanoma (KEYNOTE-151). *Transl. Oncol.* **2019**, *12*, 828–835. [CrossRef] [PubMed]
44. Weiss, S.A.; Djureinovic, D.; Jessel, S.; Krykbaeva, I.; Zhang, L.; Jilaveanu, L.; Ralabate, A.; Johnson, B.; Levit, N.S.; Anderson, G.; et al. A Phase I Study of APX005M and Cabiralizumab with or without Nivolumab in Patients with Melanoma, Kidney Cancer, or Non-Small Cell Lung Cancer Resistant to Anti-PD-1/PD-L1. *Clin. Cancer Res.* **2021**, *27*, 4757–4767. [CrossRef] [PubMed]
45. Tawbi, H.A.; Schadendorf, D.; Lipson, E.J.; Ascierto, P.A.; Matamala, L.; Castillo Gutierrez, E.; Rutkowski, P.; Gogas, H.J.; Lao, C.D.; De Menezes, J.J.; et al. Relatlimab and Nivolumab versus Nivolumab in Untreated Advanced Melanoma. *N. Engl. J. Med.* **2022**, *386*, 24–34. [CrossRef]
46. Ascierto, P.A.; Del Vecchio, M.; Mandalá, M.; Gogas, H.; Arance, A.M.; Dalle, S.; Cowey, C.L.; Schenker, M.; Grob, J.J.; Chiarion-Sileni, V.; et al. Adjuvant nivolumab versus ipilimumab in resected stage IIIB-C and stage IV melanoma (CheckMate 238): 4-year results from a multicentre, double-blind, randomised, controlled, phase 3 trial. *Lancet Oncol.* **2020**, *21*, 1465–1477. [CrossRef]
47. Larkin, J.; Del Vecchio, M.; Mandalá, M.; Gogas, H.; Arance Fernandez, A.M.; Dalle, S.; Cowey, C.L.; Schenker, M.; Grob, J.J.; Chiarion-Sileni, V.; et al. Adjuvant Nivolumab versus Ipilimumab in Resected Stage III/IV Melanoma: 5-Year Efficacy and Biomarker Results from CheckMate 238. *Clin. Cancer Res.* **2023**, *29*, 3352–3361. [CrossRef]
48. Lin, C.C.; Garralda, E.; Schöffski, P.; Hong, D.S.; Siu, L.L.; Martin, M.; Maur, M.; Hui, R.; Soo, R.A.; Chiu, J.; et al. A phase 2, multicenter, open-label study of anti-LAG-3 ieramilimab in combination with anti-PD-1 spartalizumab in patients with advanced solid malignancies. *Oncoimmunology* **2024**, *13*, 2290787. [CrossRef]
49. Ziogas, D.C.; Theocharopoulos, C.; Koutouratsas, T.; Haanen, J.; Gogas, H. Mechanisms of resistance to immune checkpoint inhibitors in melanoma: What we have to overcome? *Cancer Treat. Rev.* **2023**, *113*, 102499. [CrossRef]
50. Lim, S.Y.; Shklovskaya, E.; Lee, J.H.; Pedersen, B.; Stewart, A.; Ming, Z.; Irvine, M.; Shivalingam, B.; Saw, R.P.M.; Menzies, A.M.; et al. The molecular and functional landscape of resistance to immune checkpoint blockade in melanoma. *Nat. Commun.* **2023**, *14*, 1516. [CrossRef]
51. Sharma, P.; Hu-Lieskovan, S.; Wargo, J.A.; Ribas, A. Primary, Adaptive, and Acquired Resistance to Cancer Immunotherapy. *Cell* **2017**, *168*, 707–723. [CrossRef] [PubMed]
52. Spranger, S.; Bao, R.; Gajewski, T.F. Melanoma-intrinsic β-catenin signalling prevents anti-tumour immunity. *Nature* **2015**, *523*, 231–235. [CrossRef] [PubMed]
53. Li, X.; Xiang, Y.; Li, F.; Yin, C.; Li, B.; Ke, X. WNT/β-Catenin Signaling Pathway Regulating T Cell-Inflammation in the Tumor Microenvironment. *Front. Immunol.* **2019**, *10*, 2293. [CrossRef] [PubMed]
54. Trujillo, J.A.; Sweis, R.F.; Bao, R.; Luke, J.J. T Cell-Inflamed versus Non-T Cell-Inflamed Tumors: A Conceptual Framework for Cancer Immunotherapy Drug Development and Combination Therapy Selection. *Cancer Immunol. Res.* **2018**, *6*, 990–1000. [CrossRef] [PubMed]
55. Hugo, W.; Zaretsky, J.M.; Sun, L.; Song, C.; Moreno, B.H.; Hu-Lieskovan, S.; Berent-Maoz, B.; Pang, J.; Chmielowski, B.; Cherry, G.; et al. Genomic and Transcriptomic Features of Response to Anti-PD-1 Therapy in Metastatic Melanoma. *Cell* **2017**, *168*, 542. [CrossRef]
56. Campbell, K.M.; Amouzgar, M.; Pfeiffer, S.M.; Howes, T.R.; Medina, E.; Travers, M.; Steiner, G.; Weber, J.S.; Wolchok, J.D.; Larkin, J.; et al. Prior anti-CTLA-4 therapy impacts molecular characteristics associated with anti-PD-1 response in advanced melanoma. *Cancer Cell* **2023**, *41*, 791–806.e794. [CrossRef]
57. Lax, B.M.; Palmeri, J.R.; Lutz, E.A.; Sheen, A.; Stinson, J.A.; Duhamel, L.; Santollani, L.; Kennedy, A.; Rothschilds, A.M.; Spranger, S.; et al. Both intratumoral regulatory T cell depletion and CTLA-4 antagonism are required for maximum efficacy of anti-CTLA-4 antibodies. *Proc. Natl. Acad. Sci. USA* **2023**, *120*, e230089512010. [CrossRef]
58. Xiao, W.; Du, N.; Huang, T.; Guo, J.; Mo, X.; Yuan, T.; Chen, Y.; Ye, T.; Xu, C.; Wang, W.; et al. TP53 Mutation as Potential Negative Predictor for Response of Anti-CTLA-4 Therapy in Metastatic Melanoma. *EBioMedicine* **2018**, *32*, 119–124. [CrossRef]
59. Portela, A.; Esteller, M. Epigenetic modifications and human disease. *Nat. Biotechnol.* **2010**, *28*, 1057–1068. [CrossRef] [PubMed]
60. Pang, L.; Zhou, F.; Liu, Y.; Ali, H.; Khan, F.; Heimberger, A.B.; Chen, P. Epigenetic regulation of tumor immunity. *J. Clin. Investig.* **2024**, *134*, e178540. [CrossRef]
61. Zhong, F.; Lin, Y.; Zhao, L.; Yang, C.; Ye, Y.; Shen, Z. Reshaping the tumour immune microenvironment in solid tumours via tumour cell and immune cell DNA methylation: From mechanisms to therapeutics. *Br. J. Cancer* **2023**, *129*, 24–37. [CrossRef] [PubMed]
62. Emran, A.A.; Chatterjee, A.; Rodger, E.J.; Tiffen, J.C.; Gallagher, S.J.; Eccles, M.R.; Hersey, P. Targeting DNA Methylation and EZH2 Activity to Overcome Melanoma Resistance to Immunotherapy. *Trends Immunol.* **2019**, *40*, 328–344. [CrossRef] [PubMed]
63. Xiao, Q.; Nobre, A.; Piñeiro, P.; Berciano-Guerrero, M.; Alba, E.; Cobo, M.; Lauschke, V.M.; Barragán, I. Genetic and Epigenetic Biomarkers of Immune Checkpoint Blockade Response. *J. Clin. Med.* **2020**, *9*, 286. [CrossRef] [PubMed]
64. Peng, D.; Kryczek, I.; Nagarsheth, N.; Zhao, L.; Wei, S.; Wang, W.; Sun, Y.; Zhao, E.; Vatan, L.; Szeliga, W.; et al. Epigenetic silencing of TH1-type chemokines shapes tumour immunity and immunotherapy. *Nature* **2015**, *527*, 249–253. [CrossRef] [PubMed]
65. Jung, H.; Kim, H.S.; Kim, J.Y.; Sun, J.M.; Ahn, J.S.; Ahn, M.J.; Park, K.; Esteller, M.; Lee, S.H.; Choi, J.K. DNA methylation loss promotes immune evasion of tumours with high mutation and copy number load. *Nat. Commun.* **2019**, *10*, 4278. [CrossRef]
66. Hoevenaar, W.H.M.; Janssen, A.; Quirindongo, A.I.; Ma, H.; Klaasen, S.J.; Teixeira, A.; van Gerwen, B.; Lansu, N.; Morsink, F.H.M.; Offerhaus, G.J.A.; et al. Degree and site of chromosomal instability define its oncogenic potential. *Nat. Commun.* **2020**, *11*, 1501. [CrossRef]

67. Li, J.; Duran, M.A.; Dhanota, N.; Chatila, W.K.; Bettigole, S.E.; Kwon, J.; Sriram, R.K.; Humphries, M.P.; Salto-Tellez, M.; James, J.A.; et al. Metastasis and immune evasion from extracellular cGAMP hydrolysis. *Cancer Discov.* **2020**, *11*, 1212–1227. [CrossRef]
68. Wu, L.; Cao, J.; Cai, W.L.; Lang, S.M.; Horton, J.R.; Jansen, D.J.; Liu, Z.Z.; Chen, J.F.; Zhang, M.; Mott, B.T.; et al. KDM5 histone demethylases repress immune response via suppression of STING. *PLoS Biol.* **2018**, *16*, e2006134. [CrossRef]
69. Ye, M.; Goudot, C.; Hoyler, T.; Lemoine, B.; Amigorena, S.; Zueva, E. Specific subfamilies of transposable elements contribute to different domains of T lymphocyte enhancers. *Proc. Natl. Acad. Sci. USA* **2020**, *117*, 7905–7916. [CrossRef]
70. Smith, C.C.; Beckermann, K.E.; Bortone, D.S.; De Cubas, A.A.; Bixby, L.M.; Lee, S.J.; Panda, A.; Ganesan, S.; Bhanot, G.; Wallen, E.M.; et al. Endogenous retroviral signatures predict immunotherapy response in clear cell renal cell carcinoma. *J. Clin. Investig.* **2018**, *128*, 4804–4820. [CrossRef]
71. Roulois, D.; Loo Yau, H.; Singhania, R.; Wang, Y.; Danesh, A.; Shen, S.Y.; Han, H.; Liang, G.; Jones, P.A.; Pugh, T.J.; et al. DNA-Demethylating Agents Target Colorectal Cancer Cells by Inducing Viral Mimicry by Endogenous Transcripts. *Cell* **2015**, *162*, 961–973. [CrossRef]
72. Kong, Y.; Rose, C.M.; Cass, A.A.; Williams, A.G.; Darwish, M.; Lianoglou, S.; Haverty, P.M.; Tong, A.J.; Blanchette, C.; Albert, M.L.; et al. Transposable element expression in tumors is associated with immune infiltration and increased antigenicity. *Nat. Commun.* **2019**, *10*, 5228. [CrossRef] [PubMed]
73. Lin, D.Y.; Huang, C.C.; Hsieh, Y.T.; Lin, H.C.; Pao, P.C.; Tsou, J.H.; Lai, C.Y.; Hung, L.Y.; Wang, J.M.; Chang, W.C.; et al. Analysis of the interaction between Zinc finger protein 179 (Znf179) and promyelocytic leukemia zinc finger (Plzf). *J. Biomed. Sci.* **2013**, *20*, 98. [CrossRef] [PubMed]
74. Jackson, C.M.; Choi, J.; Lim, M. Mechanisms of immunotherapy resistance: Lessons from glioblastoma. *Nat. Immunol.* **2019**, *20*, 1100–1109. [CrossRef]
75. Pieniazek, M.; Matkowski, R.; Donizy, P. Macrophages in skin melanoma-the key element in melanomagenesis. *Oncol. Lett.* **2018**, *15*, 5399–5404. [CrossRef]
76. Zaretsky, J.M.; Garcia-Diaz, A.; Shin, D.S.; Escuin-Ordinas, H.; Hugo, W.; Hu-Lieskovan, S.; Torrejon, D.Y.; Abril-Rodriguez, G.; Sandoval, S.; Barthly, L.; et al. Mutations Associated with Acquired Resistance to PD-1 Blockade in Melanoma. *New Engl. J. Med.* **2016**, *375*, 819–829. [CrossRef]
77. Naama, H.A.; Mack, V.E.; Smyth, G.P.; Stapleton, P.P.; Daly, J.M. Macrophage effector mechanisms in melanoma in an experimental study. *Arch. Surg.* **2001**, *136*, 804–809. [CrossRef] [PubMed]
78. Adams, R.; Osborn, G.; Mukhia, B.; Laddach, R.; Willsmore, Z.; Chenoweth, A.; Geh, J.L.C.; MacKenzie Ross, A.D.; Healy, C.; Barber, L.; et al. Influencing tumor-associated macrophages in malignant melanoma with monoclonal antibodies. *Oncoimmunology* **2022**, *11*, 2127284. [CrossRef]
79. Jensen, T.O.; Schmidt, H.; Møller, H.J.; Høyer, M.; Maniecki, M.B.; Sjoegren, P.; Christensen, I.J.; Steiniche, T. Macrophage markers in serum and tumor have prognostic impact in American Joint Committee on Cancer stage I/II melanoma. *J. Clin. Oncol. Off. J. Am. Soc. Clin. Oncol.* **2009**, *27*, 3330–3337. [CrossRef]
80. Deligne, C.; Midwood, K.S. Macrophages and Extracellular Matrix in Breast Cancer: Partners in Crime or Protective Allies? *Front. Oncol.* **2021**, *11*, 620773. [CrossRef]
81. Deligne, C.; Murdamoothoo, D.; Gammage, A.N.; Gschwandtner, M.; Erne, W.; Loustau, T.; Marzeda, A.M.; Carapito, R.; Paul, N.; Velazquez-Quesada, I.; et al. Matrix-Targeting Immunotherapy Controls Tumor Growth and Spread by Switching Macrophage Phenotype. *Cancer Immunol. Res.* **2020**, *8*, 368–382. [CrossRef]
82. Sung, J.; Rajendraprasad, S.S.; Philbrick, K.L.; Bauer, B.A.; Gajic, O.; Shah, A.; Laudanski, K.; Bakken, J.S.; Skalski, J.; Karnatovskaia, L.V. The human gut microbiome in critical illness: Disruptions, consequences, and therapeutic frontiers. *J. Crit. Care* **2024**, *79*, 154436. [CrossRef] [PubMed]
83. Levy, M.; Kolodziejczyk, A.A.; Thaiss, C.A.; Elinav, E. Dysbiosis and the immune system. *Nat. Rev. Immunol.* **2017**, *17*, 219–232. [CrossRef] [PubMed]
84. Li, K.; Ly, K.; Mehta, S.; Braithwaite, A. Importance of crosstalk between the microbiota and the neuroimmune system for tissue homeostasis. *Clin. Transl. Immunol.* **2022**, *11*, e1394. [CrossRef]
85. Lu, Y.Q.; Qiao, H.; Tan, X.R.; Liu, N. Broadening oncological boundaries: The intratumoral microbiota. *Trends Microbiol.* **2024**, *32*, 807–822. [CrossRef]
86. Kim, M.; Vogtmann, E.; Ahlquist, D.A.; Devens, M.E.; Kisiel, J.B.; Taylor, W.R.; White, B.A.; Hale, V.L.; Sung, J.; Chia, N.; et al. Fecal Metabolomic Signatures in Colorectal Adenoma Patients Are Associated with Gut Microbiota and Early Events of Colorectal Cancer Pathogenesis. *mBio* **2020**, *11*, e03186-19. [CrossRef] [PubMed]
87. Peters, B.A.; Wilson, M.; Moran, U.; Pavlick, A.; Izsak, A.; Wechter, T.; Weber, J.S.; Osman, I.; Ahn, J. Relating the gut metagenome and metatranscriptome to immunotherapy responses in melanoma patients. *Genome Med.* **2019**, *11*, 61. [CrossRef]
88. Gao, F.; Yu, B.; Rao, B.; Sun, Y.; Yu, J.; Wang, D.; Cui, G.; Ren, Z. The effect of the intratumoral microbiome on tumor occurrence, progression, prognosis and treatment. *Front. Immunol.* **2022**, *13*, 1051987. [CrossRef]
89. Liu, Z.; Zhang, Q.; Zhang, H.; Yi, Z.; Ma, H.; Wang, X.; Wang, J.; Liu, Y.; Zheng, Y.; Fang, W.; et al. Colorectal cancer microbiome programs DNA methylation of host cells by affecting methyl donor metabolism. *Genome Med.* **2024**, *16*, 77. [CrossRef]
90. Zhou, Y.; Liu, Z.; Chen, T. Gut Microbiota: A Promising Milestone in Enhancing the Efficacy of PD1/PD-L1 Blockade Therapy. *Front. Oncol.* **2022**, *12*, 847350. [CrossRef]

91. Xu, X.; Lv, J.; Guo, F.; Li, J.; Jia, Y.; Jiang, D.; Wang, N.; Zhang, C.; Kong, L.; Liu, Y.; et al. Gut Microbiome Influences the Efficacy of PD-1 Antibody Immunotherapy on MSS-Type Colorectal Cancer via Metabolic Pathway. *Front. Microbiol.* **2020**, *11*, 814. [CrossRef] [PubMed]
92. Yi, M.; Qin, S.; Chu, Q.; Wu, K. The role of gut microbiota in immune checkpoint inhibitor therapy. *Hepatobiliary Surg. Nutr.* **2018**, *7*, 481–483. [CrossRef] [PubMed]
93. Alves Costa Silva, C.; Piccinno, G.; Suissa, D.; Bourgin, M.; Schreibelt, G.; Durand, S.; Birebent, R.; Fidelle, M.; Sow, C.; Aprahamian, F.; et al. Influence of microbiota-associated metabolic reprogramming on clinical outcome in patients with melanoma from the randomized adjuvant dendritic cell-based MIND-DC trial. *Nat. Commun.* **2024**, *15*, 1633. [CrossRef] [PubMed]
94. Luu, M.; Riester, Z.; Baldrich, A.; Reichardt, N.; Yuille, S.; Busetti, A.; Klein, M.; Wempe, A.; Leister, H.; Raifer, H.; et al. Microbial short-chain fatty acids modulate CD8(+) T cell responses and improve adoptive immunotherapy for cancer. *Nat. Commun.* **2021**, *12*, 4077. [CrossRef]
95. Puig-Saus, C.; Sennino, B.; Peng, S.; Wang, C.L.; Pan, Z.; Yuen, B.; Purandare, B.; An, D.; Quach, B.B.; Nguyen, D.; et al. Neoantigen-targeted CD8(+) T cell responses with PD-1 blockade therapy. *Nature* **2023**, *615*, 697–704. [CrossRef]
96. Wang, M.; Rousseau, B.; Qiu, K.; Huang, G.; Zhang, Y.; Su, H.; Le Bihan-Benjamin, C.; Khati, I.; Artz, O.; Foote, M.B.; et al. Killing tumor-associated bacteria with a liposomal antibiotic generates neoantigens that induce anti-tumor immune responses. *Nat. Biotechnol.* **2024**, *42*, 1263–1274. [CrossRef]
97. Boesch, M.; Baty, F.; Rothschild, S.I.; Tamm, M.; Joerger, M.; Früh, M.; Brutsche, M.H. Tumour neoantigen mimicry by microbial species in cancer immunotherapy. *Br. J. Cancer* **2021**, *125*, 313–323. [CrossRef]
98. Gopalakrishnan, V.; Spencer, C.N.; Nezi, L.; Reuben, A.; Andrews, M.C.; Karpinets, T.V.; Prieto, P.A.; Vicente, D.; Hoffman, K.; Wei, S.C.; et al. Gut microbiome modulates response to anti-PD-1 immunotherapy in melanoma patients. *Science* **2018**, *359*, 97–103. [CrossRef]
99. Sivan, A.; Corrales, L.; Hubert, N.; Williams, J.B.; Aquino-Michaels, K.; Earley, Z.M.; Benyamin, F.W.; Lei, Y.M.; Jabri, B.; Alegre, M.L.; et al. Commensal Bifidobacterium promotes antitumor immunity and facilitates anti-PD-L1 efficacy. *Science* **2015**, *350*, 1084–1089. [CrossRef]
100. Bender, M.J.; McPherson, A.C.; Phelps, C.M.; Pandey, S.P.; Laughlin, C.R.; Shapira, J.H.; Medina Sanchez, L.; Rana, M.; Richie, T.G.; Mims, T.S.; et al. Dietary tryptophan metabolite released by intratumoral Lactobacillus reuteri facilitates immune checkpoint inhibitor treatment. *Cell* **2023**, *186*, 1846–1862.e1826. [CrossRef]
101. Zhu, G.; Su, H.; Johnson, C.H.; Khan, S.A.; Kluger, H.; Lu, L. Intratumour microbiome associated with the infiltration of cytotoxic CD8+ T cells and patient survival in cutaneous melanoma. *Eur. J. Cancer* **2021**, *151*, 25–34. [CrossRef] [PubMed]
102. Kim, Y.; Kim, G.; Kim, S.; Cho, B.; Kim, S.Y.; Do, E.J.; Bae, D.J.; Kim, S.; Kweon, M.N.; Song, J.S.; et al. Fecal microbiota transplantation improves anti-PD-1 inhibitor efficacy in unresectable or metastatic solid cancers refractory to anti-PD-1 inhibitor. *Cell Host Microbe* **2024**, *32*, 1380–1393.e1389. [CrossRef] [PubMed]
103. Routy, B.; Le Chatelier, E.; Derosa, L.; Duong, C.P.M.; Alou, M.T.; Daillère, R.; Fluckiger, A.; Messaoudene, M.; Rauber, C.; Roberti, M.P.; et al. Gut microbiome influences efficacy of PD-1-based immunotherapy against epithelial tumors. *Science* **2018**, *359*, 91–97. [CrossRef]
104. Nejman, D.; Livyatan, I.; Fuks, G.; Gavert, N.; Zwang, Y.; Geller, L.T.; Rotter-Maskowitz, A.; Weiser, R.; Mallel, G.; Gigi, E.; et al. The human tumor microbiome is composed of tumor type-specific intracellular bacteria. *Science* **2020**, *368*, 973–980. [CrossRef]
105. Ivleva, E.A.; Grivennikov, S.I. Microbiota-driven mechanisms at different stages of cancer development. *Neoplasia* **2022**, *32*, 100829. [CrossRef] [PubMed]
106. Choi, Y.; Lichterman, J.N.; Coughlin, L.A.; Poulides, N.; Li, W.; Del Valle, P.; Palmer, S.N.; Gan, S.; Kim, J.; Zhan, X.; et al. Immune checkpoint blockade induces gut microbiota translocation that augments extraintestinal antitumor immunity. *Sci. Immunol.* **2023**, *8*, eabo2003. [CrossRef] [PubMed]
107. Morrison, C.; Pabla, S.; Conroy, J.M.; Nesline, M.K.; Glenn, S.T.; Dressman, D.; Papanicolau-Sengos, A.; Burgher, B.; Andreas, J.; Giamo, V.; et al. Predicting response to checkpoint inhibitors in melanoma beyond PD-L1 and mutational burden. *J. Immunother. Cancer* **2018**, *6*, 32. [CrossRef]
108. Wong, P.F.; Wei, W.; Smithy, J.W.; Acs, B.; Toki, M.I.; Blenman, K.R.M.; Zelterman, D.; Kluger, H.M.; Rimm, D.L. Multiplex Quantitative Analysis of Tumor-Infiltrating Lymphocytes and Immunotherapy Outcome in Metastatic Melanoma. *Clin. Cancer Res.* **2019**, *25*, 2442–2449. [CrossRef]
109. Mukherjee, N.; Katsnelson, E.; Brunetti, T.M.; Michel, K.; Couts, K.L.; Lambert, K.A.; Robinson, W.A.; McCarter, M.D.; Norris, D.A.; Tobin, R.P.; et al. MCL1 inhibition targets Myeloid Derived Suppressors Cells, promotes antitumor immunity and enhances the efficacy of immune checkpoint blockade. *Cell Death Dis.* **2024**, *15*, 198. [CrossRef]
110. Shui, I.M.; Liu, X.Q.; Zhao, Q.; Kim, S.T.; Sun, Y.; Yearley, J.H.; Choudhury, T.; Webber, A.L.; Krepler, C.; Cristescu, R.; et al. Baseline and post-treatment biomarkers of resistance to anti-PD-1 therapy in acral and mucosal melanoma: An observational study. *J. Immunother. Cancer* **2022**, *10*, e004879. [CrossRef]
111. Wei, Y.; Gao, L.; Yang, X.; Xiang, X.; Yi, C. Inflammation-Related Genes Serve as Prognostic Biomarkers and Involve in Immunosuppressive Microenvironment to Promote Gastric Cancer Progression. *Front. Med.* **2022**, *9*, 801647. [CrossRef] [PubMed]
112. Xie, F.; Huang, X.; He, C.; Wang, R.; Li, S. An Inflammatory Response-Related Gene Signature Reveals Distinct Survival Outcome and Tumor Microenvironment Characterization in Pancreatic Cancer. *Front. Mol. Biosci.* **2022**, *9*, 876607. [CrossRef] [PubMed]

113. Hodi, F.S.; Wolchok, J.D.; Schadendorf, D.; Larkin, J.; Long, G.V.; Qian, X.; Saci, A.; Young, T.C.; Srinivasan, S.; Chang, H.; et al. TMB and Inflammatory Gene Expression Associated with Clinical Outcomes following Immunotherapy in Advanced Melanoma. *Cancer Immunol. Res.* **2021**, *9*, 1202–1213. [CrossRef] [PubMed]
114. Moeckel, C.; Bakhl, K.; Georgakopoulos-Soares, I.; Zaravinos, A. The Efficacy of Tumor Mutation Burden as a Biomarker of Response to Immune Checkpoint Inhibitors. *Int. J. Mol. Sci.* **2023**, *24*, 6710. [CrossRef] [PubMed]
115. McGrail, D.J.; Pilié, P.G.; Rashid, N.U.; Voorwerk, L.; Slagter, M.; Kok, M.; Jonasch, E.; Khasraw, M.; Heimberger, A.B.; Lim, B.; et al. High tumor mutation burden fails to predict immune checkpoint blockade response across all cancer types. *Ann. Oncol.* **2021**, *32*, 661–672. [CrossRef]
116. Ressler, J.M.; Tomasich, E.; Hatziioannou, T.; Ringl, H.; Heller, G.; Silmbrod, R.; Gottmann, L.; Starzer, A.M.; Zila, N.; Tschandl, P.; et al. DNA Methylation Signatures Correlate with Response to Immune Checkpoint Inhibitors in Metastatic Melanoma. *Target. Oncol.* **2024**, *19*, 263–275. [CrossRef]
117. Limeta, A.; Ji, B.; Levin, M.; Gatto, F.; Nielsen, J. Meta-analysis of the gut microbiota in predicting response to cancer immunotherapy in metastatic melanoma. *JCI Insight* **2020**, *5*, e140940. [CrossRef]
118. McCulloch, J.A.; Davar, D.; Rodrigues, R.R.; Badger, J.H.; Fang, J.R.; Cole, A.M.; Balaji, A.K.; Vetizou, M.; Prescott, S.M.; Fernandes, M.R.; et al. Intestinal microbiota signatures of clinical response and immune-related adverse events in melanoma patients treated with anti-PD-1. *Nat. Med.* **2022**, *28*, 545–556. [CrossRef]
119. Björk, J.R.; Bolte, L.A.; Maltez Thomas, A.; Lee, K.A.; Rossi, N.; Wind, T.T.; Smit, L.M.; Armanini, F.; Asnicar, F.; Blanco-Miguez, A.; et al. Longitudinal gut microbiome changes in immune checkpoint blockade-treated advanced melanoma. *Nat. Med.* **2024**, *30*, 785–796. [CrossRef]
120. Boutros, A.; Croce, E.; Ferrari, M.; Gili, R.; Massaro, G.; Marconcini, R.; Arecco, L.; Tanda, E.T.; Spagnolo, F. The treatment of advanced melanoma: Current approaches and new challenges. *Crit. Rev. Oncol. Hematol.* **2024**, *196*, 104276. [CrossRef]
121. Xue, X.; Li, R.; Chen, Z.; Li, G.; Liu, B.; Guo, S.; Yue, Q.; Yang, S.; Xie, L.; Zhang, Y.; et al. The role of the symbiotic microecosystem in cancer: Gut microbiota, metabolome, and host immunome. *Front. Immunol.* **2023**, *14*, 1235827. [CrossRef] [PubMed]
122. Jiang, S.; Ma, W.; Ma, C.; Zhang, Z.; Zhang, W.; Zhang, J. An emerging strategy: Probiotics enhance the effectiveness of tumor immunotherapy via mediating the gut microbiome. *Gut Microbes* **2024**, *16*, 2341717. [CrossRef] [PubMed]

International Journal of *Molecular Sciences*

MDPI

Review

Genomic and Epigenomic Biomarkers of Immune Checkpoint Immunotherapy Response in Melanoma: Current and Future Perspectives

Sultana Mehbuba Hossain [1,2], Carien Carpenter [1] and Michael R. Eccles [1,2,*]

1 Department of Pathology, Dunedin School of Medicine, University of Otago, Dunedin 9016, New Zealand; mehbuba.hossain@otago.ac.nz (S.M.H.); carca489@student.otago.ac.nz (C.C.)
2 Maurice Wilkins Centre for Molecular Biodiscovery, Level 2, 3A Symonds Street, Auckland 1010, New Zealand
* Correspondence: michael.eccles@otago.ac.nz

Abstract: Immune checkpoint inhibitors (ICIs) demonstrate durable responses, long-term survival benefits, and improved outcomes in cancer patients compared to chemotherapy. However, the majority of cancer patients do not respond to ICIs, and a high proportion of those patients who do respond to ICI therapy develop innate or acquired resistance to ICIs, limiting their clinical utility. The most studied predictive tissue biomarkers for ICI response are PD-L1 immunohistochemical expression, DNA mismatch repair deficiency, and tumour mutation burden, although these are weak predictors of ICI response. The identification of better predictive biomarkers remains an important goal to improve the identification of patients who would benefit from ICIs. Here, we review established and emerging biomarkers of ICI response, focusing on epigenomic and genomic alterations in cancer patients, which have the potential to help guide single-agent ICI immunotherapy or ICI immunotherapy in combination with other ICI immunotherapies or agents. We briefly review the current status of ICI response biomarkers, including investigational biomarkers, and we present insights into several emerging and promising epigenomic biomarker candidates, including current knowledge gaps in the context of ICI immunotherapy response in melanoma patients.

Keywords: melanoma; immunotherapy; PD-L1 expression; mutation burden; neoantigens; DNA methylation; m6A RNA methylation; long non-coding RNAs

1. Introduction

Firstline therapy for cancer patients involving immune checkpoint inhibitors (ICIs) is now the standard of care for several late-stage cancers, such as melanoma, colorectal cancer, head and neck cancers, as well as non-small cell lung cancer (NSCLC) [1–3]. Generally, ICI therapies disrupt cancer immune tolerance through immune regulatory checkpoints and strengthen the anti-tumour immune response [1]. Ipilimumab (an anti-CTLA-4 antibody), Nivolumab and Pembrolizumab (both anti-PD-1 antibodies), and Atezolizumab (an anti-PD-L1 antibody) act by targeting specific immunosuppressive checkpoints [4]. Ipilimumab targets cytotoxic T lymphocyte antigen 4 (CTLA-4) on T cells, while Nivolumab and Pembrolizumab target programmed cell death protein 1 (PD-1) on T cells, and Atezolizumab targets programmed cell death ligand 1 (PD-L1) on tumour cells and tumour-infiltrating immune cells [4]. T cells can be divided into two main groups: CD4+ T cells, which are highly versatile and polyfunctional, and CD8+ cytotoxic T lymphocytes (CTLs). CTLA-4 is an inhibitory protein receptor expressed by both CD4+ and CD8+ T cells that directly competes with CD28 for the ligands CD80 and CD86 and interrupts T-cell priming, leading to immunosuppression [5–8]. The binding of anti-PD1 or anti-PD-L1 antibodies to PD-1 or PD-L1, respectively, prevents the interaction between PD-1 and PD-L1 and results in the prolonged activation of T-cell responses, including potent tumour-specific immune responses [9].

Anti-PD-1 therapy in melanoma promotes the increased presence of tumour-infiltrating lymphocytes (TILs), as well as restoring functionality in exhausted T cells [9]. However, cancer immunotherapy has several limitations, including an inability to predict the efficacy or response to treatment, the development of cancer immunotherapy resistance, inadequate measures to reduce toxicity, and overall high treatment costs [10]. Nevertheless, combining immune checkpoint (e.g., CTLA-4 and PD-1) blockers has a synergistic effect in increasing the patient response by activating anti-tumour immune responses in dual pathways. Clinical data show that 20–40% of melanoma patients respond to these monotherapies, whereas around 60% of patients respond to treatment with a combination of CTLA4 and PD-1 blockers [11]. Anti-CTLA-4 activates Treg cells (Tregs), which suppress dendritic cells (DCs) in lymph nodes, and simultaneous anti-PD-1 treatment inhibits effector T cell (Teff) and natural killer cell (NK) activation in peripheral tissues, inducing regulatory T cell (Treg) differentiation, meanwhile facilitating anti-tumour response rates. The combination of Ipilimumab and Nivolumab therapy has accordingly been approved for the treatment of melanoma and several other cancers, including tumours with microsatellite instability [12].

Diagnostic, prognostic, and predictive biomarkers are essential tools used in the clinical management of melanoma patients. Diagnostic biomarkers such as fluorescence in situ hybridization (FISH), comparative genomic hybridization (CGH), and myPath (Myriad Genetics, Salt Lake City, UT, USA) are used to assist in melanoma diagnosis [13]. Prognostic biomarkers help to estimate whether the tumour is likely to progress or remain indolent in the absence of treatment. Predictive biomarkers help to predict how well a patient will respond to treatment [14].

One important predictive biomarker, known as PD-L1, CD274, or B7–H1, is a transmembrane protein that is frequently expressed on tumour cells. PD-L1 interacts with the PD-1 receptor on T cells, leading to host immune system evasion [7]. However, as a single biomarker, PD-L1 expression is imperfect and has marked limitations in predicting the response to ICI anti-PD1/PD-L1 therapy [15]. The expression of PD-L1 on at least 50% of tumour cells in immunohistochemistry (IHC) on formalin-fixed, paraffin-embedded (FFPE) tissue sections is a mandatory test used in some medical centres for prescribing Pembrolizumab as first-line monotherapy in NSCLC [16].

Additional investigations on PD-L1 expression and its role in tumour biology were reviewed elsewhere [17–20]. As a PD-1 blockade is dependent on T-cell recognition of tumour antigens, it may prove ineffective in cases where T cells lack TCRs corresponding to tumour antigens, where tumours fail to present antigens via their MHC, or where there is a lack of tumour-infiltrating lymphocytes (TILs) [21]. Furthermore, focal PD-L1 expression in IHC may sometimes be overlooked in small biopsy samples such as needle biopsies. PD-L1 expression can vary among different tumour lesions in the same patient over time and depending on the location. Additionally, PD-L1 can be expressed by various cell types within the tumour microenvironment, complicating the scoring and interpretation process [22]; therefore, it has been recommended that PD-L1 expression should not be used to guide the choice of combined (anti-CTLA-4 and anti-PD-1) ICI therapy for patients [23].

To improve the prediction of patient responses to ICI treatment, additional information regarding indicators or markers in patients who respond positively is required. Molecular biomarkers are considered a powerful tool for the prediction of treatment response in patients, because they potentially correlate strongly with pathological changes occurring in cells [23,24]. Identifying effective biomarkers for metastatic melanoma immunotherapy has become a primary challenge and remains a critical priority to optimize personalized medication with ICI therapy for patients who are responsive to treatment, while patients not responsive to ICI treatment could proceed with other therapies to receive significant treatment outcomes, avoiding severe side effects and minimizing treatment costs [11]. A recent study conducted a systematic review on the most recent findings on the development or validation of prognostic biomarkers in malignant melanoma treatments [25]. In the present review, we are focused exclusively on cutaneous melanoma tissue-based biomarker studies related to ICI therapy.

In the following sections we discuss the genomic biomarkers associated with the response to ICI therapy, after which we discuss the growing field of epigenomic biomarkers of response to ICI therapy, including DNA and RNA methylation and non-coding RNAs, and how these could impact patient outcomes associated with ICI therapy (Table 1).

Table 1. Biomarkers for predicting the response to immunotherapy treatment in metastatic melanoma patients.

Biomarkers	Mechanistic Insights	Ref.
Genomic Biomarkers		
PD-L1 expression in IHC	Epithelial cells can be induced to express PD-L1 in response to inflammatory cytokines, such as interferon-gamma, thus protecting these cells at sites of immune activation. PD-L1 may be expressed on tumour cells as well as inflammatory cells. The binding of PD-L1 with PD-1 or CD80 downregulates the response of activated T cells by inhibiting T-cell proliferation, cytokine production, and cytolytic activity, leading to the functional inactivation or exhaustion of T cells. Higher PD-L1 expression is often linked to better responses to ICI therapy. However, a lack of PD-L1 expression does not necessarily exclude the possibility of a response. Thus, the effectiveness of IHC detection of PD-L1, as a predictive biomarker in melanoma, is limited.	[15,16]
TMB	The evaluation of TMB is based on the hypothesis that a high number of mutations in exonic regions will lead to an increase in neoantigen production, which could then be recognized by CD8+ T cells, resulting in improved immune responses. Several variables may affect TMB determination: the depth of sequencing, length of sequencing reads, type of fixative agent, and fixation time, the latter of which influences the degree of formaldehyde-fixed, paraffin-embedded (FFPE), deamination-induced artifacts, all of which impact the analysis of TMB. In addition, a low tumour purity resulting from sampling errors may lead to reduced TMB assay sensitivity.	[26,27]
Neoantigen	Tumour types with a high TMB are theoretically often associated with a high neoantigen load. This is because a high TMB enhances the formation and presentation of immune neoantigens, leading to effective anti-tumour immune responses. It is speculated that tumours with a higher mutation burden possess more tumour-specific neoantigens, which in turn stimulates an increase in TILs due to the overexpression of immune checkpoint modulators such as PD-1 or PD-L1. However, TMB is not equivalent to a neoantigen load. One study found that half of oncogenic mutations did not result in neoantigens, indicating that TMB alone is not a reliable surrogate marker of immunogenic neoantigens.	[28–30]
dMMR and MSI-H	Tumours with mismatch repair deficiency (dMMR), either due to an inherited mutation or sporadic mutation, have a defect in one of the MMR genes (*MLH1*, *PMS2*, *MSH2*, or *MSH6*), resulting in the failure to repair errors in DNA replication. These errors are particularly prevalent in regions of repetitive DNA sequences known as microsatellites, resulting in high levels of microsatellite instability (MSI-H).	[31]
Epigenomic Biomarkers		
DNA methylation	Aberrant DNA methylation can alter the chromatin structure and gene transcription without altering the DNA sequence. Recent work revealed that DNA methylation affects tumourigenesis by regulating the tumour microenvironment.	[32]
Non-coding RNAs	Non-coding RNAs (ncRNAs) are involved in the regulation of the transcriptional activities of single genes, transcriptional programs, as well as the cell cycle, apoptosis, and differentiation. Malfunctions of ncRNAs could be involved in cancer progression, tumour growth, metastasis, and resistance to therapy by controlling the downregulation or upregulation of numerous genes. In general, ncRNAs are frequently altered in cancer tissues and are involved in innate and adaptive immunity in cancer.	[33–35]
RNA methylation	RNA methylation is a biologically reversible process and has been found to occur frequently in the mRNAs responsible for immune regulation. Moreover, RNA methylation influences immunogenicity, innate immune components, and regulates tumour immunity, making it a potential candidate as a predictive biomarker for ICI immunotherapy response.	[36]

2. Genomic Biomarkers of ICI Treatment Response in Melanoma Patients

Genomic characteristics that are associated with an improved ICI response in cancer patients help to distinguish biomarkers for an improved prediction of the response to immunotherapy. In this section, we discuss three widely studied genomic biomarkers associated with ICI response: tumour mutational burden, neoantigen expression, and mismatch repair deficiency/high microsatellite instability.

2.1. Tumour Mutational Burden (TMB)

ICI therapy exhibits a higher efficacy in tumours with enriched clonal genetic abnormalities and a higher mutation burden, which suggests that tumour mutational burden (TMB) acts as a potential biomarker for predicting responses to ICIs [37]. TMB is defined as the total number of somatic mutations per megabase of DNA or of non-synonymous mutations in tumour tissues, including replacement and insertion–deletion mutations [38]. The relevance of this biomarker is based on the hypothesis that an elevated number of exonic mutations in tumours leads to an increase in neoantigen production, which could then be recognized by CD8+ T cells, resulting in improved immune responses [26,27]. This phenomenon is thought to be evident in melanoma, where high levels of UV-induced mutations are thought to lead to an increased level of tumour neoantigens, thereby contributing to a higher immunogenic tumour microenvironment [39].

However, TMB is limited as a predictive biomarker for differentiating a complete or partial response from a progressive disease. The interplay between the T-cell response and neoantigens generated from clonal mutations [40] and the copy number alterations (CNAs) [41,42] significantly influences this limitation. For instance, driver mutations and CNAs can activate or suppress pathways that interact with tumour–immune signalling channels [43] such as the IFN-γ signalling pathway, resulting in acquired resistance to anti-PD1 therapy in metastatic melanoma [44].

Miao et al. (2018) [42] correlated gene-specific mutations and response or resistance to ICI therapy within a cohort of 249 ICI therapy-treated patients with multiple cancer types, revealing an association between *KRAS* and *EGFR* mutation statuses. This study demonstrated that a response to immunotherapy is influenced not only by mutational burden but also by mutational signature and mutational clonality [42]. Furthermore, immune activity against cancer cells depends on various factors, including mutations in the transporter associated with antigen processing (TAP) protein or in β-2-microglobulin, which may affect optimal peptide presentation to HLA class I molecules, thereby reducing the efficacy of ICI therapy despite a high TMB [40].

Additionally, an HLA-I genotype with two alleles with divergent sequences can enable the presentation of an increased diversity of neoantigens, suggesting that the HLA type also influences ICI efficacy [45]. A dominant mutational signature (such as dMMR) could be responsible for enhanced intra-tumoural heterogeneity, as it generates a large proportion of the mutational burden. Thus, the TMB itself might not directly mediate the ICI response, but may serve as a proxy for an underlying biological process that increases tumour immunogenicity and promotes the accumulation of somatic mutations [42].

Although associations between a high TMB and a response to ICIs have been reported in various cancer types, some studies fail to demonstrate a clear correlation between the TMB and ICI response. Therefore, further studies focusing on defining a predictive TMB cutoff, establishing sequencing strategies for comparable TMB detection across different laboratories, and exploring combinations of TMB with other potential markers are necessary to facilitate its routine clinical implementation.

2.2. Neoantigen Expression

The presence of somatic mutations in metastatic melanoma is widely acknowledged. These mutations, particularly if they are nonsynonymous mutations, result in amino acid sequence changes in proteins, leading to the generation of neoantigens. Thus, tumours with higher TMBs carry a larger number of neoantigens that theoretically increase tumour immunogenicity, thereby improving the likelihood of patient response and survival following treatment with ICI therapy [27,46,47].

Neoantigen formation begins when polypeptides are transported into the endoplasmic reticulum (ER) via a TAP complex. These peptides then bind to major histocompatibility complex (MHC) class I molecules with different affinities in the ER, and finally, the peptide-MHC class I complex gets recognized by CD8+ cytotoxic T cells, initiating the host anti-tumour immune response [30]. Various factors such as somatic mutations, alternative splicing, fusion genes, non-coding RNAs, and circular RNAs can produce tumour-specific antigen polypeptides, which, when mutated, become highly immunogenic and are expressed in malignant tumour cells [48,49].

However, the efficacy of treatment for patients with a high mutational load also depends on the subsequent recruitment of T cells into the tumour microenvironment (TME) [50]. While a high TMB increases the likelihood of tumour-specific neoantigen formation [39] and augments the number of TILs [30], it is important to note that the TMB alone (frequency per non-synonymous mutation) is not equivalent to the presence of neoantigens [27], since many oncogenic mutations do not give rise to neoantigens, underscoring the significance of neoantigen prediction as a distinct biomarker [29].

Nevertheless, the relationship between the neoantigen load and clinical outcomes from ICI therapy is not consistent among multiple cancer types. This inconsistency may arise because certain gene expression changes or genomic alterations, such as the upregulation of immune checkpoints [51], loss of HLA haplotypes [52], and somatic mutations in HLA or *JAK1/JAK2* genes, which reduce neoantigen presentation [44] during ICI therapy, can lead to potential changes in the neoantigen load and ultimately contribute to resistance to anti-PD1 therapy [53].

2.3. Mismatch Repair Deficiency (dMMR) and High Microsatellite Instability (MSI-H)

Microsatellite instability (MSI) is a rare event in most solid tumour types, except colorectal and endometrial carcinomas. MSI is characterized by variability in repetitive DNA sequences known as microsatellites and is caused by the inactivation of genes involved in the DNA mismatch repair (MMR) pathway, either through germline or somatic mutations [54]. The MMR system is crucial for maintaining DNA integrity by repairing base mismatches and other DNA errors [55]. Mismatch repair is necessary when nucleotide bases are mis-incorporated, leading to non-complementary base pairs, or when chemically damaged nucleotides are incorporated opposite undamaged ones, causing sequence misalignment.

The MMR system comprises DNA mismatch repair enzymes and four key genes: methylguanine methyltransferase (*MLH1*), postmeiotic segregation increased 2 (*PMS2*), mutS homologue 2 (*MSH2*), and mutS homolog 6 (*MSH6*) [56]. Errors detected by the MMR system may occur through strand slippage or the formation of secondary structures within repetitive sequences during replication, recombination, or repair [57]. Generally, MMR detects and repairs these anomalies and activates damage signalling pathways to initiate cell cycle arrest and apoptosis when the DNA damage is irreparable [58].

Defects in MMR are associated with an increase in mismatch errors and are responsible for MSI [59]. Microsatellite sequences, abundant and heterogeneous throughout the genome, are valuable for gene mapping and allele discrimination analyses due to their distinctive lengths [60]. MSI is associated with sporadic colorectal cancer and can result from the hypermethylation of the promoter region CpG islands in the DNA repair gene, *MLH1*, leading to its epigenetic silencing [60]. Thus, sporadic MMR-deficient tumours may be caused by either somatic mutation or epigenetic silencing of *MLH1* [61,62].

Tumours exhibiting mismatch repair deficiency (dMMR), whether due to an inherited or sporadic mutation, have a defect in one of the MMR genes (*MLH1*, *PMS2*, *MSH2*, or *MSH6*), resulting in the failure to repair errors in DNA replication. These errors are particularly prevalent in regions of repetitive DNA sequences known as microsatellites, resulting in high levels of MSI (MSI-H) [31]. MMR deficiency results in a 10- to 100-fold increase in somatic mutations [63,64], which in turn results in a high TMB and elevated tumour neoantigens [37,65]. This promotes the release of proinflammatory cytokines, eliciting the recruitment and activity of cytotoxic T cells [66,67].

Moreover, tumours with MSI-H/dMMR are associated with higher levels of CD8+ tumour-infiltrating lymphocytes, and they express higher levels of immune checkpoint proteins, including PD-1, PD-L1, CTLA-4, and LAG3, compared to microsatellite stable tumours [31]. MSI-H and dMMR are often used interchangeably due to a high consistency (90–95%) between dMMR and MSI-H in many tumours [68]. In this context, the FDA accelerated the approval of Pembrolizumab in 2017 as a second- or first-line treatment option for patients with unresectable or metastatic dMMR/MSI-H-positive solid tumours, irrespective of the tumour type or site [56]. Nivolumab is also approved for patients with dMMR/MSI-H metastatic colorectal cancer [69]. (see Figure 1).

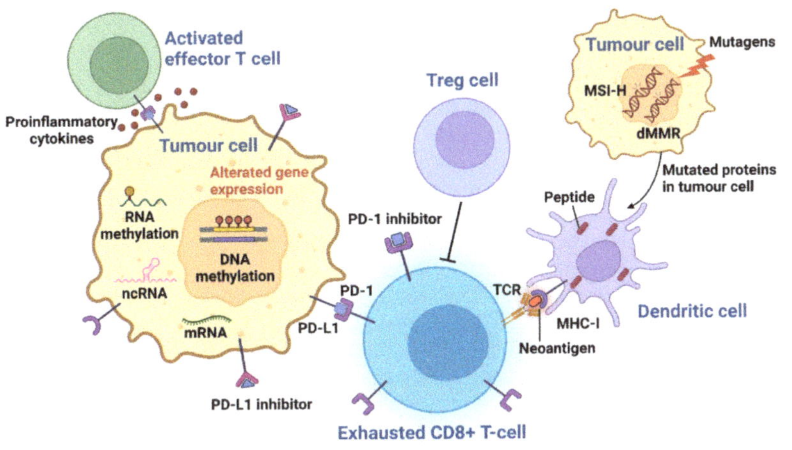

Figure 1. Depiction of epigenomic and genomic features in tumour cells that may impact the response to ICI therapy. As a result of exposure to mutagens, tumour cells generate mutations, including dMMR/MSI-H, which are incorporated into proteins and cause neoantigen production. Dendritic cells capture these neoantigens and activate naïve T cells through the presentation of neoantigens onto the major histocompatibility complex (MHC) and the subsequent binding with T-cell receptors (TCRs). Tumour cells frequently express PD-L1, which inhibits the immune activity by binding to PD-1. Tumour cells may also undergo epigenetic changes, including DNA and RNA methylation, which can influence non-coding RNA (ncRNA) and mRNA expression, leading to innate or acquired resistance to ICI therapy. Regulatory T cells (Tregs) may also inhibit T-cell activity and lead to "exhausted" effector T-cell (Teff) phenotypes. PD-1 inhibitors and PD-L1 inhibitors enhance the anti-tumour immune response by interrupting binding between tumour cell PD-L1 ligands and T-cell PD-1 receptors. This image was generated using BioRender.com (accessed on 1 April 2024).

3. Epigenomic Biomarkers with the Potential to Predict ICI Therapy Response

Emerging evidence suggests that epigenetic regulation plays a central role in tumour immunosurveillance, including tumour antigen production, the interaction between tumour cells and immune cells, and T-cell development, priming, activation, and exhaustion. On the other hand, tumours commonly hijack various epigenetic mechanisms to evade immune detection [70], therefore highlighting the potential for manipulating or modulating epigenetic regulators to normalize impaired immunosurveillance and/or induce anti-tumour immune responses.

Epigenetic modifications often produce stable changes in gene expression without disrupting the DNA sequence, and they can remain preserved after cell division [71]. Epigenetic modifications include DNA or RNA methylation, post-translational modifications of histone proteins, and altered chromatin remodelling, as well as non-coding RNA (ncRNA) or microRNA (miRNA) expression, which can interact at all stages of cancer development and cancer progression [71]. In addition to the comprehensive modifications observed in the tumour cell epigenome, the reconfiguration of the TME and the tumour-driven rewiring of immune cell chromatin landscapes play pivotal roles in modulating the magnitude and efficacy of the anti-tumour immune response. These alterations can substantially impact the potential response of a patient to immunotherapy and ultimately influence the overall disease outcome [72].

The long-term maintenance of transcription factor accessibility to gene regulatory elements is partly regulated by covalent modifications to histones and DNA which, in turn, affects the chromatin structure, resulting in an "epigenetic memory" of gene expression programs in dividing cell populations [73]. A recent study demonstrated that T-cell exhaustion is associated with a general increase in chromatin accessibility, with many accessible regions retained after PD-1 blockade therapy [74]. Additionally, several studies demonstrated that changes in epigenetic programming are coupled to transcriptional reprogramming during CD8+ T-cell effector and memory differentiation [73,75]. However, it remains unclear whether these reprogramming events play a direct role in regulating the effector properties in functional and exhausted CD8+ T cells. Ghoneim et al. (2017) demonstrated that progressive genome-wide de novo DNA methylation programming is critical for establishing T-cell exhaustion. Such DNA-methylation programming reinforces the repression of key genes involved in the effector function, proliferation, metabolic activity, and tissue homing in exhausted T cells. This study also revealed that these long-lived, exhaustion-associated epigenetic programs serve as a major cell-intrinsic barrier limiting the rejuvenation of antigen-specific CD8+ T cells during anti-PD1 therapy, highlighting epigenetic programs among exhausted T cells as a potential mechanism to cause anti-PD1 therapeutic failures [73]. Furthermore, DNA methylation enzymes, such as DNMT1 and DNMT3B, are upregulated in exhausted CD8+ T cells, and DNMT3A-mediated genome-wide de novo methylation can promote terminal exhaustion [73]. However, it is important to note that most studies to date describe biomarkers in bulk tissue preparations, and further investigation is required to elucidate biomarkers at the cellular level.

4. Understanding the Tumour Microenvironment from an Epigenetics Perspective

Carcinogenesis is a multifaceted process driven by genetic and/or epigenetic alterations within specific cells, as well as by the microenvironment in which the cells reside. The TME comprises an extracellular matrix enriched in stromal and immune cells embedded within a network of cytokines and chemokines. It has significance as a reactive platform, composing various aspects of tumour initiation, progression, metastatic spread, altered immune response, therapeutic resistance, and cancer recurrence.

At the cellular level, the process of carcinogenesis involves evading T cell-mediated immune surveillance by creating an immune-suppressive environment. Briefly, dendritic cells (DCs) capture the human leukocyte antigens (HLAs) generated by cancer cells and present them on major histocompatibility complex (MHC, MHCI, and MHCII) molecules to antigen-presenting cells (APCs). This causes the priming and activation of effector T cells (Teffs), while the regulatory T cells (Tregs) can regulate an immune response against tumour cells [76,77]. CD4+ T cells secrete different tumouricidal cytokines, such as interferon-γ (IFNγ) and TNFα to support CTLs in the disruption of primary tumour cells [78]. Epigenetic mechanisms such as DNA methylation are essential for CTL differentiation, with the transition from naïve CTLs to effector cells requiring a shift from the methylated to the demethylated states of biologically relevant gene promoters, enhancing the anti-tumoural effects [79].

Tumour-associated macrophages (TAMs) within the malignant stroma are a critical immune cell subpopulation responsible for cancer-associated inflammation, matrix remodelling, tumour immune escape, growth, invasion, angiogenesis, metastasis, cancer cell stemness, and drug resistance. Macrophage polarization between M1 (pro-inflammatory and tumouricidal) and M2 (anti-inflammatory and protumourigenic) phenotypes is regulated by distinct TMEs [80]. Pro-inflammatory CD16+ macrophages (M1) release T-cell recruiting chemokines, interact with anti-CTLA-4 antibodies, and have been associated with a positive response to combination immune therapy (anti-PD-1 and anti-CTLA-4) [81,82].

Moreover, M1 macrophages, which are PD-L1+ and localized close to cytotoxic T cells, are highly correlated to ICI-responsive patients [83]. Additionally, M1 macrophages are enriched in melanocytic "hot" melanomas, whereas M2 macrophages are enriched in neural crest-like "cold" melanomas [84], where "hot" versus "cold" tumours are characterized by a high infiltration of TILs. Notably, epigenetic regulation also influences macrophage activation and polarization, with DNMT3B knockdown promoting an alternatively activated M2 phenotype and DNMT3B overexpression acting as a negative regulator of M2 macrophage polarization [85]. Ishii et al. [86] reported that chromatin remodelling is mechanistically important in the acquisition of the M2-macrophage phenotype. M2-macrophage marker genes are epigenetically regulated by reciprocal changes in histone H3 lysine-4 (H3K4) and histone H3 lysine-27 (H3K27) methylation; the latter methylation marks are removed by the H3K27 demethylase Jumonji domain-containing 3 (Jmjd3).

Cytokines and chemokines are critical for immune cell communication and TME recruitment, and their promoters are often epigenetically regulated. For instance, the overexpression of HDAC11 inhibits IL-10 expression and induces inflammatory APCs that can prime naïve T cells and restore the responsiveness of tolerant CD4+ T cells; conversely, a lack of HDAC11 causes the impairment of antigen-specific T cell responses [87]. More recently, HDAC11 was described as an essential regulator of IL-10 levels in myeloid cells in MDSC expansion [88]. Chemokines such as CXCL9, CXCL10, and CXCL11, which recruit CD8+ T cells, have been associated with improved responses to ICI therapy and better overall patient survival [82]. Epigenetic regulation of chemokine production can establish an immune-suppressive TME. For instance, trimethylation at H3K27 represses the production of CXCL9 and CXCL10 in ovarian cancer, establishing an immune-suppressive TME [89], while DNMT1 is responsible for the decreased CXCL12 in osteosarcomas, resulting in reduced CTL recruitment at the cancer site [90].

These findings indicate that exploring epigenetic biomarkers to predict responses to immune checkpoint inhibitor therapy potentially holds significant promise in improving patient outcomes.

5. Currently Studied Epigenomic Biomarkers of ICI Response

In the previous paragraphs, we described the crosstalk between epigenetic alterations and the immune system in cancer. Since it is possible that epigenetic predisposition and immune response translate into a favorable tumourigenic environment and outcome, the search for and identification of epigenomic alterations could provide an approach to identify biomarkers of response to ICI treatment strategies. Moreover, epigenetic biomarkers such as DNA methylation are often more stable in fluids and formalin-fixed, paraffin-embedded (FFPE) biospecimens as compared to mRNAs [35].

5.1. DNA Methylation and Epigenomic Signatures

DNA methylation plays an important role in modulating gene activity and gene silencing [91], as well as maintaining genomic stability. DNA methylation also facilitates genomic imprinting, X-chromosome inactivation, chromosome stabilization, and the repression of transposable elements [92–94]. However, cancer cells often exhibit global hypomethylation and promoter-specific hypermethylation of tumour suppressor genes during tumourigenesis, which is associated with gene silencing [95]. For example, the promoter of tumour suppressor gene *CDKN2A*, encoding p16^{INK4a}, has been shown to be hypermethylated in metastatic melanoma, leading to p16 silencing [96]. Furthermore, methylation within the gene itself can induce mutational events [95]. Thus, sites of CpG DNA hypermethylation or hypomethylation in cancer [97] could be potential epigenetic signatures or biomarkers for evaluating the prognosis, diagnosis, or response to treatment in different types of cancer [92].

The comprehensive profiling of DNA methylation can be achieved using either microarrays (e.g., Infinium HumanMethylation450 BeadChip and Illumina MethylationEPIC BeadChip) or next generation sequencing (e.g., WGBS and RRBS). The MethylationEPIC BeadChip is capable of quantitatively analyzing the methylation levels at over

850,000 methylation sites across the genome with single-nucleotide resolution. This high-throughput approach provides comprehensive coverage of the methylome and offers the advantage of not being restricted to fresh tissue samples; it can also be effectively applied to formalin-fixed, paraffin-embedded (FFPE) tissue specimens. This capability is particularly advantageous for retrospective studies or when access to fresh tissue samples is limited.

Filipski et al. (2021) [98] used the Illumina MethylationEPIC BeadChip technology to investigate methylation signatures across the genomes of 61 stage IV melanoma patients who were treated with anti-PD-1-ICI during the course of their disease, along with Illumina 450 K methylation bead chip array data from a further 396 melanoma patients (stages I–IV, skin, soft tissue, central nervous system, peripheral, non-central nervous system organs, and lymph nodes) from The Cancer Genome Atlas (TCGA). This study performed a reference-free latent methylation components (LMC)-based DNA methylation data analysis technique. The authors showed that LMC proportion-based clustering in ICI-treated melanomas could predict durable long-term outcomes from ICI therapy. Moreover, since genome-wide methylation undergoes slower and sustained transformations within a dynamic tumour microenvironment, DNA methylation is thought to denote comparatively more stable signatures. This study also performed the deconvolution of DNA methylation data to identify immune cell methylation patterns that may serve as reliable biomarkers for the prediction of a successful ICI therapy response. However, this study was associated with several limitations, probably the most important of which was that the cutaneous melanoma tissues were collected after the ICI treatment had started, and so the tissues used for analysis had very likely undergone molecular alterations in response to the treatment. These molecular alterations could represent a confounding factor towards the identification of a biomarker for predicting the response to ICI therapy prior to starting treatment.

In another study, Ressler et al. [99] addressed this limitation by performing a similar approach to identify a set of CpG sites using pre-treated samples from metastatic melanoma patients to predict the response to ICI therapy. This study identified specific DNA methylation signatures, which revealed three distinct clusters based on the 500 most differentially methylated genes. These clusters allowed for the identification of responders (cluster 1 and cluster 2) from non-responders (cluster 3), and the findings from this study underscored the potential of DNA methylation profiling as an efficient predictive tool in the context of immunotherapy for metastatic melanoma.

Another group [100] conducted single methylation analysis of the CTLA-4 promoter using samples from 50 patients with metastasized malignant melanoma who were treated with anti-PD-1/CTLA-4 therapy. These authors used a methylation-specific quantitative real-time PCR technique. The findings revealed a significant correlation between low CTLA-4 methylation levels and both the response to therapy and overall survival.

5.2. Non-Coding RNAs

The ENCODE database reveals that the majority (~76%) of the human genome is transcribed, while only 2–3% of the genome consists of protein-coding genes; the remaining transcribed sequences comprise non-coding RNAs (ncRNAs) such as microRNAs (miRNA), small RNAs, PIWI-interacting RNAs, and various classes of long non-coding RNAs (lncRNAs). These ncRNAs are not only involved in the regulation of the transcriptional activities of single genes but also of entire transcriptional programs [33] as well as the cell cycle, apoptosis, and differentiation through acting as signals, scaffolds, molecular decoys, and sponges [34]. Malfunctions of ncRNAs could be involved in cancer progression, tumour growth, metastasis, and resistance to therapy by controlling the downregulation or upregulation of numerous genes [35], and indeed, ncRNAs are frequently altered in cancer tissues and are involved in innate and adaptive immunity in cancer. For example, lncRNAs interact with several immune microenvironment components, such as nuclear factor (NF)-κB, in the case of NF-κB-interacting lncRNA (*NKILA*), in tumour-specific cytotoxic T-lymphocytes (CTLs), or in tumour cells. Another example is a hypoxia-inducible factor 1α-stabilizing lncRNA in tumour-associated macrophages that is responsible for poor prognosis [101,102].

Yu et al. (2020) [103] identified novel lncRNA-based immune classes associated with cancer immunotherapy, and they recommended that immunotherapy would be more beneficial for patients in the active immune group. A cohort of 419 cancer patients from the TCGA (IMvigor210 trial cohort) was used to predict the association between lncRNAs and ICI therapy. Patients were grouped into four different classes such as "immune active", "immune exclusion", "immune dysfunctional", and "immune desert" based on the presence of CTLs and lncRNA signatures. Patients with low lncRNA scores had longer survival compared to patients with high lncRNA scores. The "immune dysfunctional" class showed that dysfunctional lncRNAs were associated with closed interactions and, ultimately, immune escape, while, for example, *NKILA* expression involved an interaction with the NF-κB pathway, promoting an immunosuppressive microenvironment. This study therefore identified the potential of non-coding RNAs (particularly lncRNAs) as biomarkers for immunotherapy.

Chromatin modifications are associated with altered coding or non-coding RNA expression but aside from EZH2 and ARID2, relatively few chromatin modifiers have been investigated as biomarkers of ICI response in melanoma to date [97–99].

5.3. RNA Methylation

The most common post-transcriptional mRNA modification, N6-methyladenosine (m6A), regulates RNA splicing, nuclear export, stability, translation, DNA damage repair, the initiation of miRNA biogenesis, and immunogenicity. These processes affect cellular differentiation, embryonic development, spermatogenesis, sex determination, learning and memory, the immune response, and the occurrence and development of cancer [104]. RNA methylation is a biologically reversible process [36], occurring mostly in the mRNAs responsible for immune regulation. Moreover, RNA methylation influences immunogenicity and innate immune components and regulates tumour immunity, making it a potential candidate as a predictive biomarker for immunotherapy response. For example, by affecting inhibitor proteins in Tregs, m6A-modified mRNAs were found to help maintain the inhibitory function of Tregs [105]; without m6A modification, the Tregs lost their ability to inhibit T-cell proliferation [105].

In melanoma, m6A-marked mRNAs regulate neoantigen-specific immunity through YTH N6-Methyladenosine RNA Binding Protein 1 (YTHDF1) present in DCs. The binding of YTHDF1 to these transcripts increased the translation of lysosomal cathepsins in DCs, and the inhibition of cathepsins markedly enhanced cross-presentation by wild-type DCs. Therefore m6A plays an important role in the efficacy of tumour immunotherapy [39]. The loss of YTHDF1 was shown to increase neoantigen-specific CD8+ T cells and enhance the anti-tumour response of anti-PD1 therapy [106].

The inactivation of m6A regulators is associated with cancer metastasis in the liver, colon, kidney, and pancreas [107]. In addition, hypoxic conditions in breast cancer induce m6A demethylation and stabilize pluripotency factor NANOG, thereby promoting breast cancer stem cell phenotypes [108].

6. Limitations and Future Directions

Several studies have been carried out over the past few years to stratify patients as responders and non-responders to ICI therapy and to facilitate personalized medicine approaches in melanoma patients [98–100]. Understanding the dynamic nature of biomarkers in relation to ICI therapy response patterns could provide novel insights into overcoming resistance and tailoring treatment strategies for melanoma. Dynamic events occurring in the TME underpin the dynamic nature of predictive biomarkers, for which greater understanding is needed.

The TME plays a vital role in driving melanoma cells to switch their phenotype. Within the same melanoma tumour bed, melanoma can coexist in a range of phenotypic states; some cells may be differentiated and reflect the specialized function of the cell of origin [109]. A proportion of tumour cells may be actively cycling and, thus, fuel tumour growth, and a third class of cells may be invasive, some of which may have the potential to seed new metastases. Finally, dormant cells may lie quiescent for many years before their reactivation, when they may initiate a new tumour (i.e., metastatic lesion) or give rise to relapse after an apparently successful therapy [109,110]. Simultaneously, the immune components in the TME can also adapt to extrinsic stimuli, based on oxygen tension, glucose availability, or oxidoreduction pathways [111], leading to reprogramming of the TME [112].

The phenotypic status of melanoma cells in the melanoma tumour bed is influenced by and can influence the TME through interactions that involve both local and systemic effects. For example, local interactions through the regulation of melanin expression [113,114] result in the secretion of melanin into the TME, which can inhibit immune cell function, and lead to formation of cancer-associated fibroblasts, contributing to melanoma progression and aggressiveness [115]. The expression of melanin is characteristic of relatively differentiated melanoma cells, but ultimately, it promotes tumour progression. At a systemic level, TME interactions can occur through the secretion of neuroendocrine hormones from tumour cells [116]. For example, alpha melanocyte stimulating hormone (α-MSH) is a molecule highly expressed by melanoma cells, with autoregulatory effects mediated through its binding to melanocortin type 1 receptor (MC1R) [117]. Ultimately, neuroendocrine factors, as well as other extrinsic environmental factors including ultraviolet radiation [118], can influence the immune system, which may then impact melanoma progression.

To address our limited understanding of the TME, it is important to determine how different melanoma phenotypic states are initiated and maintained, how they influence tumour progression, and whether they exhibit any unique therapeutic vulnerabilities. Multi-faceted lines of enquiry in the future are likely to impact the prediction of ICI immunotherapy response in melanoma patients. More research is needed to better understand the implicit tumour heterogeneity in the TME. With further research, biomarkers present in the TME could significantly correlate with outcomes of melanoma ICI immunotherapy response. Investigating biomarkers in individual cells in the TME could further help in identifying aggressive emerging tumour cell subpopulations [119]. While initially rare, these aggressive melanoma cells could expand significantly. For this sort of approach, methodologies like single-cell sequencing [119], including single-cell DNA methylation sequencing, would be useful.

Ultimately, an integrated approach to evaluate both genomic and epigenomic biomarkers simultaneously, whereby an optimal combination of genomic and epigenomic biomarkers may improve the precision of ICI response prediction, could generate the most useful biomarker panels. However, irrespective of the development of genomic, epigenomic, or integrated genomic/epigenomic panels, the findings derived from biomarker studies should be validated in larger patient cohorts to ensure the development of the most robust biomarker panels that are both sensitive and accurate. Furthermore, mechanistic underpinnings of biomarkers that are eventually chosen to undergo development should be explored to enhance their clinical utility.

7. Conclusions

In summary, the most promising candidate predictive biomarkers for ICI response have not yet been identified. In this review, we outlined the published biomarkers for ICI therapy response, with a focus on genomic and epigenomic markers. This review highlights knowledge gaps in the potential identification of candidate biomarkers, which could be addressed in future research. The key reason for the limitations associated with currently available biomarkers is an absence of a proper understanding of the complex network of interactions of the TME that influence the efficacy of ICI response. The lack of an effective predictive biomarker impacts a significant fraction of patients who experience innate and acquired resistance followed by hyper-progression.

Despite evidence that epigenetic drugs like Decitabine, when used in combination with ICI therapies, lead to improved cancer patient outcomes, and also the potential promise regarding epigenetic regulation (involving both DNA and RNA modifications) for reprogramming events occurring during tumour immune evasion, few studies to date have reported the identification of either chromatin-associated or CpG-site- or m6A mRNA-specific epigenetic biomarkers of ICI response in human melanoma patients [120,121]. In this regard, DNA methylation stands out as a putative mechanism for the maintenance of the exhaustion of immune cells during ICI therapy. Detailed investigations into epigenetic regulators and their association with the clinical outcomes of ICIs in future work could reveal new biomarkers, while additionally, a greater understanding of the mechanisms of action of ICI therapy would also support the identification of new predictive biomarkers.

Author Contributions: Conceptualization, S.M.H. and M.R.E.; writing—original draft preparation, S.M.H., C.C. and M.R.E.; writing—review and editing, S.M.H. and M.R.E. All authors have read and agreed to the published version of the manuscript.

Funding: S.M.H. is supported by a Postdoctoral Fellowship from the New Zealand Institute for Cancer Research Trust. Additionally, the authors received funding support from the Maurice Wilkins Centre for Molecular Biodiscovery and the Dunedin School of Medicine, University of Otago.

Data Availability Statement: No new data were generated in this work.

Acknowledgments: Figure 1 was produced using Biorender software (www.biorender.com; licence granted 9 January 2023).

Conflicts of Interest: The authors declare no conflicts of interest.

References

1. Passarelli, A.; Mannavola, F.; Stucci, L.S.; Tucci, M.; Silvestris, F. Immune system and melanoma biology: A balance between immunosurveillance and immune escape. *Oncotarget* **2017**, *8*, 106132–106142. [CrossRef] [PubMed]
2. Gong, J.; Chehrazi-Raffle, A.; Reddi, S.; Salgia, R. Development of PD-1 and PD-L1 inhibitors as a form of cancer immunotherapy: A comprehensive review of registration trials and future considerations. *J. Immunother. Cancer* **2018**, *6*, 8. [CrossRef] [PubMed]
3. Vaddepally, R.K.; Kharel, P.; Pandey, R.; Garje, R.; Chandra, A.B. Review of Indications of FDA-Approved Immune Checkpoint Inhibitors per NCCN Guidelines with the Level of Evidence. *Cancers* **2020**, *12*, 738. [CrossRef] [PubMed]
4. Grigg, C.; Rizvi, N.A. PD-L1 biomarker testing for non-small cell lung cancer: Truth or fiction? *J. Immunother. Cancer* **2016**, *4*, 48. [CrossRef] [PubMed]
5. Marconcini, R.; Spagnolo, F.; Stucci, L.S.; Ribero, S.; Marra, E.; Rosa, F.; Picasso, V.; Di Guardo, L.; Cimminiello, C.; Cavalieri, S.; et al. Current status and perspectives in immunotherapy for metastatic melanoma. *Oncotarget* **2018**, *9*, 12452–12470. [CrossRef] [PubMed]
6. Sharpe, A.H.; Pauken, K.E. The diverse functions of the PD1 inhibitory pathway. *Nat. Rev. Immunol.* **2018**, *18*, 153–167. [CrossRef] [PubMed]
7. Chatterjee, A.; Rodger, E.J.; Ahn, A.; Stockwell, P.A.; Parry, M.; Motwani, J.; Gallagher, S.J.; Shklovskaya, E.; Tiffen, J.; Eccles, M.R.; et al. Marked Global DNA Hypomethylation Is Associated with Constitutive PD-L1 Expression in Melanoma. *iScience* **2018**, *4*, 312–325. [CrossRef] [PubMed]
8. Hossain, S.M.; Lynch-Sutherland, C.F.; Chatterjee, A.; Macaulay, E.C.; Eccles, M.R. Can Immune Suppression and Epigenome Regulation in Placenta Offer Novel Insights into Cancer Immune Evasion and Immunotherapy Resistance? *Epigenomes* **2021**, *5*, 16. [CrossRef] [PubMed]
9. Koppolu, V.; Rekha Vasigala, V.K. Checkpoint immunotherapy by nivolumab for treatment of metastatic melanoma. *J. Cancer Res. Ther.* **2018**, *14*, 1167–1175. [CrossRef]
10. Ventola, C.L. Cancer Immunotherapy, Part 3: Challenges and Future Trends. *P T* **2017**, *42*, 514–521.
11. Jessurun, C.A.C.; Vos, J.A.M.; Limpens, J.; Luiten, R.M. Biomarkers for Response of Melanoma Patients to Immune Checkpoint Inhibitors: A Systematic Review. *Front. Oncol.* **2017**, *7*, 233. [CrossRef] [PubMed]
12. Rotte, A. Combination of CTLA-4 and PD-1 blockers for treatment of cancer. *J. Exp. Clin. Cancer Res.* **2019**, *38*, 255. [CrossRef] [PubMed]
13. Ankeny, J.S.; Labadie, B.; Luke, J.; Hsueh, E.; Messina, J.; Zager, J.S. Review of diagnostic, prognostic, and predictive biomarkers in melanoma. *Clin. Exp. Metastasis* **2018**, *35*, 487–493. [CrossRef]
14. Maher, N.G.; Vergara, I.A.; Long, G.V.; Scolyer, R.A. Prognostic and predictive biomarkers in melanoma. *Pathology* **2024**, *56*, 259–273. [CrossRef]
15. Paver, E.C.; Cooper, W.A.; Colebatch, A.J.; Ferguson, P.M.; Hill, S.K.; Lum, T.; Shin, J.S.; O'Toole, S.; Anderson, L.; Scolyer, R.A.; et al. Programmed death ligand-1 (PD-L1) as a predictive marker for immunotherapy in solid tumours: A guide to immunohistochemistry implementation and interpretation. *Pathology* **2021**, *53*, 141–156. [CrossRef]

16. Lantuejoul, S.; Sound-Tsao, M.; Cooper, W.A.; Girard, N.; Hirsch, F.R.; Roden, A.C.; Lopez-Rios, F.; Jain, D.; Chou, T.Y.; Motoi, N.; et al. PD-L1 Testing for Lung Cancer in 2019: Perspective From the IASLC Pathology Committee. *J. Thorac. Oncol.* **2020**, *15*, 499–519. [CrossRef]
17. Cha, J.H.; Chan, L.C.; Li, C.W.; Hsu, J.L.; Hung, M.C. Mechanisms Controlling PD-L1 Expression in Cancer. *Mol. Cell* **2019**, *76*, 359–370. [CrossRef]
18. Jiang, Y.; Chen, M.; Nie, H.; Yuan, Y. PD-1 and PD-L1 in cancer immunotherapy: Clinical implications and future considerations. *Hum. Vaccines Immunother.* **2019**, *15*, 1111–1122. [CrossRef] [PubMed]
19. Patel, S.P.; Kurzrock, R. PD-L1 Expression as a Predictive Biomarker in Cancer Immunotherapy. *Mol. Cancer Ther.* **2015**, *14*, 847–856. [CrossRef]
20. Maleki Vareki, S.; Garrigos, C.; Duran, I. Biomarkers of response to PD-1/PD-L1 inhibition. *Crit. Rev. Oncol./Hematol.* **2017**, *116*, 116–124. [CrossRef]
21. Madore, J.; Vilain, R.E.; Menzies, A.M.; Kakavand, H.; Wilmott, J.S.; Hyman, J.; Yearley, J.H.; Kefford, R.F.; Thompson, J.F.; Long, G.V.; et al. PD-L1 expression in melanoma shows marked heterogeneity within and between patients: Implications for anti-PD-1/PD-L1 clinical trials. *Pigment. Cell Melanoma Res.* **2015**, *28*, 245–253. [CrossRef] [PubMed]
22. Topalian, S.L.; Taube, J.M.; Anders, R.A.; Pardoll, D.M. Mechanism-driven biomarkers to guide immune checkpoint blockade in cancer therapy. *Nat. Rev. Cancer* **2016**, *16*, 275–287. [CrossRef] [PubMed]
23. Kamel, H.F.M.; Al-Amodi, H. Exploitation of Gene Expression and Cancer Biomarkers in Paving the Path to Era of Personalized Medicine. *Genom. Proteom. Bioinform.* **2017**, *15*, 220–235. [CrossRef] [PubMed]
24. Goossens, N.; Nakagawa, S.; Sun, X.; Hoshida, Y. Cancer biomarker discovery and validation. *Transl. Cancer Res.* **2015**, *4*, 256–269. [CrossRef] [PubMed]
25. Roccuzzo, G.; Bongiovanni, E.; Tonella, L.; Pala, V.; Marchisio, S.; Ricci, A.; Senetta, R.; Bertero, L.; Ribero, S.; Berrino, E.; et al. Emerging prognostic biomarkers in advanced cutaneous melanoma: A literature update. *Expert. Rev. Mol. Diagn.* **2024**, *24*, 49–66. [CrossRef] [PubMed]
26. Fumet, J.D.; Truntzer, C.; Yarchoan, M.; Ghiringhelli, F. Tumour mutational burden as a biomarker for immunotherapy: Current data and emerging concepts. *Eur. J. Cancer* **2020**, *131*, 40–50. [CrossRef] [PubMed]
27. Rizvi, N.A.; Hellmann, M.D.; Snyder, A.; Kvistborg, P.; Makarov, V.; Havel, J.J.; Lee, W.; Yuan, J.; Wong, P.; Ho, T.S.; et al. Cancer immunology. Mutational landscape determines sensitivity to PD-1 blockade in non-small cell lung cancer. *Science* **2015**, *348*, 124–128. [CrossRef] [PubMed]
28. Maleki Vareki, S. High and low mutational burden tumors versus immunologically hot and cold tumors and response to immune checkpoint inhibitors. *J. Immunother. Cancer* **2018**, *6*, 157. [CrossRef]
29. Gong, L.; He, R.; Xu, Y.; Luo, T.; Jin, K.; Yuan, W.; Zheng, Z.; Liu, L.; Liang, Z.; Li, A.; et al. Neoantigen load as a prognostic and predictive marker for stage II/III non-small cell lung cancer in Chinese patients. *Thorac. Cancer* **2021**, *12*, 2170–2181. [CrossRef]
30. Zou, X.L.; Li, X.B.; Ke, H.; Zhang, G.Y.; Tang, Q.; Yuan, J.; Zhou, C.J.; Zhang, J.L.; Zhang, R.; Chen, W.Y. Prognostic Value of Neoantigen Load in Immune Checkpoint Inhibitor Therapy for Cancer. *Front. Immunol.* **2021**, *12*, 689076. [CrossRef]
31. Maio, M.; Ascierto, P.A.; Manzyuk, L.; Motola-Kuba, D.; Penel, N.; Cassier, P.A.; Bariani, G.M.; De Jesus Acosta, A.; Doi, T.; Longo, F.; et al. Pembrolizumab in microsatellite instability high or mismatch repair deficient cancers: Updated analysis from the phase II KEYNOTE-158 study. *Ann. Oncol.* **2022**, *33*, 929–938. [CrossRef]
32. Xue, G.; Cui, Z.J.; Zhou, X.H.; Zhu, Y.X.; Chen, Y.; Liang, F.J.; Tang, D.N.; Huang, B.Y.; Zhang, H.Y.; Hu, Z.H.; et al. DNA Methylation Biomarkers Predict Objective Responses to PD-1/PD-L1 Inhibition Blockade. *Front. Genet.* **2019**, *10*, 724. [CrossRef] [PubMed]
33. Kugel, J.F.; Goodrich, J.A. Non-coding RNAs: Key regulators of mammalian transcription. *Trends Biochem. Sci.* **2012**, *37*, 144–151. [CrossRef]
34. Yang, X.; Liu, M.; Li, M.; Zhang, S.; Hiju, H.; Sun, J.; Mao, Z.; Zheng, M.; Feng, B. Epigenetic modulations of noncoding RNA: A novel dimension of Cancer biology. *Mol. Cancer* **2020**, *19*, 64. [CrossRef]
35. García-Giménez, J.L.; Ushijima, T.; Tollefsbol, T.O. Chapter 1—Epigenetic Biomarkers: New Findings, Perspectives, and Future Directions in Diagnostics. In *Epigenetic Biomarkers and Diagnostics*; Academic Press: Cambridge, MA, USA, 2016.
36. Chen, X.Y.; Zhang, J.; Zhu, J.S. The role of m(6)A RNA methylation in human cancer. *Mol. Cancer* **2019**, *18*, 103. [CrossRef] [PubMed]
37. Schwitalle, Y.; Kloor, M.; Eiermann, S.; Linnebacher, M.; Kienle, P.; Knaebel, H.P.; Tariverdian, M.; Benner, A.; von Knebel Doeberitz, M. Immune response against frameshift-induced neopeptides in HNPCC patients and healthy HNPCC mutation carriers. *Gastroenterology* **2008**, *134*, 988–997. [CrossRef]
38. Yamashita, H.; Nakayama, K.; Ishikawa, M.; Nakamura, K.; Ishibashi, T.; Sanuki, K.; Ono, R.; Sasamori, H.; Minamoto, T.; Iida, K.; et al. Microsatellite instability is a biomarker for immune checkpoint inhibitors in endometrial cancer. *Oncotarget* **2018**, *9*, 5652–5664. [CrossRef]
39. Yarchoan, M.; Hopkins, A.; Jaffee, E.M. Tumor Mutational Burden and Response Rate to PD-1 Inhibition. *N. Engl. J. Med.* **2017**, *377*, 2500–2501. [CrossRef] [PubMed]
40. McGranahan, N.; Furness, A.J.; Rosenthal, R.; Ramskov, S.; Lyngaa, R.; Saini, S.K.; Jamal-Hanjani, M.; Wilson, G.A.; Birkbak, N.J.; Hiley, C.T.; et al. Clonal neoantigens elicit T cell immunoreactivity and sensitivity to immune checkpoint blockade. *Science* **2016**, *351*, 1463–1469. [CrossRef]

41. Miao, D.; Margolis, C.A.; Gao, W.; Voss, M.H.; Li, W.; Martini, D.J.; Norton, C.; Bosse, D.; Wankowicz, S.M.; Cullen, D.; et al. Genomic correlates of response to immune checkpoint therapies in clear cell renal cell carcinoma. *Science* **2018**, *359*, 801–806. [CrossRef]
42. Miao, D.; Margolis, C.A.; Vokes, N.I.; Liu, D.; Taylor-Weiner, A.; Wankowicz, S.M.; Adeegbe, D.; Keliher, D.; Schilling, B.; Tracy, A.; et al. Genomic correlates of response to immune checkpoint blockade in microsatellite-stable solid tumors. *Nat. Genet.* **2018**, *50*, 1271–1281. [CrossRef] [PubMed]
43. Gao, J.; Shi, L.Z.; Zhao, H.; Chen, J.; Xiong, L.; He, Q.; Chen, T.; Roszik, J.; Bernatchez, C.; Woodman, S.E.; et al. Loss of IFN-gamma Pathway Genes in Tumor Cells as a Mechanism of Resistance to Anti-CTLA-4 Therapy. *Cell* **2016**, *167*, 397–404.e399. [CrossRef] [PubMed]
44. Zaretsky, J.M.; Garcia-Diaz, A.; Shin, D.S.; Escuin-Ordinas, H.; Hugo, W.; Hu-Lieskovan, S.; Torrejon, D.Y.; Abril-Rodriguez, G.; Sandoval, S.; Barthly, L.; et al. Mutations Associated with Acquired Resistance to PD-1 Blockade in Melanoma. *N. Engl. J. Med.* **2016**, *375*, 819–829. [CrossRef] [PubMed]
45. Chowell, D.; Krishna, C.; Pierini, F.; Makarov, V.; Rizvi, N.A.; Kuo, F.; Morris, L.G.T.; Riaz, N.; Lenz, T.L.; Chan, T.A. Evolutionary divergence of HLA class I genotype impacts efficacy of cancer immunotherapy. *Nat. Med.* **2019**, *25*, 1715–1720. [CrossRef] [PubMed]
46. Snyder, A.; Makarov, V.; Merghoub, T.; Yuan, J.; Zaretsky, J.M.; Desrichard, A.; Walsh, L.A.; Postow, M.A.; Wong, P.; Ho, T.S.; et al. Genetic basis for clinical response to CTLA-4 blockade in melanoma. *N. Engl. J. Med.* **2014**, *371*, 2189–2199. [CrossRef] [PubMed]
47. Brown, S.D.; Warren, R.L.; Gibb, E.A.; Martin, S.D.; Spinelli, J.J.; Nelson, B.H.; Holt, R.A. Neo-antigens predicted by tumor genome meta-analysis correlate with increased patient survival. *Genome Res.* **2014**, *24*, 743–750. [CrossRef] [PubMed]
48. Mauriello, A.; Zeuli, R.; Cavalluzzo, B.; Petrizzo, A.; Tornesello, M.L.; Buonaguro, F.M.; Ceccarelli, M.; Tagliamonte, M.; Buonaguro, L. High Somatic Mutation and Neoantigen Burden Do Not Correlate with Decreased Progression-Free Survival in HCC Patients not Undergoing Immunotherapy. *Cancers* **2019**, *11*, 1824. [CrossRef] [PubMed]
49. Karpanen, T.; Olweus, J. The Potential of Donor T-Cell Repertoires in Neoantigen-Targeted Cancer Immunotherapy. *Front. Immunol.* **2017**, *8*, 1718. [CrossRef]
50. Koster, B.D.; de Gruijl, T.D.; van den Eertwegh, A.J. Recent developments and future challenges in immune checkpoint inhibitory cancer treatment. *Curr. Opin. Oncol.* **2015**, *27*, 482–488. [CrossRef]
51. Koyama, S.; Akbay, E.A.; Li, Y.Y.; Herter-Sprie, G.S.; Buczkowski, K.A.; Richards, W.G.; Gandhi, L.; Redig, A.J.; Rodig, S.J.; Asahina, H.; et al. Adaptive resistance to therapeutic PD-1 blockade is associated with upregulation of alternative immune checkpoints. *Nat. Commun.* **2016**, *7*, 10501. [CrossRef]
52. Maeurer, M.J.; Gollin, S.M.; Storkus, W.J.; Swaney, W.; Karbach, J.; Martin, D.; Castelli, C.; Salter, R.; Knuth, A.; Lotze, M.T. Tumor escape from immune recognition: Loss of HLA-A2 melanoma cell surface expression is associated with a complex rearrangement of the short arm of chromosome 6. *Clin. Cancer Res.* **1996**, *2*, 641–652.
53. Gettinger, S.N.; Horn, L.; Gandhi, L.; Spigel, D.R.; Antonia, S.J.; Rizvi, N.A.; Powderly, J.D.; Heist, R.S.; Carvajal, R.D.; Jackman, D.M.; et al. Overall Survival and Long-Term Safety of Nivolumab (Anti-Programmed Death 1 Antibody, BMS-936558, ONO-4538) in Patients With Previously Treated Advanced Non-Small-Cell Lung Cancer. *J. Clin. Oncol.* **2015**, *33*, 2004–2012. [CrossRef]
54. Trabucco, S.E.; Gowen, K.; Maund, S.L.; Sanford, E.; Fabrizio, D.A.; Hall, M.J.; Yakirevich, E.; Gregg, J.P.; Stephens, P.J.; Frampton, G.M.; et al. A Novel Next-Generation Sequencing Approach to Detecting Microsatellite Instability and Pan-Tumor Characterization of 1000 Microsatellite Instability-High Cases in 67,000 Patient Samples. *J. Mol. Diagn.* **2019**, *21*, 1053–1066. [CrossRef]
55. Modrich, P. Mechanisms in eukaryotic mismatch repair. *J. Biol. Chem.* **2006**, *281*, 30305–30309. [CrossRef]
56. Zhao, P.; Li, L.; Jiang, X.; Li, Q. Mismatch repair deficiency/microsatellite instability-high as a predictor for anti-PD-1/PD-L1 immunotherapy efficacy. *J. Hematol. Oncol.* **2019**, *12*, 54. [CrossRef]
57. Iyer, R.R.; Pluciennik, A.; Burdett, V.; Modrich, P.L. DNA mismatch repair: Functions and mechanisms. *Chem. Rev.* **2006**, *106*, 302–323. [CrossRef] [PubMed]
58. Negureanu, L.; Salsbury, F.R., Jr. The molecular origin of the MMR-dependent apoptosis pathway from dynamics analysis of MutSalpha-DNA complexes. *J. Biomol. Struct. Dyn.* **2012**, *30*, 347–361. [CrossRef] [PubMed]
59. Lynch, H.T.; Jascur, T.; Lanspa, S.; Boland, C.R. Making sense of missense in Lynch syndrome: The clinical perspective. *Cancer Prev. Res.* **2010**, *3*, 1371–1374. [CrossRef] [PubMed]
60. Boland, C.R.; Goel, A. Microsatellite instability in colorectal cancer. *Gastroenterology* **2010**, *138*, 2073–2087.e3. [CrossRef]
61. Beggs, A.D.; Domingo, E.; Abulafi, M.; Hodgson, S.V.; Tomlinson, I.P. A study of genomic instability in early preneoplastic colonic lesions. *Oncogene* **2013**, *32*, 5333–5337. [CrossRef]
62. Funkhouser, W.K., Jr.; Lubin, I.M.; Monzon, F.A.; Zehnbauer, B.A.; Evans, J.P.; Ogino, S.; Nowak, J.A. Relevance, pathogenesis, and testing algorithm for mismatch repair-defective colorectal carcinomas: A report of the association for molecular pathology. *J. Mol. Diagn.* **2012**, *14*, 91–103. [CrossRef] [PubMed]
63. Timmermann, B.; Kerick, M.; Roehr, C.; Fischer, A.; Isau, M.; Boerno, S.T.; Wunderlich, A.; Barmeyer, C.; Seemann, P.; Koenig, J.; et al. Somatic mutation profiles of MSI and MSS colorectal cancer identified by whole exome next generation sequencing and bioinformatics analysis. *PLoS ONE* **2010**, *5*, e15661. [CrossRef] [PubMed]
64. Hsieh, P.; Yamane, K. DNA mismatch repair: Molecular mechanism, cancer, and ageing. *Mech. Ageing Dev.* **2008**, *129*, 391–407. [CrossRef] [PubMed]

65. Llosa, N.J.; Cruise, M.; Tam, A.; Wicks, E.C.; Hechenbleikner, E.M.; Taube, J.M.; Blosser, R.L.; Fan, H.; Wang, H.; Luber, B.S.; et al. The vigorous immune microenvironment of microsatellite instable colon cancer is balanced by multiple counter-inhibitory checkpoints. *Cancer Discov.* **2015**, *5*, 43–51. [CrossRef] [PubMed]
66. Saeterdal, I.; Bjørheim, J.; Lislerud, K.; Gjertsen, M.K.; Bukholm, I.K.; Olsen, O.C.; Nesland, J.M.; Eriksen, J.A.; Møller, M.; Lindblom, A.; et al. Frameshift-mutation-derived peptides as tumor-specific antigens in inherited and spontaneous colorectal cancer. *Proc. Natl. Acad. Sci. USA* **2001**, *98*, 13255–13260. [CrossRef] [PubMed]
67. Boissière-Michot, F.; Lazennec, G.; Frugier, H.; Jarlier, M.; Roca, L.; Duffour, J.; Du Paty, E.; Laune, D.; Blanchard, F.; Le Pessot, F.; et al. Characterization of an adaptive immune response in microsatellite-instable colorectal cancer. *Oncoimmunology* **2014**, *3*, e29256. [CrossRef]
68. Cicek, M.S.; Lindor, N.M.; Gallinger, S.; Bapat, B.; Hopper, J.L.; Jenkins, M.A.; Young, J.; Buchanan, D.; Walsh, M.D.; Le Marchand, L.; et al. Quality assessment and correlation of microsatellite instability and immunohistochemical markers among population- and clinic-based colorectal tumors results from the Colon Cancer Family Registry. *J. Mol. Diagn.* **2011**, *13*, 271–281. [CrossRef] [PubMed]
69. Overman, M.J.; McDermott, R.; Leach, J.L.; Lonardi, S.; Lenz, H.J.; Morse, M.A.; Desai, J.; Hill, A.; Axelson, M.; Moss, R.A.; et al. Nivolumab in patients with metastatic DNA mismatch repair-deficient or microsatellite instability-high colorectal cancer (CheckMate 142): An open-label, multicentre, phase 2 study. *Lancet Oncol.* **2017**, *18*, 1182–1191. [CrossRef] [PubMed]
70. Sun, H.; Huang, B.; Cao, J.; Yan, Q.; Yin, M. Editorial: Epigenetic Regulation and Tumor Immunotherapy. *Front. Oncol.* **2022**, *12*, 893157. [CrossRef]
71. Sharma, S.; Kelly, T.K.; Jones, P.A. Epigenetics in cancer. *Carcinogenesis* **2010**, *31*, 27–36. [CrossRef]
72. Villanueva, L.; Álvarez-Errico, D.; Esteller, M. The Contribution of Epigenetics to Cancer Immunotherapy. *Trends Immunol.* **2020**, *41*, 676–691. [CrossRef]
73. Ghoneim, H.E.; Fan, Y.; Moustaki, A.; Abdelsamed, H.A.; Dash, P.; Dogra, P.; Carter, R.; Awad, W.; Neale, G.; Thomas, P.G.; et al. De Novo Epigenetic Programs Inhibit PD-1 Blockade-Mediated T Cell Rejuvenation. *Cell* **2017**, *170*, 142–157.e119. [CrossRef]
74. Pauken, K.E.; Sammons, M.A.; Odorizzi, P.M.; Manne, S.; Godec, J.; Khan, O.; Drake, A.M.; Chen, Z.; Sen, D.R.; Kurachi, M.; et al. Epigenetic stability of exhausted T cells limits durability of reinvigoration by PD-1 blockade. *Science* **2016**, *354*, 1160–1165. [CrossRef]
75. Crompton, J.G.; Narayanan, M.; Cuddapah, S.; Roychoudhuri, R.; Ji, Y.; Yang, W.; Patel, S.J.; Sukumar, M.; Palmer, D.C.; Peng, W.; et al. Lineage relationship of CD8(+) T cell subsets is revealed by progressive changes in the epigenetic landscape. *Cell. Mol. Immunol.* **2016**, *13*, 502–513. [CrossRef]
76. Hackl, H.; Charoentong, P.; Finotello, F.; Trajanoski, Z. Computational genomics tools for dissecting tumour-immune cell interactions. *Nat. Rev. Genet.* **2016**, *17*, 441–458. [CrossRef]
77. Chen, D.S.; Mellman, I. Oncology meets immunology: The cancer-immunity cycle. *Immunity* **2013**, *39*, 1–10. [CrossRef]
78. Tay, R.E.; Richardson, E.K.; Toh, H.C. Revisiting the role of CD4(+) T cells in cancer immunotherapy-new insights into old paradigms. *Cancer Gene Ther.* **2021**, *28*, 5–17. [CrossRef]
79. Scharer, C.D.; Barwick, B.G.; Youngblood, B.A.; Ahmed, R.; Boss, J.M. Global DNA methylation remodeling accompanies CD8 T cell effector function. *J. Immunol.* **2013**, *191*, 3419–3429. [CrossRef]
80. Lewis, C.E.; Pollard, J.W. Distinct role of macrophages in different tumor microenvironments. *Cancer Res.* **2006**, *66*, 605–612. [CrossRef]
81. Lee, H.; Ferguson, A.L.; Quek, C.; Vergara, I.A.; Pires daSilva, I.; Allen, R.; Gide, T.N.; Conway, J.W.; Koufariotis, L.T.; Hayward, N.K.; et al. Intratumoral CD16+ Macrophages Are Associated with Clinical Outcomes of Patients with Metastatic Melanoma Treated with Combination Anti-PD-1 and Anti-CTLA-4 Therapy. *Clin. Cancer Res.* **2023**, *29*, 2513–2524. [CrossRef]
82. House, I.G.; Savas, P.; Lai, J.; Chen, A.X.Y.; Oliver, A.J.; Teo, Z.L.; Todd, K.L.; Henderson, M.A.; Giuffrida, L.; Petley, E.V.; et al. Macrophage-Derived CXCL9 and CXCL10 Are Required for Antitumor Immune Responses Following Immune Checkpoint Blockade. *Clin. Cancer Res.* **2020**, *26*, 487–504. [CrossRef]
83. Antoranz, A.; Van Herck, Y.; Bolognesi, M.M.; Lynch, S.M.; Rahman, A.; Gallagher, W.M.; Boecxstaens, V.; Marine, J.C.; Cattoretti, G.; van den Oord, J.J.; et al. Mapping the Immune Landscape in Metastatic Melanoma Reveals Localized Cell-Cell Interactions That Predict Immunotherapy Response. *Cancer Res.* **2022**, *82*, 3275–3290. [CrossRef]
84. Hossain, S.M.; Gimenez, G.; Stockwell, P.A.; Tsai, P.; Print, C.G.; Rys, J.; Cybulska-Stopa, B.; Ratajska, M.; Harazin-Lechowska, A.; Almomani, S.; et al. Innate immune checkpoint inhibitor resistance is associated with melanoma sub-types exhibiting invasive and de-differentiated gene expression signatures. *Front. Immunol.* **2022**, *13*, 955063. [CrossRef]
85. Yang, X.; Wang, X.; Liu, D.; Yu, L.; Xue, B.; Shi, H. Epigenetic regulation of macrophage polarization by DNA methyltransferase 3b. *Mol. Endocrinol.* **2014**, *28*, 565–574. [CrossRef]
86. Ishii, M.; Wen, H.; Corsa, C.A.; Liu, T.; Coelho, A.L.; Allen, R.M.; Carson, W.F.t.; Cavassani, K.A.; Li, X.; Lukacs, N.W.; et al. Epigenetic regulation of the alternatively activated macrophage phenotype. *Blood* **2009**, *114*, 3244–3254. [CrossRef]
87. Villagra, A.; Cheng, F.; Wang, H.W.; Suarez, I.; Glozak, M.; Maurin, M.; Nguyen, D.; Wright, K.L.; Atadja, P.W.; Bhalla, K.; et al. The histone deacetylase HDAC11 regulates the expression of interleukin 10 and immune tolerance. *Nat. Immunol.* **2009**, *10*, 92–100. [CrossRef]

88. Sahakian, E.; Powers, J.J.; Chen, J.; Deng, S.L.; Cheng, F.; Distler, A.; Woods, D.M.; Rock-Klotz, J.; Sodre, A.L.; Youn, J.I.; et al. Histone deacetylase 11: A novel epigenetic regulator of myeloid derived suppressor cell expansion and function. *Mol. Immunol.* **2015**, *63*, 579–585. [CrossRef]
89. Peng, D.; Kryczek, I.; Nagarsheth, N.; Zhao, L.; Wei, S.; Wang, W.; Sun, Y.; Zhao, E.; Vatan, L.; Szeliga, W.; et al. Epigenetic silencing of TH1-type chemokines shapes tumour immunity and immunotherapy. *Nature* **2015**, *527*, 249–253. [CrossRef]
90. Li, B.; Wang, Z.; Wu, H.; Xue, M.; Lin, P.; Wang, S.; Lin, N.; Huang, X.; Pan, W.; Liu, M.; et al. Epigenetic Regulation of CXCL12 Plays a Critical Role in Mediating Tumor Progression and the Immune Response In Osteosarcoma. *Cancer Res.* **2018**, *78*, 3938–3953. [CrossRef]
91. Papaiz, D.D.; Rius, F.E.; Ayub, A.L.P.; Origassa, C.S.; Gujar, H.; Pessoa, D.O.; Reis, E.M.; Nsengimana, J.; Newton-Bishop, J.; Mason, C.E.; et al. Genes regulated by DNA methylation are involved in distinct phenotypes during melanoma progression and are prognostic factors for patients. *Mol. Oncol.* **2022**, *16*, 1913–1930. [CrossRef]
92. Micevic, G.; Theodosakis, N.; Bosenberg, M. Aberrant DNA methylation in melanoma: Biomarker and therapeutic opportunities. *Clin. Epigenetics* **2017**, *9*, 34. [CrossRef]
93. Huan, T.; Joehanes, R.; Song, C.; Peng, F.; Guo, Y.; Mendelson, M.; Yao, C.; Liu, C.; Ma, J.; Richard, M.; et al. Genome-wide identification of DNA methylation QTLs in whole blood highlights pathways for cardiovascular disease. *Nat. Commun.* **2019**, *10*, 4267. [CrossRef]
94. Schinke, C.; Mo, Y.; Yu, Y.; Amiri, K.; Sosman, J.; Greally, J.; Verma, A. Aberrant DNA methylation in malignant melanoma. *Melanoma Res.* **2010**, *20*, 253–265. [CrossRef]
95. Wajed, S.A.; Laird, P.W.; DeMeester, T.R. DNA methylation: An alternative pathway to cancer. *Ann. Surg.* **2001**, *234*, 10–20. [CrossRef]
96. Zhao, R.; Choi, B.Y.; Lee, M.H.; Bode, A.M.; Dong, Z. Implications of Genetic and Epigenetic Alterations of CDKN2A (p16(INK4a)) in Cancer. *EBioMedicine* **2016**, *8*, 30–39. [CrossRef]
97. Torano, E.G.; Petrus, S.; Fernandez, A.F.; Fraga, M.F. Global DNA hypomethylation in cancer: Review of validated methods and clinical significance. *Clin. Chem. Lab. Med.* **2012**, *50*, 1733–1742. [CrossRef]
98. Filipski, K.; Scherer, M.; Zeiner, K.N.; Bucher, A.; Kleemann, J.; Jurmeister, P.; Hartung, T.I.; Meissner, M.; Plate, K.H.; Fenton, T.R.; et al. DNA methylation-based prediction of response to immune checkpoint inhibition in metastatic melanoma. *J. Immunother. Cancer* **2021**, *9*, e002226. [CrossRef]
99. Ressler, J.M.; Tomasich, E.; Hatziioannou, T.; Ringl, H.; Heller, G.; Silmbrod, R.; Gottmann, L.; Starzer, A.M.; Zila, N.; Tschandl, P.; et al. DNA Methylation Signatures Correlate with Response to Immune Checkpoint Inhibitors in Metastatic Melanoma. *Target. Oncol.* **2024**, *19*, 263–275. [CrossRef]
100. Goltz, D.; Gevensleben, H.; Vogt, T.J.; Dietrich, J.; Golletz, C.; Bootz, F.; Kristiansen, G.; Landsberg, J.; Dietrich, D. CTLA4 methylation predicts response to anti-PD-1 and anti-CTLA-4 immunotherapy in melanoma patients. *JCI Insight* **2018**, *3*, e96793. [CrossRef]
101. Huang, D.; Chen, J.; Yang, L.; Ouyang, Q.; Li, J.; Lao, L.; Zhao, J.; Liu, J.; Lu, Y.; Xing, Y.; et al. NKILA lncRNA promotes tumor immune evasion by sensitizing T cells to activation-induced cell death. *Nat. Immunol.* **2018**, *19*, 1112–1125. [CrossRef]
102. Chen, F.; Chen, J.; Yang, L.; Liu, J.; Zhang, X.; Zhang, Y.; Tu, Q.; Yin, D.; Lin, D.; Wong, P.P.; et al. Extracellular vesicle-packaged HIF-1alpha-stabilizing lncRNA from tumour-associated macrophages regulates aerobic glycolysis of breast cancer cells. *Nat. Cell Biol.* **2019**, *21*, 498–510. [CrossRef]
103. Yu, Y.; Zhang, W.; Li, A.; Chen, Y.; Ou, Q.; He, Z.; Zhang, Y.; Liu, R.; Yao, H.; Song, E. Association of Long Noncoding RNA Biomarkers With Clinical Immune Subtype and Prediction of Immunotherapy Response in Patients With Cancer. *JAMA Netw. Open* **2020**, *3*, e202149. [CrossRef]
104. Zhang, M.; Song, J.; Yuan, W.; Zhang, W.; Sun, Z. Roles of RNA Methylation on Tumor Immunity and Clinical Implications. *Front. Immunol.* **2021**, *12*, 641507. [CrossRef]
105. Tong, J.; Cao, G.; Zhang, T.; Sefik, E.; Amezcua Vesely, M.C.; Broughton, J.P.; Zhu, S.; Li, H.; Li, B.; Chen, L.; et al. m^6A mRNA methylation sustains Treg suppressive functions. *Cell Res.* **2018**, *28*, 253–256. [CrossRef]
106. Han, D.; Liu, J.; Chen, C.; Dong, L.; Liu, Y.; Chang, R.; Huang, X.; Liu, Y.; Wang, J.; Dougherty, U.; et al. Anti-tumour immunity controlled through mRNA m^6A methylation and YTHDF1 in dendritic cells. *Nature* **2019**, *566*, 270–274. [CrossRef]
107. Liang, Y.; Zhang, X.; Ma, C.; Hu, J. m^6A Methylation Regulators Are Predictive Biomarkers for Tumour Metastasis in Prostate Cancer. *Cancers* **2022**, *14*, 4035. [CrossRef]
108. Zhang, C.; Samanta, D.; Lu, H.; Bullen, J.W.; Zhang, H.; Chen, I.; He, X.; Semenza, G.L. Hypoxia induces the breast cancer stem cell phenotype by HIF-dependent and ALKBH5-mediated m^6A-demethylation of NANOG mRNA. *Proc. Natl. Acad. Sci. USA* **2016**, *113*, E2047–E2056. [CrossRef]
109. Giancotti, F.G. Mechanisms governing metastatic dormancy and reactivation. *Cell* **2013**, *155*, 750–764. [CrossRef]
110. Sosa, M.S.; Bragado, P.; Aguirre-Ghiso, J.A. Mechanisms of disseminated cancer cell dormancy: An awakening field. *Nat. Rev. Cancer* **2014**, *14*, 611–622. [CrossRef]
111. Milotti, E.; Fredrich, T.; Chignola, R.; Rieger, H. Oxygen in the Tumor Microenvironment: Mathematical and Numerical Modeling. *Adv. Exp. Med. Biol.* **2020**, *1259*, 53–76. [CrossRef]
112. Reinfeld, B.I.; Madden, M.Z.; Wolf, M.M.; Chytil, A.; Bader, J.E.; Patterson, A.R.; Sugiura, A.; Cohen, A.S.; Ali, A.; Do, B.T.; et al. Cell-programmed nutrient partitioning in the tumour microenvironment. *Nature* **2021**, *593*, 282–288. [CrossRef]

113. Slominski, A.; Zmijewski, M.A.; Pawelek, J. L-tyrosine and L-dihydroxyphenylalanine as hormone-like regulators of melanocyte functions. *Pigment. Cell Melanoma Res.* **2012**, *25*, 14–27. [CrossRef]
114. Slominski, A.; Tobin, D.J.; Shibahara, S.; Wortsman, J. Melanin pigmentation in mammalian skin and its hormonal regulation. *Physiol. Rev.* **2004**, *84*, 1155–1228. [CrossRef]
115. Cabaço, L.C.; Tomás, A.; Pojo, M.; Barralm, D.C. The Dark Side of Melanin Secretion in Cutaneous Melanoma Aggressiveness. *Front. Oncol.* **2022**, *12*, 887366. [CrossRef]
116. Slominski, R.M.; Raman, C.; Chen, J.Y.; Slominski, A.T. How cancer hijacks the body's homeostasis through the neuroendocrine system. *Trends Neurosci.* **2023**, *46*, 263–275. [CrossRef]
117. Dall'Olmo, L.; Papa, N.; Surdo, N.C.; Marigo, I.; Mocellin, S. Alpha-melanocyte stimulating hormone (α-MSH): Biology, clinical relevance and implication in melanoma. *J. Transl. Med.* **2023**, *21*, 562. [CrossRef]
118. Slominski, R.M.; Chen, J.Y.; Raman, C.; Slominski, A.T. Photo-neuro-immuno-endocrinology: How the ultraviolet radiation regulates the body, brain, and immune system. *Proc. Natl. Acad. Sci. USA* **2024**, *121*, e2308374121. [CrossRef]
119. Niebel, D.; Fröhlich, A.; Zarbl, R.; Fietz, S.; de Vos, L.; Vogt, T.J.; Dietrich, J.; Sirokay, J.; Kuster, P.; Saavedra, G.; et al. DNA methylation regulates TIGIT expression within the melanoma microenvironment, is prognostic for overall survival, and predicts progression-free survival in patients treated with anti-PD-1 immunotherapy. *Clin. Epigenetics* **2022**, *14*, 50. [CrossRef]
120. Xu, Y.; Li, P.; Liu, Y.; Xin, D.; Lei, W.; Liang, A.; Han, W.; Qian, W. Epi-immunotherapy for cancers: Rationales of epi-drugs in combination with immunotherapy and advances in clinical trials. *Cancer Commun.* **2022**, *42*, 493–516. [CrossRef]
121. Hogg, S.J.; Beavis, P.A.; Dawson, M.A.; Johnstone, R.W. Targeting the epigenetic regulation of antitumour immunity. *Nat. Rev. Drug Discov.* **2020**, *19*, 776–800. [CrossRef]

International Journal of
Molecular Sciences

MDPI

Review

Genetic Concordance in Primary Cutaneous Melanoma and Matched Metastasis: A Systematic Review and Meta-Analysis

Thamila Kerkour [1], Catherine Zhou [1], Loes Hollestein [1] and Antien Mooyaart [2,*]

[1] Department of Dermatology, Erasmus MC Cancer Institute, 3015 GD Rotterdam, The Netherlands; t.kerkour@erasmusmc.nl (T.K.); c.zhou@erasmusmc.nl (C.Z.); l.hollestein@erasmusmc.nl (L.H.)
[2] Department of Pathology, Erasmus MC Cancer Institute, 3015 GD Rotterdam, The Netherlands
* Correspondence: a.mooyaart@erasmusmc.nl; Tel.: +31-6-3010-2590

Abstract: Studying primary melanoma and its corresponding metastasis has twofold benefits. Firstly, to better understand tumor biology, and secondly, to determine which sample should be examined in assessing drug targets. This study systematically analyzed all the literature on primary melanoma and its matched metastasis. Following PRISMA guidelines, we searched multiple medical databases for relevant publications from January 2000 to December 2022, assessed the quality of the primary-level studies using the QUIPS tool, and summarized the concordance rate of the most reported genes using the random-effects model. Finally, we evaluated the inter-study heterogeneity using the subgroup analysis. Thirty-one studies investigated the concordance of *BRAF* and *NRAS* in 1220 and 629 patients, respectively. The pooled concordance rate was 89.4% [95% CI: 84.5; 93.5] for *BRAF* and 97.8% [95% CI: 95.8; 99.4] for *NRAS*. When high-quality studies were considered, only *BRAF* mutation status consistency increased. Five studies reported the concordance status of c-*KIT* (93%, 44 patients) and *TERT* promoter (64%, 53 patients). Lastly, three studies analyzed the concordance of cancer genes involved in the signaling pathways, apoptosis, and proliferation, such as *CDKN2A* (25%, four patients), *TP53* (44%, nine patients), and *PIK3CA* (20%, five patients). Our study found that the concordance of known drug targets (mainly *BRAF*) during melanoma progression is higher than in previous meta-analyses, likely due to advances in molecular techniques. Furthermore, significant heterogeneity exists in the genes involved in the melanoma genetic makeup; although our results are based on small patient samples, more research is necessary for validation.

Keywords: concordance; primary cutaneous melanoma; metastasis; *BRAF*; *NRAS*; *c-KIT*

1. Introduction

Cutaneous melanoma (CM) is an aggressive tumor arising from the pigment-producing cells (melanocytes) located in the skin. The incidence of melanoma has steadily increased in many susceptible populations over the past five decades [1]. Patients diagnosed with localized disease undergo surgical resection with a favorable prognosis [2]. However, 40% of those patients develop metastatic disease, reducing the 5-year overall survival to less than 30% [3,4]. Unraveling the molecular biology of CM has revolutionized treatment with targeted therapy (BRAF and MEK inhibitors) and immunotherapy (anti-PD1 and anti-CTLA-4 agents) [5–10]. Patients with metastatic tumors undergo molecular testing for the *BRAF* V600 mutation to determine treatment options with BRAF/MEK inhibitors [7,11,12]. With the discovery of additional melanoma driver genes, strong efforts were made to develop targeted therapies for BRAF wild-type tumors [13]. Several researchers investigated potential targeted treatments for *NRAS* Q61 mutant melanomas. Ongoing clinical trials tested the new treatments with MEK and CD147i inhibitors in advanced melanoma after immunotherapy failure [14,15]. Moreover, further inhibitors are also available for melanoma harboring an amplified *c-KIT* gene [16,17]. The mutations in *BRAF* V600, *NRAS* Q61, and *c-KIT* occur early in melanoma development [18,19]. Consequently, if a patient develops a metastasis, the absence of these alterations in the primary tumor may be sufficient to exclude the patient from the targeted therapies. Otherwise, an invasive biopsy of the metastatic deposit needs to be performed. However, a meta-analysis conducted in 2017 showed an overall discrepancy rate of 13.4% of the *BRAF* status between the primary melanoma and the matched metastasis [20]. Hence, it is advised to determine the *BRAF* status in the metastasis deposit [21].

With advances in sequencing techniques for mutation detection, additional studies addressed the concordance of the mutation status of primary CM and matched metastasis in multiple cancer genes. However, the sensitivity of these methods for mutation detection has not yet been compared to older techniques. Therefore, collecting up-to-date information on the concordance status of *BRAF* and additional driver genes, along with assessing the quality of the new studies, may help to redirect the diagnosis and therapeutic decisions for CM patients. Additionally, understanding how CM tumors evolve and differ between primary and metastatic sites is important. Thus, in this study, we aimed to systematically review all the literature and undertake the meta-analysis where appropriate in order to determine the mutation concordance rate between primary CM and its matched metastatic sites.

2. Methods

We conducted this systematic review and meta-analysis in accordance with the Preferred Reporting Items for Systematic Review and Meta-Analysis (PRISMA) guidelines. The preregistered protocol is available at PROSPERO under the protocol number CRD42022327641, accessed on 15 May 2022 and available from: https://www.crd.york.ac.uk/prospero/display_record.php?ID=CRD42022327641.

2.1. Search Strategy and Eligibility Criteria

A comprehensive search strategy was employed to ensure the inclusion of relevant studies. We performed an initial search in Embase to detect the relevant keywords in the titles and the abstracts. The primary search terms used in Embase were "genetic features", "primary cutaneous melanoma" and "metastatic melanoma". The obtained synonymous terms from Embase were then added to enhance the search strategy. Articles published from 2000 to December 2022 were searched in the following databases: Medline, Embase, Web of Science, and the Cochrane Central Register of Controlled Trials. The search strategies are available in Supplementary Material Table S1. Two independent reviewers (C.Z. and T.K.) evaluated the titles and abstracts of the identified studies in separate EndNote libraries. Discrepancies were discussed with a third reviewer (A.M.). Inclusion criteria consisted of studies that compared the genetic patterns between primary CM and the matched metastasis within the same patient. Studies that only included uveal and mucosal melanoma were excluded, as well as conference abstracts and case studies.

2.2. Data Extraction and Quality Assessment

Full-text screening of all the relevant articles was conducted by two reviewers (C.Z. and T.K.). Data extraction was independently performed by the two reviewers (C.Z. and T.K.) using a customized data extraction Excel sheet. The following information was extracted from each study: The first author's name and their affiliated country, the year of the publication, the technique used to determine the mutation status, the analyzed genes, the total number of patients, and the number of patients with concordant status for each gene. To assess the quality of each included study, one reviewer (T.K.) used the Quality in Prognosis Studies (QUIPS) tool [22] and discussed the outcomes with a second reviewer (A.M.) to ensure consensus. This tool consists of six domains: Study participation, study attrition, prognosis actor measurement, study confounding, statistical analysis, and reporting. For each domain, the score was assigned: High risk of bias = 0, moderate risk of bias = 0.5, and low risk of bias = 1. Studies with a total score of $\geq$4 were considered high quality, whereas studies with a total score of <4 were considered low quality.

2.3. Outcome of Interest

The outcome of interest in the meta-analysis is defined as the concordance rate of the mutation status between the primary cutaneous melanoma and their paired distant metastasis in each single gene. For this study, we considered meta-analysis only for the genes that were reported in more than ten studies. Therefore, we conducted the meta-analysis for *BRAF* V600 and *NRAS* Q61 mutations. We reported the available data regarding additional genes in a systematic manner.

2.4. Pathway Analysis

To determine if the mutations are associated with pathways that may be involved in the metastasis progression, we used the web-free server g:profiler [23] to identify the possible pathways associated with the mutated genes that we mutated in both primary and metastasis. We selected the top three pathways with the highest *p*-value. g:profiler output list details are presented in Supplementary Material Figure S1.

2.5. Statistical Analysis

Differences in the concordance of *BRAF* status between male and female patients were assessed using a Student's *t*-test. Random-effects meta-analysis models were used to pool the concordance rate and the confidence interval (CI) across all the studies for each gene (*BRAF* and *NRAS*) because combining all the genes may be biased. Freeman–Tukey double arcsine transformation was applied to weigh the individual studies [24]. To assess the heterogeneity across the studies, we performed a chi-square test to estimate the I^2 statistic (0–100%, 0% indicated no heterogeneity).

To explain potential sources of heterogeneity, pre-specified potential effect modifiers, such as the technique of detecting the mutation (molecular vs. immunohistochemistry) and the study quality (QUIPS total score), were considered. Subgroup analyses were used to calculate the concordance rates for each group. Small study effects and publication bias were assessed using funnel plots and Egger's test (Supplementary Material Figure S2). The analyses were performed using the meta [25] and the metaphor packages [26]. All the analyses were done in R version 4.2.13.

3. Results

3.1. Search Results and Studies Characteristics

The PRISMA flowchart of the selection process is presented in Figure 1. A total of 2466 studies (after excluding duplicates) were identified from the selected databases. Screening and evaluation of eligibility criteria resulted in 40 studies being considered for qualitative assessment, with 31 included in the quantitative assessment. The majority of studies included in the meta-analysis (25) focused mainly on *BRAF* concordance status. For the studies that included mucosal or uveal melanomas, we only extrapolated the mutation data of patients with CM.

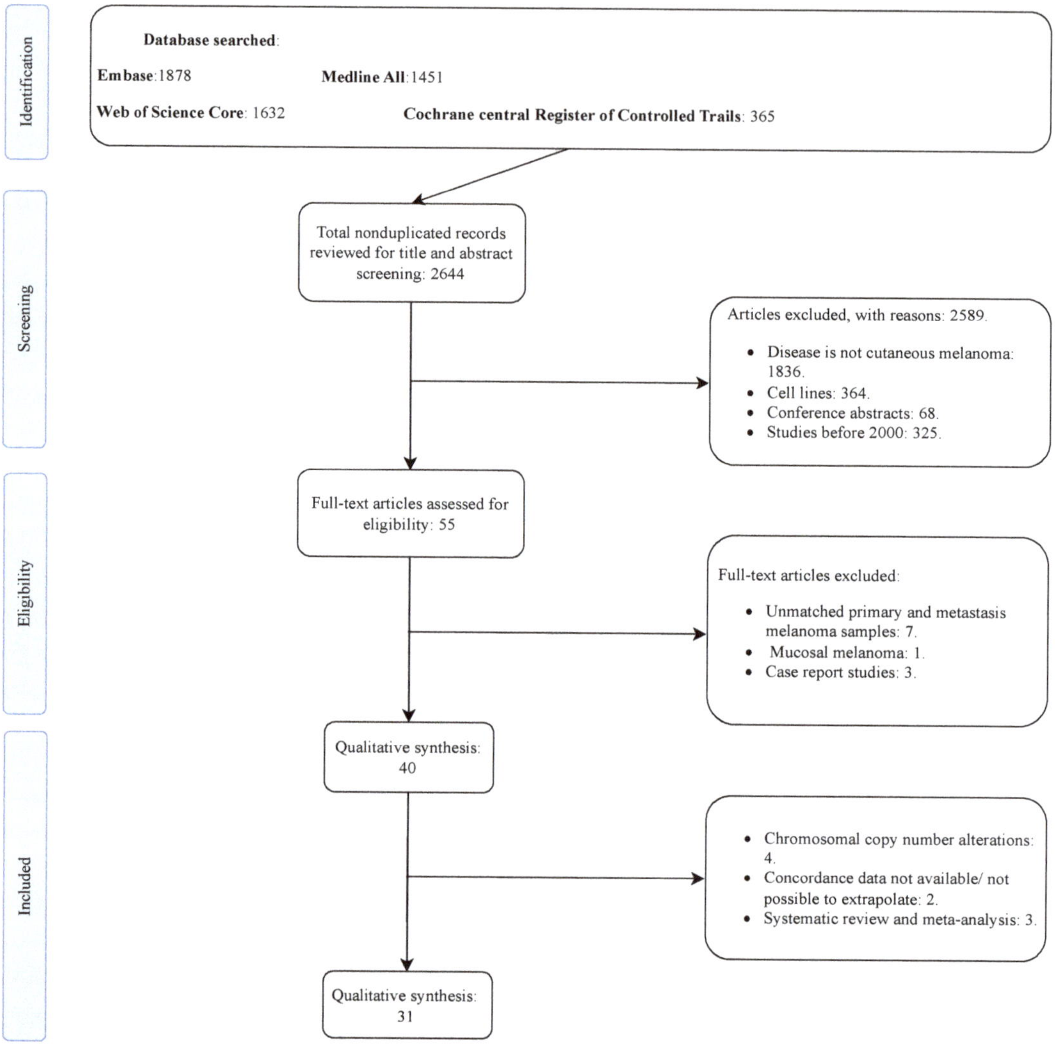

Figure 1. PRISMA flow diagram of the literature search.

3.2. The Genetic Concordance between Primary Cutaneous Melanoma and Matched Distant Metastasis

The concordance in patients with cutaneous melanoma was reported mainly in the melanoma driver genes. Twenty-five studies [27–51] compared the mutation status of *BRAF* with the median concordance rate of 88% (range 56–100, total patients = 1220) (Table 1). *BRAF* was mainly reported as either muted in position V600 or wild type. *NRAS* status was the second most highly reported gene in 14 studies [28,30,32,38,43,45,48–55] (Table 2), with a median concordance of 97% (range 85–100, total patients = 629), and the mutation site was mainly focused on the protein position Q61. *c-KIT* concordance was reported in 3 studies [32,38,49] with a median concordance rate of 100% (range 88–100, total patients = 44) (Table 3). Finally, the concordance of the *TERT* promoter was reported in two studies [45,50], and the media concordance was 64% (range 55–68, total patients = 53) (Table 4).

Table 1. Characteristics of the studies included in the meta-analysis for *BRAF* concordance rate.

Study	Country	Technique	Total Cohort (*n*)	Patients with Concordant Status (*n*)	Risk of Bias Score (Study Quality)
Omholt et al., 2003 [27]	Sweden	PCR	50	48	5 (high)
Yancovitz et al., 2012 [29]	USA	MS-PCR	18	10	4 (high)
Colombino et al., 2012 [28]	Italy	ADS	99	87	2.5 (low)
Heinzerling et al., 2013 [31]	Germany	PCR	11	7	1 (low)
Zebary et al., 2013 [32]	Sweden	PCR	16	16	4 (high)
Colombino et al., 2013 [30]	Italy	ADS	236	208	3 (low)
Saroufim et al., 2014 [33]	Lebanon	PCR	27	20	4.5 (high)
Nardin et al., 2015 [36]	France	Pyrosequencing	25	23	6 (high)
Satzger et al., 2015 [39]	Germany	Ultra-deep NGS	75	71	6 (high)
Riveiro-Falkenbach et al., 2015 [37]	Spain	Cobas + IHC	140	117	5 (high)
Bradish et al., 2015 [34]	USA	PCR	25	21	5 (high)
Eriksson et al., 2015 [35]	Sweden	IHC	63	59	4 (high)
Sakaizwa et al., 2015 [38]	Japan	DS	25	22	3 (low)
Yaman et al., 2016 [40]	Turkey	Pyrosequencing + IHC	47	40	5 (high)
Bruno et al., 2017 [41]	Italy	PNA, IHC, capillary seq	14	9	2 (low)
Hannan et al.,2017 [42]	Ireland	PCR and IHC	42	36	5.5 (high)
Kaji et al., 2017 [43]	Japan	MassARRAY	17	9	3.5 (low)
Yang et al., 2018 [45]	USA	IHC and direct + Sanger sequencing	43	42	6 (high)
Cormican et al., 2018 [46]	Ireland	PCR and IHC	53	53	5.5 (high)
Nielsen et al., 2018 [44]	Denmark	Cobas test and IHC	80	79	5.5 (high)
Manca et al., 2019 [48]	Italy	Targeted NGS	41	39	5.5 (high)
Ito et al., 2019 [47]	Japan	IHC	31	28	4 (high)
Mejbel et al., 2019 [49]	USA	NGS	3	3	2.5 (high)
Pellergrini et al., 2020 [51]	Italy	PCR and IHC	30	26	5.5 (high)
Chang et al., 2020 [50]	USA	SNaPshot assays, Sanger sequencing, MS PCR	12	10	4 (high)

ADS: automated direct sequencing, DS: direct sequencing, IHC: immunohistochemistry, MS-PCR: methylation specific PCR, NGS: next-generation sequencing.

Three studies [43,48,49] compared the mutational status between primary melanoma and their matched metastasis tumors in multiple cancer genes. Details of each gene are described in Table 4. Most of the reported mutated genes were reported in both the primary and metastasis tissues, except *KRAS* G12A and *NEK E379K* mutations that were found in primary tumors and *CCND1* G103R in the metastasis tumor. To understand the role of these mutations, we looked at their possible association with pathways known in cancer progression. Most of the genes are involved in proliferation, cell cycle, and cellular senescence. The details of the pathways analysis are reported in Supplementary Material Figure S1.

Table 2. Characteristics of the studies included in the meta-analysis for *NRAS* concordance rate.

Study	Country	Technique	Total Cohort (*n*)	Patients with Concordant Status (*n*)	Risk of Bias Score
Demunter et al., 2001 [52]	Belgium	DOP-PCR	9	9	1
Omholtet al., 2002 [53]	Sweden	PCR and SSCP	54	53	5
Akslenet al., 2005 [54]	Germany	SSCP	15	15	3
Colombino et al., 2012 [28]	Italy	ADS	99	94	2.5
Colombino et al., 2013 [30]	Italy	ADS	233	226	3
Zebary et al., 2013 [32]	Sweden	PCR	16	16	4
Uhara et al., 2014 [55]	Japan	PCR	35	34	2.5
Sakaizawa et al., 2015 [38]	Japan	DS	25	24	3
Kaji et al., 2017 [43]	Japan	Sequenom MelaCarta MassARRAY	17	17	3.5
Yang et al., 2018 [45]	USA	Direct and Sanger sequencing + IHC	43	42	6
Manca et al., 2019 [48]	Italy	Targeted NGS	41	35	5.5
Mejbel et al., 2019 [49]	USA	NGS	3	3	2.5
Pellergrini et al., 2020 [51]	Italy	PCR and IHC	30	26	5.5
Chang et al., 2020 [50]	USA	SNaPshot assays, Sanger sequencing, MS PCR	12	12	4

ADS: automated direct sequencing, DS: direct sequencing, IHC: immunohistochemistry, DOP-PCR: degenerate oligonucleotide-primed polymerase chain reaction, MS PCR: methylation-specific polymerase chain reaction, SSCP: single-strand conformational polymorphism.

Table 3. Characteristics of the studies reporting the *c-KIT* status.

Study Name	Country	Technique	Population Cohort (*n*)	Patients with Concordant Status (*n*)	Risk of Bias Score
Zebary et al., 2013 [32]	Sweden	Sequencing	16	16	4
Sakaizawa et al., 2015 [38]	Japan	DS	25	22	3
Mejbel et al., 2019 [49]	USA	PCR	3	3	2.5

DS: direct sequencing, PCR: polymerase chain reaction.

Table 4. Reported additional genes for the concordance between the primary melanoma and matched metastasis.

Study	Total Patient	Gene	Mutation	N Mutated Primary	N Mutated Metastasis	N Mutated Samples	N Concordant Patients
Chang et al., 2020 [50]	11	*TERT*	promoter (146 C > T)	4	11 *	15	6
Yang et al., 2018 [45]	41	*TERT*	promoter	N/A	N/A	N/A	28
Kaji et al., 2017 [43]	17	*CDK4*	R24C	1	2	3	0
	17	*KRAS*	G12A	1	0	1	0
	17	*NEK10*	E379K	1	0	1	0
	17	*EPHB6*	G404S	2	1	3	1

Table 4. *Cont.*

Study	Total Patient	Gene	Mutation	N Mutated Primary	N Mutated Metastasis	N Mutated Samples	N Concordant Patients
Manca et al., 2019 [48]	41	*TP53*	V216M	0	2	2	0
	41	*TP53*	R158C	0	1	1	0
	41	*MAP2K1*	Q46Tter	0	1	1	0
	41	*MAP2K1*	Q110Ter	0	1	1	0
	41	*PTEN*	G127	0	1	1	0
	41	*PTEN*	Q110ter	0	1	1	0
	41	*CCND1*	G103R	0	1	1	0
	41	*CDKN2A*	G23S	1	0	1	0
	41	*CDKN2A*	R131H	1	0	1	0
	41	*PIK3CA*	T1031I	1	0	1	0
	41	*PIK3CA*	G1049S	1	0	1	0
	41	*TP53*	E286K	1	2	3	0
	41	*TP53*	R196L	1	0	1	0
	41	*MAP2K1*	Q383ter	1	0	1	0
	41	*MAP2K1*	Q243Ter	1	0	1	0
	41	*MAP2K1*	Q354ter	1	1	2	0
	41	*RB1*	Q354ter	1	1	2	0
	41	*PTEN*	G165R	1	0	1	0
	41	*CDKN2A*	A40V	1	1	2	1
	41	*PIK3CA*	V344M	1	1	2	1
	41	*TP53*	R196Ter	1	1	2	1
	41	*TP53*	P278L	1	1	2	1
	41	*TP53*	P278S	1	1	2	1
	41	*PIK3CA*	V344A	2	0	2	0
Mejbel et al., 2019 [49]	3	*RAC1*	P29S	0	1	1	0
	3	*CTNNB1*	S37F	1	0	1	0
	3	*HNFA1*	A269T	1	0	1	0
	3	*TP53*	H179Y	1	1 *	2	1

* (patients with multiple metastases).

3.3. The Genetic Concordance between Primary Cutaneous Melanoma and Matched Distant Metastasis According to Metastatic Site and Gender

To determine the impact of the metastatic site and gender on the concordance rate between primary melanoma and metastatic deposit, we extracted data on the tissue type of the metastasis (Table 5) and patient gender (Table 6) from each study. However, due to the unavailability of data for *NRAS* and *KIT*, we could only report the data for *BRAF*.

The lymph node (excluding sentinel lymph node) was the most commonly reported metastatic site, with eight studies encompassing 262 patients. The skin was the second most frequently reported site, with six studies comprising 84 patients. Other metastatic sites, including visceral, brain, and subcutaneous locations, were reported in limited studies, with 50, 29, and 18 patients, respectively. The concordance rates for *BRAF* according to gender were reported in 5 studies. Although males represented a slightly larger proportion, no statistically significant difference in the concordance rate between females and males was observed (p-value = 0.19).

Table 5. Concordance studies by metastatic site.

Study	Lymph Node Metastasis	Brain Metastasis	Visceral Metastasis	Subcutaneous Metastasis	Skin Metastasis/ Other Type
	Concordance Rate % (Concordant Cases/Total Cases)				
Heinzerling et al., 2013 [31]	-	-	-	-	100 (7/7)
Zebary et al., 2013 [32]	100 (15/15)	-	-	-	100 (1/1)
Colombino et al., 2013 [30]	90 (109/120)	92 (22/24)	93 (37/40)	-	77 (40/52)
Saroufim et al., 2014 [33]	89 (16/18)	-	-	67 (4/6)	50 (2/4)
Nardin et al., 2015 [36]	100 (14/14)	-	80 (4/5)	92 (11/12)	
Bradish et al., 2015 [34]	-	50 (2/4)	-	-	92 (11/12)
Yaman et al., 2016 [40]	83 (34/41)	-	-	-	-
Kaji et al., 2017 [43]	53 (9/17)	-	-	-	-
Manca et al., 2019 [48]	94 (17/18)	-	100 (3/3)	-	-
Pellergrini et al., 2020 [51]	89 (17/19)	100 (1/1)	50 (1/2)	-	88 (7/8)
Total samples in all studies	262	29	50	18	84

Table 6. *BRAF* concordance rate by gender in the reported studies.

Study	Risk of Bias Score	Total Cohort (n)	Total Females (n)	Total Males (n)	Concordant Female Patients (n)	Concordant Male Patients (n)
Heinzerling et al., 2013 [31]	1	11	7	5	4	4
Saroufim et al., 2014 [33]	4.5	27	7	19	5	15
Bradish et al., 2015 [34]	5	25	13	11	11	9
Yaman et al., 2016 [40]	5	47	18	29	14	26
Kaji et al., 2017 [43]	3.5	17	9	8	3	5
Total		127	54	72	37	59
Concordance rate % (p-value = 0.19)					68.5	81.9

3.4. Meta-Analysis of the Concordance Rate for BRAF and NRAS

We assessed the concordance rate for *BRAF* in 1220 patients and for *NRAS* in 629 patients (Figures 2 and 3). We calculated the concordance rate separately for wild-type versus mutated status for each gene. Because we focused on cutaneous melanoma in this study, we excluded uveal and mucosal melanoma patients in five studies [23,25,28,35,38].

The pooled random effects concordance rate for *BRAF* was 89.4% [95% CI: 84.5; 93.5] and 97.8% [95% CI: 95.8; 99.4] for *NRAS*. The heterogeneity between studies was high for the *BRAF* concordance rate (I^2 = 74%, $p < 0.01$). However, for *NRAS*, the risk of bias was low (I^2 = 7%, p = 0.38).

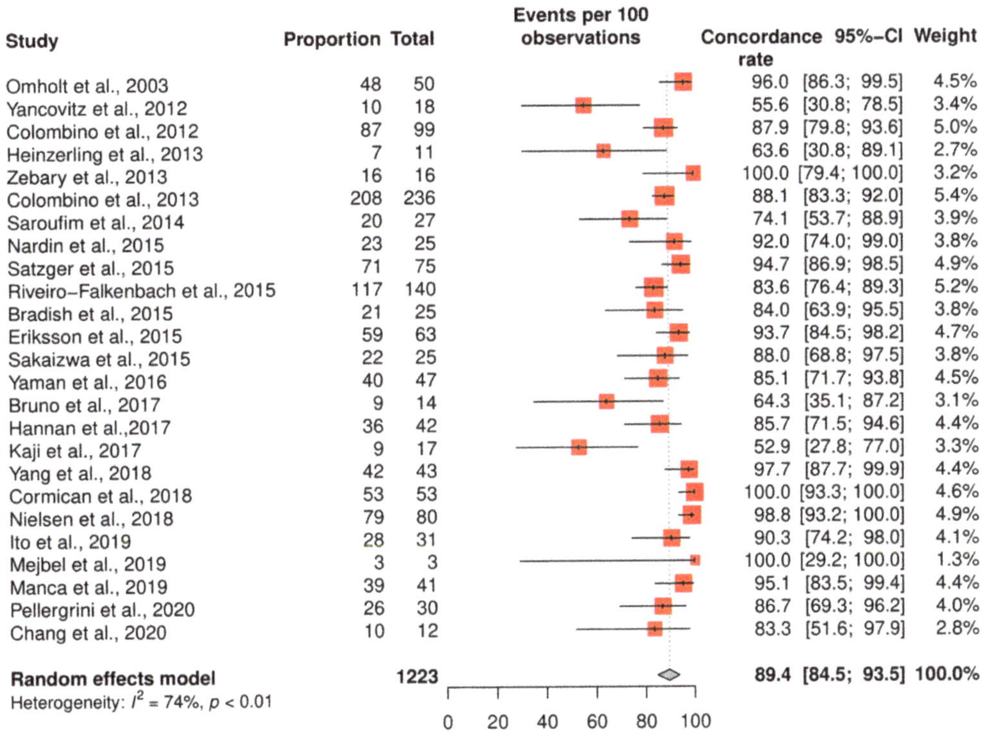

Figure 2. Results of the *BRAF* meta-analysis. Twenty-five studies were included to pool the concordance rate of *BRAF* status [27–51], red square: point estimate of each study, and grey diamond: summary estimate of the total studies.

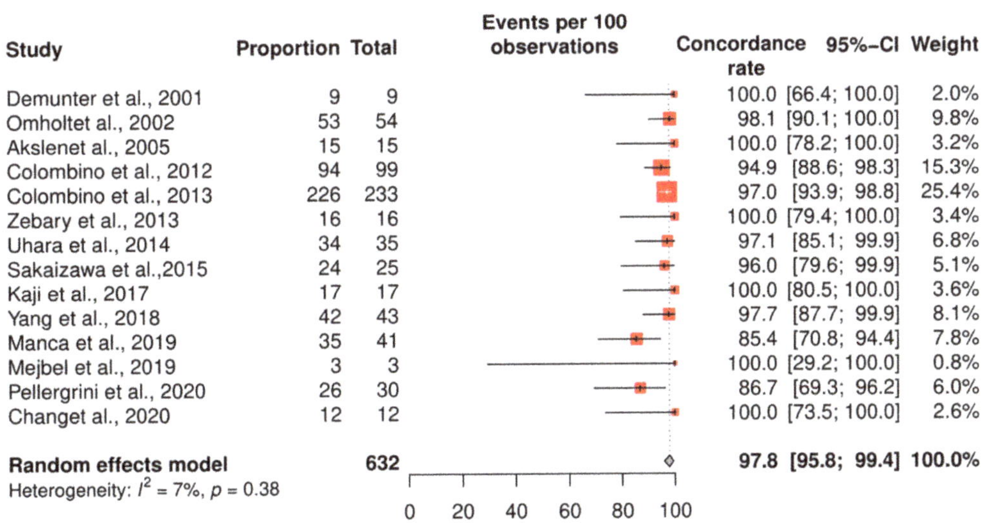

Figure 3. Results of the meta-analysis *NRAS*. Fourteen studies were included to pool the concordance rate of *NRAS* status [28,30,32,38,43,45,48–55], red square: point estimate of each study, and grey diamond: summary estimate of the total studies.

3.5. Subgroup Analysis According to the Technique and QUIPS Tool Score

The mutation status of *BRAF* and *NRAS* in the reported studies may be affected by the study design and the techniques used for mutation detection. For *BRAF* detection, 16 studies utilized molecular-based techniques, two utilized IHC, and seven used both. The pooled *BRAF* concordance rate was 86.4% [95% CI 79.6; 92.1] with a molecular-based technique, 92.8% [95% CI: 86.3; 97.5] with IHC, 81.9% [95% CI: 82.2; 98.4] with IHC, and a molecular-based technique combined. However, these differences were statistically insignificant (*p*-value = 0.24) (Figure 4). We did not perform subgroup analyses based on detection techniques on *NRAS* concordance because most of the studies used molecular-based techniques.

Study or Subgroup	Events	Total	Weight	Events per 100 observations IV, Random, 95% CI
Molecular-based				
Omholt et al., 2003	48	50	4.5%	96.0 [86.3; 99.5]
Yancovitz et al., 2012	10	18	3.4%	55.6 [30.8; 78.5]
Colombino et al., 2012	87	99	5.0%	87.9 [79.8; 93.6]
Heinzerling et al., 2013	7	11	2.7%	63.6 [30.8; 89.1]
Zebary et al., 2013	16	16	3.2%	100.0 [79.4; 100.0]
Colombino et al., 2013	208	236	5.4%	88.1 [83.3; 92.0]
Saroufim et al., 2014	20	27	3.9%	74.1 [53.7; 88.9]
Nardin et al., 2015	23	25	3.8%	92.0 [74.0; 99.0]
Satzger et al., 2015	71	75	4.9%	94.7 [86.9; 98.5]
Bradish et al., 2015	21	25	3.8%	84.0 [63.9; 95.5]
Sakaizwa et al., 2015	22	25	3.8%	88.0 [68.8; 97.5]
Yaman et al., 2016	40	47	4.5%	85.1 [71.7; 93.8]
Kaji et al., 2017	9	17	3.3%	52.9 [27.8; 77.0]
Mejbel et al., 2019	3	3	1.3%	100.0 [29.2; 100.0]
Manca et al., 2019	39	41	4.4%	95.1 [83.5; 99.4]
Chang et al., 2020	10	12	2.8%	83.3 [51.6; 97.9]
Total (95% CI)		**727**	**60.7%**	**87.2 [80.5; 92.8]**
Heterogeneity: Tau^2 = 0.0187; Chi^2 = 44.58, df = 15 (P < 0.01); I^2 = 66%				
Molecular-based + immunohistochemistry-based				
Riveiro-Falkenbach et al., 2015	117	140	5.2%	83.6 [76.4; 89.3]
Bruno et al., 2017	9	14	3.1%	64.3 [35.1; 87.2]
Hannan et al.,2017	36	42	4.4%	85.7 [71.5; 94.6]
Yang et al., 2018	42	43	4.4%	97.7 [87.7; 99.9]
Cormican et al., 2018	53	53	4.6%	100.0 [93.3; 100.0]
Nielsen et al., 2018	79	80	4.9%	98.8 [93.2; 100.0]
Pellergrini et al., 2020	26	30	4.0%	86.7 [69.3; 96.2]
Total (95% CI)		**402**	**30.5%**	**91.9 [82.2; 98.4]**
Heterogeneity: Tau^2 = 0.0295; Chi^2 = 40.59, df = 6 (P < 0.01); I^2 = 85%				
Immunohistochemistry-based				
Eriksson et al., 2015	59	63	4.7%	93.7 [84.5; 98.2]
Ito et al., 2019	28	31	4.1%	90.3 [74.2; 98.0]
Total (95% CI)		**94**	**8.8%**	**92.8 [86.3; 97.5]**
Heterogeneity: Tau^2 = 0; Chi^2 = 0.39, df = 1 (P = 0.53); I^2 = 0%				
Total (95% CI)		**1223**	**100.0%**	**89.4 [84.5; 93.5]**
Heterogeneity: Tau^2 = 0.0204; Chi^2 = 90.82, df = 24 (P < 0.01); I^2 = 74%				
Test for subgroup differences: Chi^2 = 2.77, df = 2 (P = 0.25)				

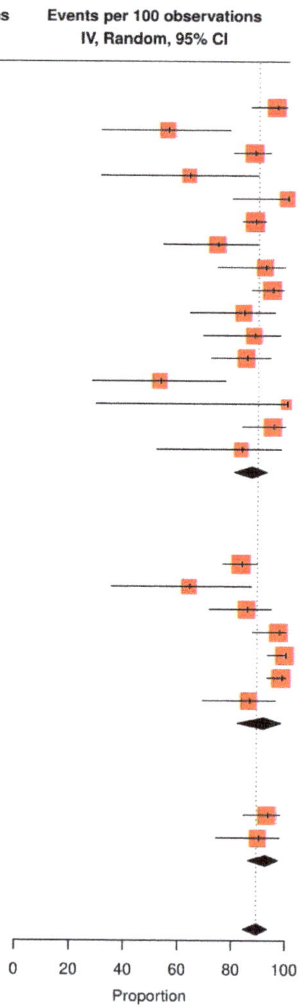

Figure 4. Subgroup analysis for *BRAF* concordance rate based on mutation detection methods. Studies with molecular-based technique only [27–34,36,38–40,43,48–50], studies with molecular-based + immunohistochemistry-based technique [37,41,42,44–46,51], studies with immunohistochemistry-based technique only [35,47], red square: point estimate of each study, and black rhomb: summary estimate of each subgroup.

Other confounders, such as sample collection, analysis interpretation, and the type of statistical tests in the individual studies, may affect the mutation detections and, subsequently, the concordance rate. Therefore, we performed a subgroup analysis based on the QUIPS score for *BRAF* and *NRAS* concordance rates (Figures 5 and 6). The pooled concordance rate for BRAF was 91.4% [95% CI: 86.7; 95.3] for studies with a high QUIPS score (≥4) and 81.0 [95% CI: 68.1; 91.6] for studies with a low QUIPS score (<4), (p-value = 0.03). The pooled concordance rate for NRAS was 95.7% [95% CI: 89.7; 99.5] for studies with a high QUIPS score (≥4) and 99.1% [95% CI: 97.3; 100] for studies with a low QUIPS score (<4). This difference was statistically insignificant (p-value = 0.38).

Study or Subgroup	Events	Total	Weight	Events per 100 observations IV, Random, 95% CI
Low risk				
Omholt et al., 2003	48	50	4.5%	96.0 [86.3; 99.5]
Yancovitz et al., 2012	10	18	3.4%	55.6 [30.8; 78.5]
Zebary et al., 2013	16	16	3.2%	100.0 [79.4; 100.0]
Saroufim et al., 2014	20	27	3.9%	74.1 [53.7; 88.9]
Nardin et al., 2015	23	25	3.8%	92.0 [74.0; 99.0]
Satzger et al., 2015	71	75	4.9%	94.7 [86.9; 98.5]
Riveiro-Falkenbach et al.,2015	117	140	5.2%	83.6 [76.4; 89.3]
Bradish et al., 2015	21	25	3.8%	84.0 [63.9; 95.5]
Eriksson et al., 2015	59	63	4.7%	93.7 [84.5; 98.2]
Yaman et al., 2016	40	47	4.5%	85.1 [71.7; 93.8]
Hannan et al.,2017	36	42	4.4%	85.7 [71.5; 94.6]
Yang et al., 2018	42	43	4.4%	97.7 [87.7; 99.9]
Cormican et al., 2018	53	53	4.6%	100.0 [93.3; 100.0]
Nielsen et al., 2018	79	80	4.9%	98.8 [93.2; 100.0]
Ito et al., 2019	28	31	4.1%	90.3 [74.2; 98.0]
Manca et al., 2019	39	41	4.4%	95.1 [83.5; 99.4]
Pellergrini et al., 2020	26	30	4.0%	86.7 [69.3; 96.2]
Chang et al., 2020	10	12	2.8%	83.3 [51.6; 97.9]
Total (95% CI)		**818**	**75.5%**	**91.4 [86.7; 95.3]**
Heterogeneity: $Tau^2 = 0.0164$; $Chi^2 = 63.94$, df = 17 (P < 0.01); $I^2 = 73\%$				
High risk				
Colombino et al., 2012	87	99	5.0%	87.9 [79.8; 93.6]
Heinzerling et al., 2013	7	11	2.7%	63.6 [30.8; 89.1]
Colombino et al., 2013	208	236	5.4%	88.1 [83.3; 92.0]
Sakaizwa et al., 2015	22	25	3.8%	88.0 [68.8; 97.5]
Bruno et al., 2017	9	14	3.1%	64.3 [35.1; 87.2]
Kaji et al., 2017	9	17	3.3%	52.9 [27.8; 77.0]
Mejbel et al., 2019	3	3	1.3%	100.0 [29.2; 100.0]
Total (95% CI)		**405**	**24.5%**	**81.0 [68.1; 91.6]**
Heterogeneity: $Tau^2 = 0.0208$; $Chi^2 = 18.49$, df = 6 (P < 0.01); $I^2 = 68\%$				
Total (95% CI)		**1223**	**100.0%**	**89.4 [84.5; 93.5]**
Heterogeneity: $Tau^2 = 0.0204$; $Chi^2 = 90.82$, df = 24 (P < 0.01); $I^2 = 74\%$				
Test for subgroup differences: $Chi^2 = 4.31$, df = 1 (P = 0.04)				

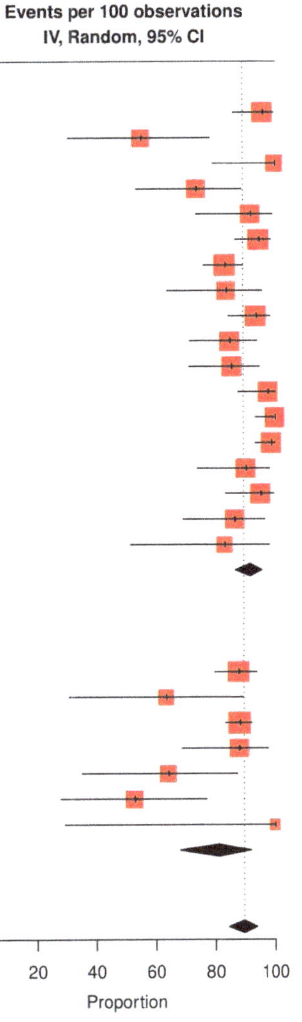

Figure 5. Subgroup analysis of the *BRAF* concordance rate based on QUIPS score. Low-risk bias studies were [27,29,32–37,39,40,42,44–48,50,51], high-risk bias studies were [28,30,31,38,41,43,49], red square: point estimate of each study, and black rhomb: summary estimate of each subgroup.

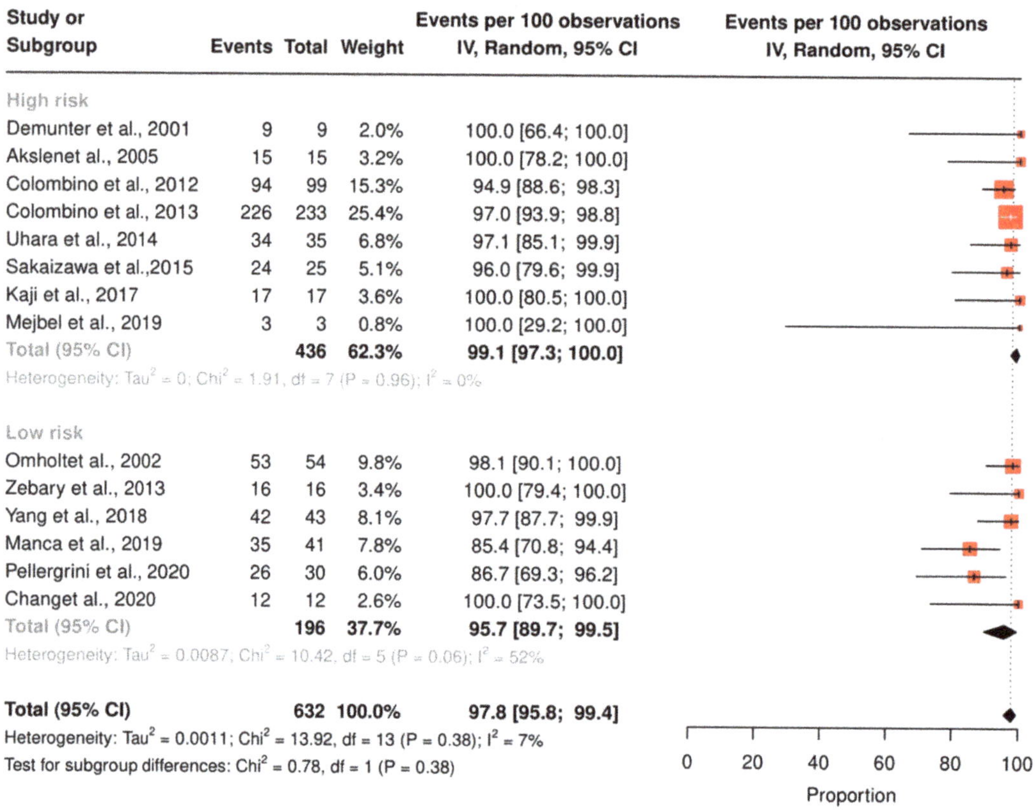

Figure 6. Subgroup analysis of the *NRAS* concordance rate based on QUIPS score. High-risk bias studies were [28,30,38,43,49,52,54,55], low-risk bias studies were [32,45,48,50,51,53], red square: point estimate of each study, and black rhomb: summary estimate of each subgroup.

4. Discussion

In this study, we comprehensively analyzed the current knowledge on the concordance of mutated genes between primary CM and their matched metastasis. Most of the reviewed studies focused on the concordance of *BRAF* mutation status because it has clinical value in the treatment decision for BRAF inhibitors. The second-most studied gene was *NRAS*. The overall pooled concordance rates for *BRAF* and *NRAS* status were high (88.8% and 97.2%, respectively). However, the reported concordance rates in the individual studies varied widely, ranging from 56% to 100% for *BRAF* and 85% to 100% for *NRAS*. Among the factors that could explain this wide range are: Mutation detection technique, gender, metastatic site type, and study quality. We observed that all these factors were of influence on the concordance rate. First, we explored the impact of mutation detection techniques. For *BRAF*, the concordance rate was higher when an IHC-based technique was used (92.8%) and lower when molecular-based techniques were used (86.4%). Although we could not explore the effects of gender and metastatic sites with significant power, we did see for *BRAF* concordance rate the most discordant cases in the direction of female sex and skin as a metastatic site.

Only five studies [43,45,48–50], with study sizes ranging from 3 to 41 participants, analyzed the variability in the mutation profiles using panel cancer driver genes. The alterations in *TERT*, *CDKN2A*, *TP53*, *RPPIK3CA*, and *EPHB6* were simultaneously detected in matched primary and metastasis tumors, albeit in only a small subset of patients. In contrast, other mutated genes were found exclusively in either primary or metastatic tumors. Predominantly, the majority of the genes displaying alterations were associated with critical pathways involved in tumor invasion, including those regulating proliferation, cell cycle, and apoptosis. This is in line with the current knowledge on melanoma progression [56–58]. In essence, investigating the sequential acquisition of mutations will be required to fully identify the key driver mutations that are responsible for the processes of invasion, adaptation, and, ultimately, melanoma metastasis dissemination [59].

CM presents cancer with a very high tumor mutational burden (TMB) [60]. This characteristic may lead to polyclonal formation within the individual primary melanoma tumor. In other words, a primary tumor can comprise a mixture of cells presenting different genetic profiles of the same gene, with the ability to metastasize to other tissue organs [61]. Two studies showed intratumoral heterogeneity within the same melanoma samples for *BRAF* and *TERT* mutation status using different micro-dissected regions of the same sample [29,50]. A meta-analysis reported similar observations when investigating *EGFR* and *KRAS* mutation status in matched primary tumors and distant metastasis of non-small cell lung cancer, which is also considered a tumor with a TMB [62]. Thus, intratumoral heterogeneity may be a common feature of high-TMB tumors. In our study, we also showed that additional mutations in genes such as *KRAS* and *NEK10* were likely to be seen in primary melanoma. In contrast, mutations in genes such as *TERT* and *CCND1* were likely present in metastasis. Thus, we highlight the need to investigate the clonality of more melanoma-specific genes, especially in the case of building metastasis risk prediction models that are based on the genetic profile of primary tumors, as the primary tumors may contain driver genes that are irrelevant for the recurrence of the metastasis. For example, Chang et al. have shown that within the same melanoma patients, the primary tumor had a *BRAF* mutant status, but the metastatic tumor had lost this mutation and acquired a new mutation in the *TERT* promoter [50]. As a result, a metastasis risk prediction model based on the *BRAF* mutation status of the primary tumor would not be accurate for this patient. Therefore, it is essential to develop metastasis risk prediction models that take into account the intratumoral heterogeneity of melanoma tumors. This could be done by sequencing multiple regions of the primary tumor or by sequencing both the primary and metastatic tumor tissues.

The accuracy of the mutation detection technique may have an effect when comparing the mutation status [63,64]. Bruno et al. tested the concordance of *BRAF* status between 25 paired primary and matched melanoma samples by applying both IHC and real-time PCR. Their study showed that IHC was more effective in detecting the signal of mutated *BRAF* V600E [41]. This finding suggested that IHC is the stable method for the *BRAF* testing method, especially for detecting the most common *BRAF* mutation, V600E. From a molecular point of view, IHC is subject to some limitations. For instance, IHC can be subjective as the pathologist's interpretation affects the results. IHC may not detect mutations in all cases, particularly when the tumor sample is small or if the mutation is present in only a small percentage of tumor cells [65]. At the same time, molecular-based techniques such as real-time PCR are more objective and sensitive than IHC [66]. In the daily practice of *BRAF* testing, molecular techniques are considered the golden standard [67].

The tumors can evolve over time, and new mutations can arise in the metastases. Thus, the time to metastasis, which is defined as the time between the primary tumor and the metastasis tumor biopsy, may also affect the mutation concordance rate. In our study, we were unable to analyze the impact of time on metastasis as there were not enough eligible studies. It is essential to mention that no new studies have reported more extensive information on the timing of metastasis since the previous meta-analysis of *BRAF* [20]. In colorectal cancer, the concordance rate of *KRAS* status decreases when the time to metastasis increases [68,69]. Thus, it is recommended to perform more frequent surveillance for patients with a longer time to metastasis, as they may be at higher risk for developing metastases with a different KRAS mutation status [68].

The metastatic site plays a crucial role in changing the mutation status between matched primary and metastasis melanoma tumors. Firstly, the microenvironment of the metastasis site can exert a unique selection pressure on the melanoma cancer site. In other words, the metastasis tissue site can offer distinct biochemical, immune, and structural conditions that differ from the skin site. This means the melanoma cells can adapt and acquire new mutations to thrive in the specific microenvironment of the metastasis site. For example, the melanoma cells that metastasize to the brain may develop mutations that evade the immune system, as the brain is an immune-privileged site [70]. Melanoma that metastases to the lung may develop mutations that allow it to resist the effects of chemotherapy, as the lung is a vascularized organ [71].

The overall study quality had no significant effect on the concordance rates of *NRAS* mutation status. Yielding that the reliability of *NRAS* mutation status determination was fairly consistent across studies, regardless of their quality ratings. However, we observed higher concordance rates for *BRAF* mutation status in studies rated as high quality compared to studies rated as low quality. These findings suggest that beyond mutation detection techniques, other factors such as patient selection and time and type of fixation, as well as improper tumor sampling, may affect the concordance rate of the mutation profile [72]. From a biological standpoint, it is worth noting that both *BRAF* and *NRAS* mutations are present in nevi, suggesting that such mutations might represent early events that could already be present in all tumor cells. This is also supported by the results seen in immunohistochemistry (IHC) [29,73]. It appears that, based on the available data, discrepancies in the current literature may be attributed to sample management and mutation detection techniques rather than being solely due to tumor heterogeneity. Refining and standardizing sample collection and analysis procedures are crucial to enhancing the accuracy and consistency of mutation profiling in melanoma cancer research. Ultimately, this leads to more reliable insights into this complex disease.

Our study has several limitations; firstly, the original studies that we included in our meta-analysis for *BRAF* and *NRAS* status were relatively small, which limited the power of our study to detect statistically significant results. Secondly, most of the included studies used different criteria to select patients, mainly for the metastasis tumor (lymph node or distant metastasis). Lastly, we did not have access to clinical data for all of the patients in the original studies, which prevented us from analyzing the effect of clinical variables, such as the tumor thickness and the presence of the ulceration, on the concordance rate. Despite these limitations, our study presents the first meta-analysis that pooled the *NRAS* concordance rate in matched primary and metastasis of cutaneous melanoma. This is an important finding, as NRAS mutations are responsible for a significant proportion of melanomas, but no well-established NRAS-targeted therapies are yet known. In addition to the updated data about the pooled *BRAF* concordance rate from the previous meta-analysis.

Our results consolidate the evidence of the mutation concordance between primary melanoma and matched metastasis. We demonstrated a high concordance for *BRAF* and *NRAS* mutation status. We observed that the *BRAF* concordance rate is higher than reported in the last systematic review. This finding may suggest that advances have been made in molecular techniques and IHC techniques. Nevertheless, further investigations are required to comprehend the intricacies of melanoma, including its genetic heterogeneity and the complex interaction of multiple genes driving the metastatic progression. Expanding the scope of our study is essential to attaining a comprehensive understanding of tumor heterogeneity and the genetic changes that take place throughout the metastatic evolution of melanoma. This should include not only a wider range of genes but also the integration of more clinical information, as these multi-faceted forms of research will aid in uncovering the complexities of the genetic landscape of melanoma.

5. Conclusions

The complete explanation of the genomic background behind melanoma pathogenesis remains elusive. This study presents a summary of current understanding regarding the clonal relatedness of mutated genes in primary cutaneous melanoma and matched tumors. We draw attention to the knowledge gap regarding the genetic heterogeneity of melanoma-specific genes, which could serve as a valuable tool in identifying suitable patients for trials testing possible new targeted therapies. Furthermore, we found that CM presents a significant concordance in *BRAF* status between primary and metastatic tumors than in previous meta-analyses, probably due to technical advances, although a minority of patients showed inconsistencies. Therefore, we propose that molecular testing in metastatic tissue is a more appropriate method for determining *BRAF* status to tailor the treatment decision, although it is still reasonable to use the primary tumor in cases of difficulty. Further research should investigate the factors causing these discrepancies and the feasibility of using other molecular markers with *BRAF* status to better stratify patients for melanoma treatment.

Supplementary Materials: The following supporting information can be downloaded at: https://www.mdpi.com/article/10.3390/ijms242216281/s1.

Author Contributions: Conceptualization, T.K., L.H. and A.M.; methodology, T.K., L.H. and A.M.; software, T.K. and C.Z.; validation, T.K. and C.Z.; formal analysis, T.K.; resources, T.K. and C.Z.; writing—original draft preparation, T.K.; writing—review and editing, L.H., T.K., A.M. and C.Z.; visualization, T.K.; supervision, A.M. and L.H. All authors have read and agreed to the published version of the manuscript.

Funding: This research received no external funding.

Institutional Review Board Statement: Not applicable.

Informed Consent Statement: Not applicable.

Data Availability Statement: All data relevant to this study are included in the manuscript.

Acknowledgments: The authors thank W.M. Bramer of the Erasmus MC Medical Library for developing the search strategy.

Conflicts of Interest: The authors declare no conflict of interest.

References

1. Whiteman, D.C.; Green, A.C.; Olsen, C.M. The growing burden of invasive melanoma: Projections of incidence rates and numbers of new cases in six susceptible populations through 2031. *J. Investig. Dermatol.* **2016**, *136*, 1161–1171. [CrossRef] [PubMed]
2. Garbe, C.; Keim, U.; Amaral, T.; Berking, C.; Eigentler, T.K.; Flatz, L.; Gesierich, A.; Leiter, U.; Stadler, R.; Sunderkötter, C. Prognosis of patients with primary melanoma stage I and II according to American Joint Committee on Cancer Version 8 Validated in two independent cohorts: Implications for adjuvant treatment. *J. Clin. Oncol.* **2022**, *40*, 3741. [CrossRef] [PubMed]
3. Ertekin, S.S.; Podlipnik, S.; Riquelme-Mc Loughlin, C.; Barreiro-Capurro, A.; Arance, A.; Carrera, C.C.; Malvehy, J.; Puig, S. Initial stage of cutaneous primary melanoma plays a key role in the pattern and timing of disease recurrence. *Acta Derm. Venereol.* **2021**, *101*, adv00502. [CrossRef] [PubMed]
4. Zhou, C.; Louwman, M.; Wakkee, M.; Van der Veldt, A.; Grünhagen, D.; Verhoef, C.; Mooyaart, A.; Nijsten, T.; Hollestein, L. Primary melanoma characteristics of metastatic disease: A nationwide cancer registry study. *Cancers* **2021**, *13*, 4431. [CrossRef]
5. Bedikian, A.Y.; DeConti, R.C.; Conry, R.; Agarwala, S.; Papadopoulos, N.; Kim, K.B.; Ernstoff, M. Phase 3 study of docosahexaenoic acid–paclitaxel versus dacarbazine in patients with metastatic malignant melanoma. *Ann. Oncol.* **2011**, *22*, 787–793. [CrossRef] [PubMed]
6. Garbe, C.; Amaral, T.; Peris, K.; Hauschild, A.; Arenberger, P.; Bastholt, L.; Bataille, V.; Del Marmol, V.; Dréno, B.; Fargnoli, M.C. European consensus-based interdisciplinary guideline for melanoma. Part 2: Treatment–Update 2019. *Eur. J. Cancer* **2020**, *126*, 159–177. [CrossRef] [PubMed]
7. Hodi, F.S.; O'Day, S.J.; McDermott, D.F.; Weber, R.W.; Sosman, J.A.; Haanen, J.B.; Gonzalez, R.; Robert, C.; Schadendorf, D.; Hassel, J.C. Improved survival with ipilimumab in patients with metastatic melanoma. *N. Engl. J. Med.* **2010**, *363*, 711–723. [CrossRef]
8. Larkin, J.; Minor, D.; D'Angelo, S.; Neyns, B.; Smylie, M.; Miller Jr, W.H.; Gutzmer, R.; Linette, G.; Chmielowski, B.; Lao, C.D. Overall survival in patients with advanced melanoma who received nivolumab versus investigator's choice chemotherapy in CheckMate 037: A randomized, controlled, open-label phase III trial. *J. Clin. Oncol.* **2018**, *36*, 383. [CrossRef]
9. Patel, P.M.; Suciu, S.; Mortier, L.; Kruit, W.H.; Robert, C.; Schadendorf, D.; Trefzer, U.; Punt, C.J.A.; Dummer, R.; Davidson, N. Extended schedule, escalated dose temozolomide versus dacarbazine in stage IV melanoma: Final results of a randomised phase III study (EORTC 18032). *Eur. J. Cancer* **2011**, *47*, 1476–1483. [CrossRef]

10. Sibaud, V. Dermatologic reactions to immune checkpoint inhibitors: Skin toxicities and immunotherapy. *Am. J. Clin. Dermatol.* **2018**, *19*, 345–361. [CrossRef]
11. Robert, C.; Thomas, L.; Bondarenko, I.; O'Day, S.; Weber, J.; Garbe, C.; Lebbe, C.; Baurain, J.-F.; Testori, A.; Grob, J.-J. Ipilimumab plus dacarbazine for previously untreated metastatic melanoma. *N. Engl. J. Med.* **2011**, *364*, 2517–2526. [CrossRef] [PubMed]
12. Sosman, J.A.; Kim, K.B.; Schuchter, L.; Gonzalez, R.; Pavlick, A.C.; Weber, J.S.; McArthur, G.A.; Hutson, T.E.; Moschos, S.J.; Flaherty, K.T. Survival in BRAF V600–mutant advanced melanoma treated with vemurafenib. *N. Engl. J. Med.* **2012**, *366*, 707–714. [CrossRef]
13. Ko, J.M.; Fisher, D.E. A new era: Melanoma genetics and therapeutics. *J. Pathol.* **2011**, *223*, 242–251. [CrossRef] [PubMed]
14. Dummer, R.; Schadendorf, D.; Ascierto, P.A.; Arance, A.; Dutriaux, C.; Di Giacomo, A.M.; Rutkowski, P.; Del Vecchio, M.; Gutzmer, R.; Mandala, M. Binimetinib versus dacarbazine in patients with advanced NRAS-mutant melanoma (NEMO): A multicentre, open-label, randomised, phase 3 trial. *Lancet Oncol.* **2017**, *18*, 435–445. [CrossRef] [PubMed]
15. Landras, A.; Reger de Moura, C.; Villoutreix, B.O.; Battistella, M.; Sadoux, A.; Dumaz, N.; Menashi, S.; Fernández-Recio, J.; Lebbé, C.; Mourah, S. Novel treatment strategy for NRAS-mutated melanoma through a selective inhibitor of CD147/VEGFR-2 interaction. *Oncogene* **2022**, *41*, 2254–2264. [CrossRef]
16. Guo, J.; Si, L.; Kong, Y.; Flaherty, K.T.; Xu, X.; Zhu, Y.; Corless, C.L.; Li, L.; Li, H.; Sheng, X. Phase II, open-label, single-arm trial of imatinib mesylate in patients with metastatic melanoma harboring c-Kit mutation or amplification. *J. Clin. Oncol.* **2011**, *29*, 2904–2909. [CrossRef]
17. Hodi, F.S.; Corless, C.L.; Giobbie-Hurder, A.; Fletcher, J.A.; Zhu, M.; Marino-Enriquez, A.; Friedlander, P.; Gonzalez, R.; Weber, J.S.; Gajewski, T.F. Imatinib for melanomas harboring mutationally activated or amplified KIT arising on mucosal, acral, and chronically sun-damaged skin. *J. Clin. Oncol.* **2013**, *31*, 3182. [CrossRef]
18. Mehnert, J.M.; Kluger, H.M. Driver mutations in melanoma: Lessons learned from bench-to-bedside studies. *Curr. Oncol. Rep.* **2012**, *14*, 449–457. [CrossRef]
19. Pham, D.D.M.; Guhan, S.; Tsao, H. KIT and melanoma: Biological insights and clinical implications. *Yonsei Med. J.* **2020**, *61*, 562. [CrossRef]
20. Valachis, A.; Ullenhag, G.J. Discrepancy in BRAF status among patients with metastatic malignant melanoma: A meta-analysis. *Eur. J. Cancer* **2017**, *81*, 106–115. [CrossRef]
21. en de Nederlandse, N.G.N. Richtlijn Melanoom: Modulaire revisie 2016. *Ned. Tijdschr. Oncol.* **2016**, *13*, 218–220.
22. Hayden, J.A.; van der Windt, D.A.; Cartwright, J.L.; Côté, P.; Bombardier, C. Assessing bias in studies of prognostic factors. *Ann. Intern. Med.* **2013**, *158*, 280–286. [CrossRef]
23. Kolberg, L.; Raudvere, U.; Kuzmin, I.; Adler, P.; Vilo, J.; Peterson, H. g: Profiler—Interoperable web service for functional enrichment analysis and gene identifier mapping (2023 update). *Nucleic Acids Res.* **2023**, *51*, gkad347. [CrossRef] [PubMed]
24. Chen, Y.; Chen, D.; Wang, Y.; Han, Y. Using Freeman-Tukey Double Arcsine Transformation in Meta-analysis of Single Proportions. *Aesthetic Plast. Surg.* **2023**, *47*, 83–84. [CrossRef] [PubMed]
25. Schwarzer, G. meta: An R package for meta-analysis. *R News* **2007**, *7*, 40–45.
26. Viechtbauer, W. Conducting meta-analyses in R with the metafor package. *J. Stat. Softw.* **2010**, *36*, 1–48. [CrossRef]
27. Omholt, K.; Platz, A.; Kanter, L.; Ringborg, U.; Hansson, J. NRAS and BRAF Mutations Arise Early during Melanoma Pathogenesis and Are Preserved throughout Tumor Progression. *Clin. Cancer Res.* **2003**, *9*, 6483–6488.
28. Colombino, M.; Capone, M.; Lissia, A.; Cossu, A.; Rubino, C.; De Giorgi, V.; Massi, D.; Fonsatti, E.; Staibano, S.; Nappi, O.; et al. BRAF/NRAS mutation frequencies among primary tumors and metastases in patients with melanoma. *J. Clin. Oncol.* **2012**, *30*, 2522–2529. [CrossRef]
29. Yancovitz, M.; Litterman, A.; Yoon, J.; Ng, E.; Shapiro, R.L.; Berman, R.S.; Pavlick, A.C.; Darvishian, F.; Christos, P.; Mazumdar, M.; et al. Intra- and inter-tumor heterogeneity of BRAFV600Emutations in primary and metastatic melanoma. *PLoS ONE* **2012**, *7*, e29336. [CrossRef]
30. Colombino, M.; Lissia, A.; Capone, M.; De Giorgi, V.; Massi, D.; Stanganelli, I.; Fonsatti, E.; Maio, M.; Botti, G.; Caracò, C.; et al. Heterogeneous distribution of BRAF/NRAS mutations among Italian patients with advanced melanoma. *J. Transl. Med.* **2013**, *11*, 202. [CrossRef]
31. Heinzerling, L.; Baiter, M.; Kühnapfel, S.; Schuler, G.; Keikavoussi, P.; Agaimy, A.; Kiesewetter, F.; Hartmann, A.; Schneider-Stock, R. Mutation landscape in melanoma patients clinical implications of heterogeneity of BRAF mutations. *Br. J. Cancer* **2013**, *109*, 2833–2841. [CrossRef] [PubMed]
32. Zebary, A.; Omholt, K.; Vassilaki, I.; Höiom, V.; Lindén, D.; Viberg, L.; Kanter-Lewensohn, L.; Johansson, C.H.; Hansson, J. KIT, NRAS, BRAF and PTEN mutations in a sample of Swedish patients with acral lentiginous melanoma. *J. Dermatol. Sci.* **2013**, *72*, 284–289. [CrossRef] [PubMed]
33. Saroufim, M.; Habib, R.H.; Gerges, R.; Saab, J.; Loya, A.; Amr, S.S.; Sheikh, S.; Satti, M.; Oberkanins, C.; Khalifeh, I. Comparing BRAF mutation status in matched primary and metastatic cutaneous melanomas: Implications on optimized targeted therapy. *Exp. Mol. Pathol.* **2014**, *97*, 315–320. [CrossRef] [PubMed]
34. Bradish, J.R.; Richey, J.D.; Post, K.M.; Meehan, K.; Sen, J.D.; Malek, A.J.; Katona, T.M.; Warren, S.; Logan, T.F.; Fecher, L.A.; et al. Discordancy in BRAF mutations among primary and metastatic melanoma lesions: Clinical implications for targeted therapy. *Mod. Pathol.* **2015**, *28*, 480–486. [CrossRef]

35. Eriksson, H.; Zebary, A.; Vassilaki, I.; Omholt, K.; Ghaderi, M.; Hansson, J. BRAFV600E protein expression in primary cutaneous malignant melanomas and paired metastases. *JAMA Dermatol.* **2015**, *151*, 410–416. [CrossRef] [PubMed]
36. Nardin, C.; Puzenat, E.; Prétet, J.L.; Algros, M.P.; Doussot, A.; Puyraveau, M.; Mougin, C.; Aubin, F. BRAF mutation screening in melanoma: Is sentinel lymph node reliable? *Melanoma Res.* **2015**, *25*, 328–334. [CrossRef] [PubMed]
37. Riveiro-Falkenbach, E.; Villanueva, C.A.; Garrido, M.C.; Ruano, Y.; García-Martín, R.M.; Godoy, E.; Ortiz-Romero, P.L.; Ríos-Martín, J.J.; Santos-Briz, A.; Rodríguez-Peralto, J.L. Intra- and inter-tumoral homogeneity of BRAF V600E mutations in melanoma tumors. *J. Investig. Dermatol.* **2015**, *135*, 3078–3085. [CrossRef]
38. Sakaizawa, K.; Ashida, A.; Uchiyama, A.; Ito, T.; Fujisawa, Y.; Ogata, D.; Matsushita, S.; Fujii, K.; Fukushima, S.; Shibayama, Y.; et al. Clinical characteristics associated with BRAF, NRAS and KIT mutations in Japanese melanoma patients. *J. Dermatol. Sci.* **2015**, *80*, 33–37. [CrossRef]
39. Satzger, I.; Marks, L.; Kerick, M.; Klages, S.; Berking, C.; Herbst, R.; Völker, B.; Schacht, V.; Timmermann, B.; Gutzmer, R. Allele frequencies of BRAFV600 mutations in primary melanomas and matched metastases and their relevance for BRAF inhibitor therapy in metastatic melanoma. *Oncotarget* **2015**, *6*, 37895–37905. [CrossRef]
40. Yaman, B.; Kandiloglu, G.; Akalin, T. BRAF-V600 Mutation Heterogeneity in Primary and Metastatic Melanoma: A Study with Pyrosequencing and Immunohistochemistry. *Am. J. Dermatopathol.* **2016**, *38*, 113–120. [CrossRef]
41. Bruno, W.; Martinuzzi, C.; Andreotti, V.; Pastorino, L.; Spagnolo, F.; Dalmasso, B.; Cabiddu, F.; Gualco, M.; Ballestrero, A.; Bianchi-Scarrà, G.; et al. Heterogeneity and frequency of BRAF mutations in primary melanoma: Comparison between molecular methods and immunohistochemistry. *Oncotarget* **2017**, *8*, 8069–8082. [CrossRef] [PubMed]
42. Hannan, E.J.; O'Leary, D.P.; Macnally, S.P.; Kay, E.W.; Farrell, M.A.; Morris, P.G.; Power, C.P.; Hill, A.D.K. The significance of BRAF V600E mutation status discordance between primary cutaneous melanoma and brain metastases. *Medicine* **2017**, *96*, e8404. [CrossRef] [PubMed]
43. Kaji, T.; Yamasaki, O.; Takata, M.; Otsuka, M.; Hamada, T.; Morizane, S.; Asagoe, K.; Yanai, H.; Hirai, Y.; Umemura, H.; et al. Comparative study on driver mutations in primary and metastatic melanomas at a single Japanese institute: A clue for intra- and inter-tumor heterogeneity. *J. Dermatol. Sci.* **2017**, *85*, 51–57. [CrossRef] [PubMed]
44. Nielsen, L.B.; Dabrosin, N.; Sloth, K.; Bønnelykke–Behrndtz, M.L.; Steiniche, T.; Lade-Keller, J. Concordance in BRAF V600E status over time in malignant melanoma and corresponding metastases. *Histopathology* **2018**, *72*, 814–825. [CrossRef] [PubMed]
45. Yang, S.; Leone, D.A.; Biswas, A.; Deng, A.; Jukic, D.; Singh, R.; Sundram, U.; Mahalingam, M. Concordance of somatic mutation profiles (BRAF, NRAS, and TERT) and tumoral PD-L1 in matched primary cutaneous and metastatic melanoma samples. *Hum. Pathol.* **2018**, *82*, 206–214. [CrossRef]
46. Cormican, D.; Kennedy, C.; Murphy, S.; Werner, R.; Power, D.G.; Heffron, C.C.B.B. High concordance of BRAF mutational status in matched primary and metastatic melanoma. *J. Cutan. Pathol.* **2019**, *46*, 117–122. [CrossRef]
47. Ito, T.; Kaku-Ito, Y.; Murata, M.; Ichiki, T.; Kuma, Y.; Tanaka, Y.; Ide, T.; Ohno, F.; Wada-Ohno, M.; Yamada, Y.; et al. Intra-and inter-tumor braf heterogeneity in acral melanoma: An immunohistochemical analysis. *Int. J. Mol. Sci.* **2019**, *20*, 6191. [CrossRef]
48. Manca, A.; Paliogiannis, P.; Colombino, M.; Casula, M.; Lissia, A.; Botti, G.; Caracò, C.; Ascierto, P.A.; Sini, M.C.; Palomba, G.; et al. Mutational concordance between primary and metastatic melanoma: A next-generation sequencing approach. *J. Transl. Med.* **2019**, *17*, 289. [CrossRef]
49. Mejbel, H.A.; Arudra, S.K.C.; Pradhan, D.; Torres-Cabala, C.A.; Nagarajan, P.; Tetzlaff, M.T.; Curry, J.L.; Ivan, D.; Duose, D.Y.; Luthra, R.; et al. Immunohistochemical and molecular features of melanomas exhibiting intratumor and intertumor histomorphologic heterogeneity. *Cancers* **2019**, *11*, 1714. [CrossRef]
50. Chang, G.A.; Wiggins, J.M.; Corless, B.C.; Syeda, M.M.; Tadepalli, J.S.; Blake, S.; Fleming, N.; Darvishian, F.; Pavlick, A.; Berman, R.; et al. TERT, BRAF, and NRAS Mutational Heterogeneity between Paired Primary and Metastatic Melanoma Tumors. *J. Investig. Dermatol.* **2020**, *140*, 1609–1618. [CrossRef]
51. Pellegrini, C.; Cardelli, L.; De Padova, M.; Di Nardo, L.; Ciciarell, V.; Rocco, T.; Cipolloni, G.; Clementi, M.; Cortellini, A.; Ventura, A.; et al. Intra-patient heterogeneity of BRAF and NRAS molecular alterations in primary melanoma and metastases. *Acta Derm. Venereol.* **2020**, *100*, adv00040. [CrossRef] [PubMed]
52. Demunter, A.; Stas, M.; Degreef, H.; De Wolf-Peeters, C.; Van den Oord, J.J. Analysis of N- and K-ras mutations in the distinctive tumor progression phases of melanoma. *J. Investig. Dermatol.* **2001**, *117*, 1483–1489. [CrossRef] [PubMed]
53. Omholt, K.; Karsberg, S.; Platz, A.; Kanter, L.; Ringborg, U.; Hansson, J. Screening of N-ras codon 61 mutations in paired primary and metastatic cutaneous melanomas: Mutations occur early and persist throughout tumor progression. *Clin. Cancer Res.* **2002**, *8*, 3468–3474. [PubMed]
54. Akslen, L.A.; Angelini, S.; Straume, O.; Bachmann, I.M.; Molven, A.; Hemminki, K.; Kumar, R. BRAF and NRAS mutations are frequent in nodular melanoma but are not associated with tumor cell proliferation or patient survival. *J. Investig. Dermatol.* **2005**, *125*, 312–317. [CrossRef] [PubMed]
55. Uhara, H.; Ashida, A.; Koga, H.; Ogawa, E.; Uchiyama, A.; Uchiyama, R.; Hayashi, K.; Kiniwa, Y.; Okuyama, R. NRAS mutations in primary and metastatic melanomas of Japanese patients. *Int. J. Clin. Oncol.* **2014**, *19*, 544–548. [CrossRef]
56. Davis, E.J.; Johnson, D.B.; Sosman, J.A.; Chandra, S. Melanoma: What do all the mutations mean? *Cancer* **2018**, *124*, 3490–3499. [CrossRef]
57. Zhang, T.; Dutton-Regester, K.; Brown, K.M.; Hayward, N.K. The genomic landscape of cutaneous melanoma. *Pigment. Cell Melanoma Res.* **2016**, *29*, 266–283. [CrossRef]

58. Vergara, I.A.; Mintoff, C.P.; Sandhu, S.; McIntosh, L.; Young, R.J.; Wong, S.Q.; Colebatch, A.; Cameron, D.L.; Kwon, J.L.; Wolfe, R. Evolution of late-stage metastatic melanoma is dominated by aneuploidy and whole genome doubling. *Nat. Commun.* **2021**, *12*, 1434. [CrossRef]
59. Cherepakhin, O.S.; Argenyi, Z.B.; Moshiri, A.S. Genomic and transcriptomic underpinnings of melanoma genesis, progression, and metastasis. *Cancers* **2021**, *14*, 123. [CrossRef]
60. Castle, J.C.; Uduman, M.; Pabla, S.; Stein, R.B.; Buell, J.S. Mutation-derived neoantigens for cancer immunotherapy. *Front. Immunol.* **2019**, *10*, 1856. [CrossRef]
61. Tímár, J.; Vizkeleti, L.; Doma, V.; Barbai, T.; Rásó, E. Genetic progression of malignant melanoma. *Cancer Metastasis Rev.* **2016**, *35*, 93–107. [CrossRef] [PubMed]
62. Wang, S.; Wang, Z. Meta-analysis of epidermal growth factor receptor and KRAS gene status between primary and corresponding metastatic tumours of non-small cell lung cancer. *Clin. Oncol.* **2015**, *27*, 30–39. [CrossRef] [PubMed]
63. Pinzani, P.; Santucci, C.; Mancini, I.; Simi, L.; Salvianti, F.; Pratesi, N.; Massi, D.; De Giorgi, V.; Pazzagli, M.; Orlando, C. BRAFV600E detection in melanoma is highly improved by COLD-PCR. *Clin. Chim. Acta* **2011**, *412*, 901–905. [CrossRef]
64. Barbano, R.; Pasculli, B.; Coco, M.; Fontana, A.; Copetti, M.; Rendina, M.; Valori, V.M.; Graziano, P.; Maiello, E.; Fazio, V.M. Competitive allele-specific TaqMan PCR (Cast-PCR) is a sensitive, specific and fast method for BRAF V600 mutation detection in Melanoma patients. *Sci. Rep.* **2015**, *5*, 18592. [CrossRef] [PubMed]
65. Colomba, E.; Hélias-Rodzewicz, Z.; Von Deimling, A.; Marin, C.; Terrones, N.; Pechaud, D.; Surel, S.; Côté, J.-F.; Peschaud, F.; Capper, D. Detection of BRAF p. V600E mutations in melanomas: Comparison of four methods argues for sequential use of immunohistochemistry and pyrosequencing. *J. Mol. Diagn.* **2013**, *15*, 94–100. [CrossRef]
66. Yakout, N.M.; Abdallah, D.M.; Abdelmonsif, D.A.; Kholosy, H.M.; Talaat, I.M.; Elsakka, O. BRAFV600E mutational status assessment in cutaneous melanocytic neoplasms in a group of the Egyptian population. *Cancer Cell Int.* **2023**, *23*, 17. [CrossRef] [PubMed]
67. Thiel, A.; Moza, M.; Kytölä, S.; Orpana, A.; Jahkola, T.; Hernberg, M.; Virolainen, S.; Ristimäki, A. Prospective immunohistochemical analysis of BRAF V600E mutation in melanoma. *Hum. Pathol.* **2015**, *46*, 169–175. [CrossRef]
68. Ardito, F.; Razionale, F.; Salvatore, L.; Cenci, T.; Vellone, M.; Basso, M.; Panettieri, E.; Calegari, M.A.; Tortora, G.; Martini, M. Discordance of KRAS mutational status between primary tumors and liver metastases in colorectal cancer: Impact on long-term survival following radical resection. *Cancers* **2021**, *13*, 2148. [CrossRef]
69. Bhullar, D.S.; Barriuso, J.; Mullamitha, S.; Saunders, M.P.; O'Dwyer, S.T.; Aziz, O. Biomarker concordance between primary colorectal cancer and its metastases. *eBioMedicine* **2019**, *40*, 363–374. [CrossRef]
70. Abate-Daga, D.; Ramello, M.C.; Smalley, I.; Forsyth, P.A.; Smalley, K.S.M. The biology and therapeutic management of melanoma brain metastases. *Biochem. Pharmacol.* **2018**, *153*, 35–45. [CrossRef]
71. Röckmann, H.; Schadendorf, D. Drug resistance in human melanoma: Mechanisms and therapeutic opportunities. *Oncol. Res. Treat.* **2003**, *26*, 581–587. [CrossRef] [PubMed]
72. Mao, C.; Wu, X.-Y.; Yang, Z.-Y.; Threapleton, D.E.; Yuan, J.-Q.; Yu, Y.-Y.; Tang, J.-L. Concordant analysis of KRAS, BRAF, PIK3CA mutations and PTEN expression between primary colorectal cancer and matched metastases. *Sci. Rep.* **2015**, *5*, 8065. [CrossRef] [PubMed]
73. Lin, J.; Takata, M.; Murata, H.; Goto, Y.; Kido, K.; Ferrone, S.; Saida, T. Polyclonality of BRAF mutations in acquired melanocytic nevi. *JNCI J. Natl. Cancer Inst.* **2009**, *101*, 1423–1427. [CrossRef] [PubMed]

International Journal of
Molecular Sciences

MDPI

Review

Development of Personalized Strategies for Precisely Battling Malignant Melanoma

Armond J. Isaak †, GeGe R. Clements †, Rand Gabriel M. Buenaventura, Glenn Merlino and Yanlin Yu *

Laboratory of Cancer Biology and Genetics, Center for Cancer Research, National Cancer Institute, National Institutes of Health, Bethesda, MD 20892, USA

* Correspondence: yuy@mail.nih.gov; Tel.: +1-(240)-760-6812

† These authors contributed equally and shared the first authorship.

Simple Summary: Precision oncology is emerging as a viable option to improve survival in patients who fail to remain disease-free even after the employment of currently available treatments. Such an alternative is particularly essential for patients with melanoma, where recurrence and progression of the disease following the development of acquired resistance are common. In this review, we aim to address the treatments available to patients diagnosed with melanoma and discuss promising treatment options that rely on specific and individualized approaches to treatment, particularly for the subset of patients who experience therapy failure due to acquired resistance.

Abstract: Melanoma is the most severe and fatal form of skin cancer, resulting from multiple gene mutations with high intra-tumor and inter-tumor molecular heterogeneity. Treatment options for patients whose disease has progressed beyond the ability for surgical resection rely on currently accepted standard therapies, notably immune checkpoint inhibitors and targeted therapies. Acquired resistance to these therapies and treatment-associated toxicity necessitate exploring novel strategies, especially those that can be personalized for specific patients and/or populations. Here, we review the current landscape and progress of standard therapies and explore what personalized oncology techniques may entail in the scope of melanoma. Our purpose is to provide an up-to-date summary of the tools at our disposal that work to circumvent the common barriers faced when battling melanoma.

Keywords: melanoma; metastatic treatment; precision oncology; targeted therapy; vaccine; immunotherapies; adoptive cell therapy; personalized medicine

1. Introduction

Cutaneous melanoma remains the most aggressive and deadliest form of skin cancer, with a survival rate of less than 10%, despite recent advances in therapy [1]. Four major subtypes of cutaneous melanoma have been established according to the presence of specific somatic mutations occurring in different oncogenes (Figure 1): (1) the B-Raf proto-oncogene serine-threonine kinase (BRAF) mutant, (2) the NRAS proto-oncogene GTPase (NRAS) mutant, (3) the neurofibromin-1 (NF1) tumor suppressor mutant, and (4) the triple BRAF/NRAS/NF1 wildtype (WT) form that does not contain mutations in any of the three oncogenes [2,3]. An overwhelming proportion of melanomas harbor hotspot mutations in either the BRAF or NRAS oncogenes—over 50% and approximately 20–25% of melanomas, respectively [4–6]. Patients with metastatic BRAF-mutant melanoma have an estimated survival of 6–10 months after diagnosis without current drug therapy intervention [7].

Each melanoma case is categorized based on the 2009 TNM (Tumor, Node, Metastasis) staging system derived by the American Joint Committee on Cancer (AJCC). The AJCC system stages disease on a scale of stage I–V, where patients may present with solely a primary tumor/local disease (I–II), node-positive disease (III), or advanced or metastatic disease (IV). These stages consider the extent of the primary tumor in terms of thickness and the possible presence of ulceration (T), an investigation of spread to nearby lymph nodes (N), and metastatic spread (M) [1,8]. Although surgical resection can successfully treat patients with melanoma in the earlier stages [3], those diagnosed with stage IV/late-stage, metastatic, or unresectable melanoma have historically faced limited treatment options and dismal prognoses. An optimal treatment strategy is based on somatic mutational status and the patient's clinical presentation (e.g., toxicity profiles, disease dissemination, serum lactate dehydrogenase) [4,9]. To date, two types of systemic therapies have been identified as the most efficacious treatment option for advanced and high-risk early-stage melanoma: targeted therapy and immune checkpoint inhibitors (ICIs). Targeted therapy employs small-molecule inhibitors, notably BRAF kinase and mitogen-activated protein kinase inhibitors (BRAFis and MAPKis), selectively designed to inhibit targets in the MAPK pathway [10]. Meanwhile, the development of ICIs allows for the pharmacological manipulation of the immune response, reactivating T cells to inhibit tumor cell evasion [9].

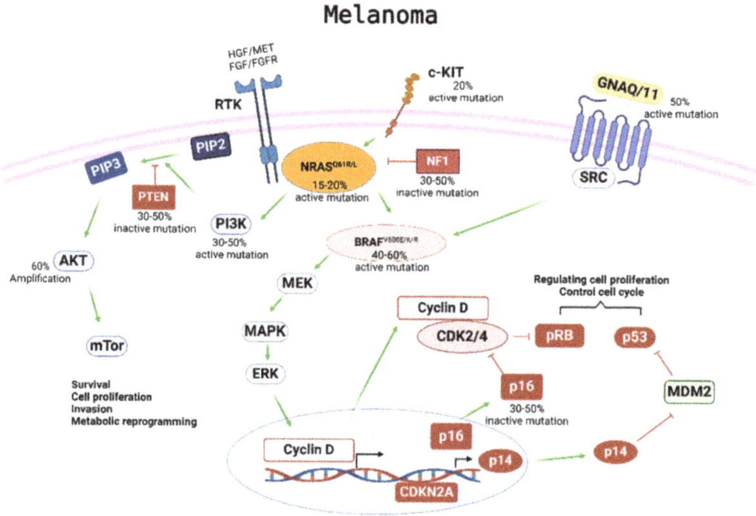

Figure 1. Melanoma development and progression are driven by multiple driver gene mutations. Four major subtypes of cutaneous melanoma have been established according to specific somatic mutations in different oncogenes, including BRAF, NRAS, NF1, c-KIT4, and GNAQ/11. These somatic mutations activate the phosphoinositide 3-kinase/protein kinase B (PI3K/AKT) and mitogen-activated protein kinase (MAPK) pathways, resulting in melanoma development and progression. Mutations in BRAF can impact the MAPK pathway and have downstream effects on cell proliferation and cell cycle control. Mutations in NRAS can affect both the MAPK and the PI3K/AKT pathways, which regulate cell survival, proliferation, invasion, and metabolic programming. Overactivation of these pathways can contribute to the tumorigenesis, proliferation, invasion, and metastasis of melanoma cells, as well as drug resistance to applied therapies.

Cutaneous melanomas have high mutational burdens, making this disease a prime candidate for adoptive cellular therapy (ACT) of either tumor-infiltrating lymphocytes (TILs) or chimeric antigen receptor T (CAR-T) cells [1,11–14]. From a treatment perspective, TIL therapy is behind MAPKi targeted therapy and ICI therapy, especially for treatment-refractory patients. CAR-T therapy may be particularly helpful for metastatic and targeted-therapy-resistant melanoma patients [1,11,12]. However, while it has higher specificity than MAPKi targeted therapy, CAR-T therapy has more dangerous potential side effects, such as cytokine release syndrome (CRS) [11,12,14]. The review aims to recapitulate an up-to-date overview of where we stand regarding the scope of precision oncology techniques, describe what we can expect in terms of the future landscape by challenging what is already known in the field, and provide recommendations for ways to circumvent the crucial dead ends we currently face in the treatment of advanced melanoma.

2. Biomarkers for Personalized Targeted Therapy

The molecular composition of the tumor and the tumor microenvironment (TME) play an important role in the progression of cutaneous melanoma. The different subtypes of melanoma can vary widely in their properties, consequently affecting treatment and patient survival benefits.

2.1. BRAF and MEK-Related Biomarkers

BRAF, along with CRAF, is a member of the Raf family protein and plays a role in the MAPK signaling pathway via downstream activation of MEK and, subsequently, ERK. BRAF is a serine-threonine-specific kinase whose most common mutation occurs at codon 600 in melanoma. Approximately 80% of these missense mutations involve the substitution of a Valine (V) for a Glutamate (E) in the activation loop, known as $BRAF^{V600E}$ mutations [4]. The remaining portion of mutations can include V600 substitutions for a Lysine (K) ($BRAF^{V600K}$) or an Arginine (R) ($BRAF^{V600R}$) [4]. Importantly, these substitutions initiate a constitutional activation of the MAPK pathway, leading to the overactive growth of BRAF-mutant melanoma cells. BRAF mutations typically develop from external environmental causes (e.g., UV radiation from the sun), and as such, it is very rare for this to be an inherited mutation [15].

Patients with BRAF-mutant melanomas have historically demonstrated an initial benefit from the pharmacological inhibition of mutant BRAF and/or MEK. Current targeted therapies include the first FDA-approved BRAF inhibitors (BRAFis) vemurafenib (PLX-4032, approved in 2011) and dabrafenib (GSK2118436, approved in 2013) [16]. These BRAFis can be taken orally and have high selective binding to the ATP-binding site of BRAF mutants V600E, V600D, V600K, and V600R [15]. Multiple studies have shown that both vemurafenib and dabrafenib improved patient outcomes when used as monotherapies against $BRAF^{V600E}$ unresectable or metastatic melanoma relative to the prior therapy standard of chemotherapy [17,18]. The most recent BRAFi to gain FDA approval was encorafenib in 2018 [19]. In tandem with BRAFis, MEK inhibitors (MEKis) have been developed to target a downstream molecule of the BRAF kinase and produce a longer-lasting effect on progression-free survival (PFS). There are currently three main FDA-approved MEKis: trametinib (2013), cobimetinib (2015), and binimetinib (2018) [16,20]. MEKis can target both forms of MEK (MEK1 and MEK2), generally through allosteric binding that inhibits MEK recruitment, phosphorylation, release, or affinity with BRAF [21]. As with BRAFi monotherapy, pharmacological inhibition by the MEKi trametinib has been shown to have a significant survival benefit compared to chemotherapy [22]. Treatment with BRAFis and MEKis is not without difficulty, as patients typically fail to remain disease-free long term due to the development of resistance to these inhibitors. Using BRAFis and MEKis in combination has yielded some improvements—common combinations include dabrafenib and trametinib, vemurafenib and cobimetinib, and encorafenib and binimetinib [23]. However, drug resistance is still prevalent and has become a critical factor in the search to develop new immunotherapies.

Furthermore, clinicians have found that having a BRAF mutation alone is insufficient to cause melanomagenesis; an inactivating PTEN (phosphatase and tensin homolog deleted from chromosome 10) mutation is also required [24,25]. PTEN, a protein that works in opposition to PI3K to dephosphorylate PIP3 to PIP2, is also known to inhibit BRAF's kinase expression and therefore regulate downstream MAPK signaling [25,26]. Evidence indicates an association between BRAF and PTEN mutations, with PTEN inactivation being one of the most common causes of resistance to BRAF inhibitors [27–30] (Figure 2). Catalanotti et al. [31] observed similar findings where patients with PTEN loss-of-function melanoma had reduced survival and response rates. Moreover, melanomas with inactivation of PTEN or activated PI3K/AKT have a higher potential of metastasis [32–34]. These results highlight the potential of PI3K inhibitors, in combination with BRAF and MEK inhibitors, to treat BRAF-mutant patients regardless of their PTEN status.

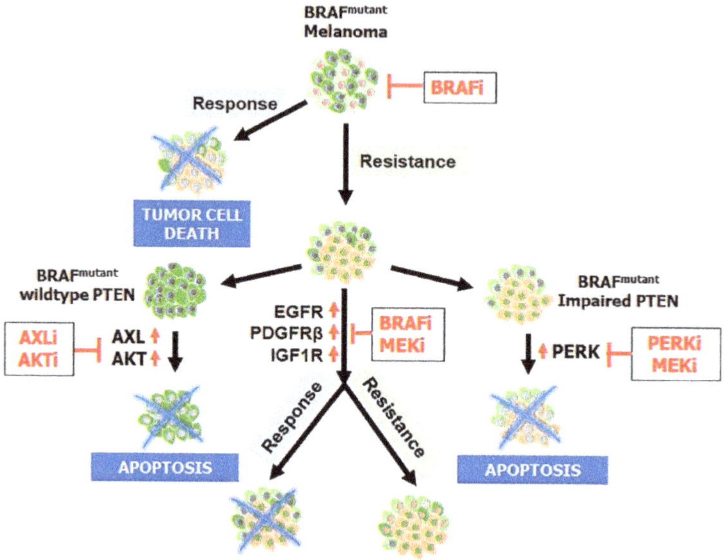

Figure 2. Targeted therapy and mechanism of resistance. Treatment with BRAFis causes programmed cell death in melanoma patients whose cancer has a BRAF^{V600E} mutation. Resistance to BRAFis can arise as tumor cells overexpress EGFR, PDGFRβ, and IGF1R, creating an alternative survival pathway. Treatment with a combination of BRAFis–MEKis can result in programmed cell death but may also lead to double resistance to these therapies. The molecular mechanism mediating resistance may depend on PTEN status in BRAF-mutant melanoma. In melanoma with wild-type PTEN, AXL and AKT activation are elevated and can confer resistance to BRAFis; treatment with AXLi and AKTi can block further tumor growth. In contrast, melanoma with impaired PTEN is associated with decreased AKT activation; the MAPK/ERK pathway is reactivated as the core drug resistance pathway and is responsive to treatment with PERKis and MEKis.

To circumvent BRAFi and MEKi double resistance, their upstream and downstream targets are also a focus for clinicians. For example, SHP2 (Src homology region 2 domain-containing phosphatase-2), linking receptor tyrosine kinases, and the MAPK signaling pathway have been reported to increase in melanoma samples [35]. Specifically, within the melanoma microenvironment, Zhang et al. [36] reported that SHP2 positively regulates ERK and AKT signaling and, therefore, melanoma proliferation and survival. When SHP2 is targeted in vivo by an inhibitor such as 11a-1, melanoma xenograft tumor growth is suppressed. SHP2 is upstream of the alternate pathways, such as AKT and mTOR, and is employed by BRAFi–MEKi double-resistant melanoma samples, suggesting that SHP2 inhibition can effectively treat BRAFi and MEKi double-resistant cells.

While BRAF and MEK inhibition is a common tactic for treating melanoma, ERK-specific targeting has been rare despite its placement downstream of both BRAF and MEK, which has a more direct effect on the genetic and proliferative effects of the MAPK signaling pathway. Some researchers have developed ERK inhibitors (ERKis), such as SCH772984, which are highly selective and can be used as a viable supplement in combination with BRAFis and MEKis or replace them in subsequent acquired BRAFi–MEKi double resistance. Morris et al. [37] noted that SCH772984 effectively treated melanoma cells with and without BRAFi and MEKi resistance because the alternate pathways used in double resistance are often associated with ERK reactivation. However, if ERKi resistance develops, the resulting melanoma samples may prove to be even more challenging to treat due to the limited knowledge of alternate pathways subsequent to ERK.

An additional factor in BRAF mutation melanoma survival is the level of autophagy present in melanoma samples. Abnormal rates of autophagy and its related genes such as *Atg5* and *Sqstm1/p62* have been found within BRAF-mutant melanoma samples [38]. For example, although both genes are known to promote autophagy, Karras et al. [39] found *Atg5* to decrease with heterozygous deletions, while *Sqstm1/p62* expression was amplified in proliferative melanoma. However, the relationship between melanoma proliferation and autophagy is not solely based on genetics. Many factors, such as ER stress, can influence autophagy. Ma et al. [40] showed that the addition of BRAF inhibitors to melanoma cells caused an increase in autophagy due to the binding of mutant BRAF to the ER stress gatekeeper GRP78. Subsequent BRAF and autophagy inhibition via hydroxychloroquine caused a reduction in tumors in BRAFi-resistant cells. Other studies have noted that autophagy may be tumor-suppressive in the early stages of tumor development and then become tumorigenic in later stages [41].

Another approach that could be considered to improve the current state of BRAF and MEK inhibitory therapies is the use of predictive biomarkers to guide treatment decisions between patients [42]. For example, markers of tumor burden, such as serum lactate dehydrogenase levels and the number of organ sites with metastatic features, were correlated with better outcomes in PFS and overall survival (OS) in patients that received combination therapy of dabrafenib and trametinib [43]. The discovery of new oncogenic driver mutations as potential biomarkers may help predict responses for targeted therapies in certain patient populations.

2.2. Non-BRAF and MEK-Related Biomarkers

Melanomas with mutations in NRAS, the second most prevalent mutated proto-oncogene in melanoma, are characteristically more aggressive and susceptible to developing resistance to treatment when compared to BRAF mutants [2,5]. Unlike BRAF mutants, melanoma harboring an NRAS mutation alters GTP hydrolysis to consequently activate the MAPK, PI3K, and RAS-like protein guanine nucleotide exchange factor (GEF) signaling pathways [5]. In total, 90% of NRAS mutations in melanomas are NRAS^{Q61R} [44]. In these melanomas, MAPK is activated via CRAF, not BRAF, and these tumors also have aberrant cyclin-dependent kinase (CDK) 4/6 expression and hyperactivated PI3K/AKT signaling. Currently, the standard of care for NRAS-mutant patients involves anti-PD-1-based immunotherapy (see below) as the first line of treatment, with the second line of treatment including MEK and CTLA-4 inhibitors, albeit with varying degrees of success [45]. The lack of druggable pockets within RAS makes it hard to develop RAS-specific inhibitors [2], although recent structural studies of mutant KRAS offer promising new therapeutic strategies [46]. Another study using the FAK inhibitor defactinib, Del Mistro et al. [47] demonstrated that the inhibition of FAK can desensitize melanoma cells regardless of BRAF/NRAS mutational status. While the efficacy of defactinib is not certain, clinical trials are currently being conducted employing defactinib to treat metastatic melanoma and other cancers in a phase II trial (NCT04270417) [48].

Other non-V600 BRAF mutants, which have been reported in up to 14% of melanoma patients, are very rare, and therefore, little is known about their available treatment [49]. Since these melanomas can often activate the MAPK pathway through uncommon means, such as CRAF, pan-RAF inhibitors, like sorafenib and AZ628, have been explored on non-V600 BRAF-mutant melanoma samples [50]. Molnár et al. [50] reported that a combination of sorafenib or AZ628 and selumetinib, an MEK inhibitor, can effectively combat non-V600 BRAF-mutant melanoma in preclinical mouse models. Furthermore, recent clinical trials, such as the phase I trial (NCT01425008) by Rasco et al. [51], investigated the safety and anti-tumor activity of tovorafenib, another pan-RAF inhibitor and showed encouraging results. In all, these studies represent promising steps forward for the use of pan-RAF inhibitors on not only BRAF^{V600E} but also BRAF-wild type and CRAF-wild type melanoma patients.

CDK4/6 is another molecule involved in the development of melanoma [52]. The common role of CDK4/6 is to bind with Cyclin-D1, enter the nucleus, and hyperphosphorylate the retinoblastoma (RB) protein; this results in the release of the transcription factor E2F, which drives the transcription of genes for cell cycle progression. In melanoma, multiple mutations can affect CDK4/6 activity and increase proliferation by promoting the G1-S transition [53]. Interestingly, CDK4/6 can be activated beyond the MAPK pathway via the estrogen receptor (ER) signaling pathway, which is common in breast cancer [54,55]. Because CDK4/6 inhibitors have already been developed and effectively used to treat breast cancer tumors, clinicians are testing the efficacy of CDK4/6 inhibitors in combination with other inhibitors to combat melanoma. For example, Yoshida et al. [56] discovered that vemurafenib-resistant tumors were still sensitive to palbociclib (a CDK4/6 inhibitor). This has been further explored by Jost et al. [57], who found that palbociclib induced cell cycle arrest in melanoma cells when used in combination with radiotherapy. These findings have identified CDK4/6 as another potential path for treating patients with BRAFi- and MEKi-resistant melanoma.

AXL, a tyrosine kinase receptor, is another potential target due to its notable elevated expression in many cancers, including melanoma [29,58]. Once bound by a ligand, AXL will activate downstream signaling pathways that affect cell cycle progression, including the PI3K/AKT pathway. AXL is involved in many crucial roles in cancer development, including cell movement, immunosuppression, and epithelial–mesenchymal transitions (EMTs) [59]. AXL expression is also correlated with acquired MAPK resistance [29], including BRAFi/MEKi double resistance, and targeting AXL cooperatively inhibited tumor growth with BRAF/MEK inhibitors in patient-derived xenografts [60]. Recent in vitro studies have shown that the knockdown of AXL by siRNA or its inhibitor bemcentinib in melanoma cells decreased migration and invasion [58,61]. A phase II study (NCT02872259) comparing the efficacy of the standard melanoma treatment of dabrafenib, trametinib, and pembrolizumab with or without bemcentinib in patients with phase III or IV melanoma is currently ongoing [62].

Notably, most of the NF1 mutations associated with melanoma result in loss of function in the NF1 gene, classifying it as a tumor suppressor [63]. Approximately 12–18% of melanoma patients have mutations in NF1, which are most common in elderly and sun-exposed individuals. This protein has a GTPase-activating protein-related domain that negatively regulates RAS-GTP to the inactive RAS-GDP form, thus inhibiting the progression of the MAPK pathway. Current treatments of NF1-mutant melanomas rely on targeting other proteins, such as MEK and anti-PD-1 therapy [64,65].

Met (mesenchymal–epithelial transition factor receptor), along with its paracrine-induced ligand HGF (hepatocyte growth factor), is another signaling pathway that has been targeted for melanoma therapy [66,67]. Like with other kinase receptors, abnormal activities of Met and HGF have been associated with cancers such as melanoma. What is unique about Met in melanoma cell lines is that HGF is secreted via autocrine and paracrine signaling [68], often leading to a positive feedback loop of growth [69]. Drug inhibitors for the Met/HGF signaling pathway, such as crizotinib, tivantinib, and quercetin, are undergoing experimental trials with promising results [70]. For example, using tumor samples from melanoma patients, Das et al. [71] demonstrated that a combination of crizotinib and a tyrosine kinase inhibitor, afatinib, reduced melanoma tumor growth, regardless of BRAF/NRAS mutational status. Additionally, PHA665752, a drug that blocks MET phosphorylation, has shown to be effective in targeting NRAS-mutant cells during in vitro studies, indicating the broader effectiveness of Met inhibitors in treating various melanoma subtypes, not only the common $BRAF^{V600E}$ mutant [72].

2.3. Melanoma-Stem-Cell (MSC)-Related Biomarkers

With recent advancements in our growing knowledge of stem cells, general biomarkers associated with melanoma stem cells (MSCs) have been elucidated, including CD133 [73], CD271 [74], and ABCB5 [75]. Targeting MSC biomarkers is expected to benefit patients with melanoma. For example, CD133, a critical biomarker of MSC to maintain stemness properties and drug resistance, is reported to be upregulated in melanoma and involved in tumor growth, angiogenesis, and metastasis via mechanisms of PI3K/AKT and MAPK activation [76], suggesting inhibition of PI3K/AKT and/or MAPK signaling pathways not only targets melanoma with BRAF and NRAS or other gene mutations but also battles MSCs [29,30,33,76]. Knockdown of CD133 expression in NRAS-mutant melanoma promoted cell apoptosis and improved trametinib efficacy in the NRAS-mutant cells [77]. A recent study reported that a vaccine against MSCs ($CD44^{+}CD133^{+}$ cells) stimulates immune response and inhibits melanoma growth and metastasis in vivo [78]. However, due to these biomarkers exhibiting other types of cancer as well as normal stem cells, studies should assess tolerability and efficacy.

2.4. Non-Genomic Biomarkers in the Melanoma Microenvironment

Beyond a high mutation rate, melanoma often rewires its metabolism program through non-genomic regulation to provide a favorable tumor microenvironment (TME) for supporting tumor cell growth and suppressing immune surveillance [11,12,79]. Targeting the vulnerabilities of metabolism may improve melanoma therapy. For example, NRAS-mutated melanoma cells reprogram a quiescent metabolic program to avoid MEK-inhibition-induced cell apoptosis [80] with increased reactive oxygen species (ROS) levels, making these cells highly sensitive to ROS induction. Thus, treatment with an ROS inducer and an MEK inhibitor inhibited tumor growth and metastasis [80]. Studies have shown that melanoma patients with high levels of lactate dehydrogenase (LDH) often have a worse prognosis and low response to checkpoint therapy, implicating that inhibition of LDH may provide an opportunity to modulate the TME favorably. Treating patient-derived melanoma with a lactate dehydrogenase A (LDHA) inhibitor, GSK2837808A, showed T-cell antitumor cytotoxicity. Recently, a compound AZD3965 developed to target MCT1 and MCT4 of LDH transporters is under investigation in a clinical trail (NCT01791595) [81]. Within the TME, fibroblasts also make functional shifts to cancer-associated fibroblasts (CAFs), which are known to support melanoma immune evasion and tumor growth via many proteins, including FBLN1 and COL5A1 [82]. Inhibiting the expression of FBLN1 and COL5A1 by mifepristone and dexamethasone drugs has potentially improved patient outcomes [82]. Furthermore, antibody–drug conjugate ABBV-085 against LRRC15 of the new CAF biomarker showed significant antitumor activity with minimal toxicity [83]. In addition to melanoma in the TME, circulating tumor cells (CTCs) are proposed to have dominant mitochondria-mediated oxidative phosphorylation (OXPHOS) [84], suggesting anti-OXPHOS may prevent melanoma metastasis.

3. Advances in Immunotherapy

3.1. Immune Checkpoint Inhibitors (ICIs)

Currently, the preference for the clinical treatment of advanced and high-risk, early-stage melanoma is ICI therapy [85]. This systemic therapy offers a unique advantage by not only inducing cancer cell eradication but also by extending survival through anti-cancer maintenance that improves overall survival with some first-line ICIs, making it the preferential treatment for most metastatic melanoma cases [86]. ICIs can ultimately block the tumor's ability to escape the immune system.

The first immune checkpoint to be identified in treating cancer was cytotoxic T lymphocyte-associated protein 4 (CTLA-4), which competes with the costimulatory molecule CD28 for ligands CD80 and/or CD86 (collectively known as B7 ligands) [19,87]. In contrast to CD28, CTLA-4 has a greater binding affinity and avidity for these two ligands. The ensuing deprivation of costimulatory signals to T cells was eventually linked to the finding that anti-CTLA-4 antibodies result in tumor regression in preclinical mouse models [88]. Ipilimumab, tremelimumab, and BCD-145 are the three major anti-CTLA-4 human monoclonal antibodies for use against metastatic melanoma and are currently undergoing preclinical and clinical trials [19,89].

Secondly, programmed cell death protein 1 (PD-1) and its ligand programmed cell death ligand 1 (PD-L1) are other immune checkpoints for standard melanoma immunotherapy. $CD8^+$ exhausted T (T_{EX}) cells lose effector function during the antigen stimulation process for malignancies. By blocking PD-1 and, by extension, PD-L1, the effector functions of $CD8^+$ T cells can be restored, resulting in improved tumor control [87]. In 2014, anti-PD-1 antibodies pembrolizumab and nivolumab were granted FDA approval for clinical use against metastatic melanoma. These ICIs have been joined by several other anti-PD-1/PD-L1 antibodies, including avelumab, durvalumab, cemiplimab, atezolizumab, and cosibelimab [19]. Additionally, while ICIs were initially approved for use as monotherapies, recent evidence has shown that combining multiple immunotherapies can result in an augmented anti-tumor response and a greater degree of long-term efficacy. Thus, there has been increasing interest in a combined anti-PD-1/PD-L1 and anti-CTLA-4 checkpoint blockade for the treatment of melanoma [90]. For example, a phase Ib/2 trial (NCT02535078) found that the combination of tebentafusp with durvalumab and/or tremelimumab is effective in treating advanced or metastatic melanoma [89]. The current landscape regarding anti-CTLA-4 and anti-PD-1/PD-L1 therapy focuses on optimizing dosages and reducing associated toxicity events, which are not insignificant in the clinic. A significant phase III trial testing the combination of ipilimumab and nivolumab indicated that it was effective in treating both advanced melanoma and melanoma that has metastasized to the brain [91]. Interestingly, patients in this study with BRAF mutations fared better than those with wild-type BRAF. van Zeijl et al. [91] report that this was most likely due to BRAF-mutant patients also receiving BRAFi and MEKi (dabrafenib and trametinib, respectively) treatment.

Success surrounding the use of the aforementioned ICIs has led to the continuing identification of novel immune checkpoint molecules. Lymphocyte activation gene-3 (LAG-3, also named CD223) is a surface inhibitory receptor with structural similarities to CD4 and is a promising new target for immune checkpoint blockade [9,87,92]. The suppressive function of LAG-3 is contributed to by its constitutive overexpression on regulatory T cells (T_{REGS}) [92]. At present, relatlimab is the most developed anti-LAG-3 antibody, and a randomized double-blind phase II/III trial (NCT03470922) is currently investigating its effectiveness in combination with anti-PD-1 antibodies, principally nivolumab, in several tumor models, including melanoma [93]. According to the study's findings, relatlimab paired with nivolumab results in improved PFS compared to nivolumab monotherapy [94]. It remains unclear which combination ICI therapy has better antitumor efficacy while simultaneously decreasing toxicity levels. Further clinical trials, such as the phase I trial (NCT04140500) investigating the effect of a bispecific anti-PD-1 and anti-LAG-3 antibody (RO7247669) on solid tumors, may validate the above conclusions and expand the treatment options for patients with melanoma [95,96].

While the management of advanced solid tumors has been significantly impacted by the increasing availability of ICIs [97], many patients either do not respond to immunotherapy or experience adverse outcomes. Thus, it is also important to explore other potential biomarkers and develop further combination treatments that may improve response rates and outcomes [97]. B7 homolog 3 protein (B7-H3) is currently being explored as a target for next-generation cancer immunotherapy, entering many clinical trials as a therapeutic target [98]. B7-H3 has been found to be overexpressed in many solid cancers (including melanoma) and is a biomarker of disease severity and recurrence [99]. MGC018, a duocarmycin-based antibody–drug conjugate targeting B7-H3, has displayed potential antitumor activity in preclinical melanoma models with a favorable pharmacokinetic safety profile [99]. In the phase I/II clinical trial, the dual blockade of B7-H3 and PD-1 with enoblituzumab and pembrolizumab has demonstrated acceptable safety and antitumor activity in patients with solid tumors [97]. However, there has been a limited response in patients with cutaneous melanoma, with only one out of thirteen patients exhibiting a partial response.

T-cell immunoreceptors with immunoglobulin and the immunoreceptor tyrosine-based inhibition motif domain (TIGIT) and its ligand CD155 are also being explored as a new immune checkpoint target for their role in delivery inhibition signals to T cells, NK cells, and regulatory T cells [100]. TIGIT expression can be closely associated with melanoma occurrence, development, and prognosis; consequently, decreased TIGIT expression is associated with inhibited tumor growth in melanoma patients. The TIGIT/CD155 axis has also been implicated in mediating resistance to ICIs, where TIGIT blockade or CD155 deletion in activated T cells has aided in overcoming ICI resistance [101]. CD96, a receptor protein that can regulate NK cell effector function and metastasis, is also of note as it can interact with CD155, and blocking CD96 can suppress primary tumor growth in mouse tumor models [102]. The addition of anti-CD96 in combination with anti-PD-1, anti-CTLA-4, anti-TIGIT, or doxorubicin chemotherapy resulted in superior antitumor responses by enhancing T-cell activity and suppressing tumor growth [102,103].

T-cell immunoglobulin domain and mucin domain-3 (TIM-3) is another biomarker of interest, as its ligand (Galectin-9), along with PD-L1, are both upregulated during tumor progression [104]. Prokopi et al. [104] found that boosting DC in combination with anti-PD-1 and anti-TIM-3 therapy improved T-cell function within tumors and delayed tumor growth. A phase I/Ib clinical trial has demonstrated that the combination treatment of sabatolimab (MBG453) and spartalizumab, monoclonal antibodies that can bind to TIM-3 and PD-1, respectively, can be well tolerated and show preliminary signs of antitumor activity in advanced solid tumors, including one patient with malignant perianal melanoma [105]. Additionally, a novel melanoma-stem-cell vaccine has been developed that can suppress the expression of CTLA-4, PD-1, and TIM-3 and delay the progression of melanoma by inducing antitumor immune responses [78].

Human leukocyte antigen G (HLA-G) is also of note as it is one of the genes found to be commonly upregulated in premetastatic brain-metastasis-initiating cells (BMICs) [106]. HLA-G was found to function in an HLA-G/SPAG9/STAT3 axis that promotes the establishment of brain metastatic lesions. Overall, identifying clinically relevant biomarkers can inform the development of next-generation immunotherapies [106]. Characterizing a patient's relevant biomarkers can reveal the optimal treatment strategy for each patient.

3.2. *Adoptive Cellular Therapy (ACT)*

In the scope of advanced cutaneous melanoma, adoptive cellular therapy (ACT) is a relatively new treatment approach that is geared toward treatment-refractory patients who have exhausted all approved therapy options [13,107–109]. ACT is a subsection of immunotherapy that relies on the internal and external manipulation of patients' immune systems to construct a personalized approach to treating metastatic or unresectable solid tumors [13,108]. In brief, endogenous immune (T or NK) cells are isolated from the patient, selected, and expanded ex vivo before reintroduction into the patient [108]. The current state of the ACT field can be broken down between the growing developments of two major techniques: tumor-infiltrating lymphocyte (TIL) and chimeric antigen receptor (CAR-T) therapies. One of the significant differences between TIL-based ACT and CAR-T therapy is the type of cells that are ultimately reintroduced to the patient. TILs express unmodified endogenous T-cell receptors (TCRs), while CAR-T therapy uses TCRs that have been synthetically modified to recognize a specific antigen [13,108].

3.2.1. Tumor-Infiltrating Lymphocytes (TILs)

The transformation from normal to malignant cells is facilitated by a multitude of genetic mutations and changes to the TME that result in heterogeneity differences between the tumors of patients, even in those diagnosed with similar malignancies [108]. Developing personalized therapies that account for these tumor-specific characteristics is of utmost importance. Recently, autologous tumor-infiltrating lymphocytes (TILs), or TIL-based ACT, have been developed based on this concept. TIL-based ACT follows a three-step workflow: (i) isolation of TILs from tumor excision, (ii) rapid ex vivo expansion of TILs, and (iii) infusion of TILs back into the lymphodepleted patient during hospitalization [13,108].

While TILs can recognize many targets in cancer and TIL-based therapy remains the preferential treatment option for most metastatic melanoma cases, some significant limitations prevent TIL-based ACT from expanding as a widely used treatment option for patients. These challenges include the manufacturing requirements of TILs, treatment-related toxicity events, and treatment resistance. First, TIL production is both labor-intensive and complex, and thus only available primarily to well-funded medical centers that can accommodate the necessary technology to handle the TIL workflow and potential treatment-emergent adverse events (TEAs) that could occur during patient hospitalization. It is imperative to centrally expand the manufacturing process of TIL products as it could allow for a widespread application of TIL-based ACT that is both cost-effective and accessible, such as Iovance Biotherapeutics and their development of a central manufacturing facility that produces Lifileucel, a cryopreserved, autologous TIL product [108,109]. Encouragingly, the FDA has recently approved lifileucel (Amtagvi) for advanced melanoma.

Second, reinfusion also requires the patient to undergo a pre-conditioning regimen—the side effects of which make up most reported treatment-related toxicities. These toxicities can either be cytokine-related toxicities, resulting from the high levels of IL-2 frequently given with TIL therapy to enhance the lymphocytes' antitumor activity, or rare autoimmune-related toxicities, commonly caused by the non-specific expression of tumor-associated antigens on non-cancer cells that can become targeted by reintroduced lymphocytes [110,111]. This preparative lymphodepleting regimen, comprising a combination of cyclophosphamide and fludarabine, has been shown to increase the effectiveness of TIL-based ACT, although the cellular mechanisms are not fully understood at this time and the tradeoff in terms of severe toxicities is substantial [13].

Finally, the use of TILs, as in many cases, is vulnerable to resistance. Both innate and acquired resistance are prevalent, where innate resistance refers to observed unresponsiveness following the initial therapy administration, and acquired resistance refers to a developed resistance that presents itself after a patient's previous positive response [108]. The mechanisms resulting in these resistance types can be broken down into four main distinctions: (1) curated T cells fail to recognize tumor cells effectively, (2) interference from immunosuppressive cells in the TME, (3) TME-driven T-cell dysfunction and/or exhaustion, and (4) restrictions in T-cell migration to the tumor [13,108]. While the mechanisms underlying these resistance phenomena are becoming better understood, work remains to be done to further optimize the curation of TILs. Promisingly, current work has focused on combining TIL therapy with other therapies, such as the prospective randomized phase II trial (NCT02621021) currently in progress that seeks to understand if the addition of pembrolizumab with TIL/IL-2 therapy can improve response rates in metastatic melanoma patients [112].

3.2.2. Chimeric Antigen Receptor (CAR) T-Cell Therapy

Chimeric antigen receptor (CAR) T-cell therapy, one of the first personalized techniques commercially available to the clinical population, involves three main stages to generate clinically utilizable CAR T cells: selection, expansion, and harvesting [113]. During the selection stage, T cells collected from the patient via leukapheresis undergo monocyte elutriation to remove other cell types (e.g., myeloid, natural killer, erythroid, and malignant cells) and allow for efficient extraction and isolation [113]. The selected T-cell product is then activated and genetically transduced with a viral vector that encodes for the tumor-antigen-specific CAR construct. The T-cell product is then expanded ex vivo to generate a high yield of engineered cells before being harvested to form the final CAR-T cell product that is reinfused back into the patient [113]. Like TIL-based ACT, patients must receive conditioning chemotherapy to deplete autologous lymphocytes and immunosuppressive cells [114]. Two CAR-T cell constructs for the CD19 protein—tisagenlecleucel (Kymriah, Novartis, Basel, Switzerland) and axicabtagene ciloleucel (Yescarta, Kite, Foster City, CA, USA)—have recently been approved for the treatment of B cell lymphoma. Axicabtagene was noted to have a slightly higher 12-month overall survival than tisagenlecleucel (51% and 47%, respectively), but they both had similar efficacy [115].

CAR-T cell research currently focuses on translating this success to solid cancer tumors. CAR constructs can recognize whole surface proteins on cancer cells without relying on the presentation of the major histocompatibility complex (MHC) and antigen processing [1]. The ability of these constructs to function in a non-MHC-restricted manner makes this subset of adoptive cell therapy a promising option for the immunogenic features of melanoma [116]. CAR constructs express chimeric antigen receptors with three main domains of interest: extracellular, transmembrane, and intracellular. The extracellular domain houses the single-chain variable fragment (scFv), which is composed of an antibody-variable heavy chain (V_H) and an antibody-variable light chain (V_L) that have been fused together by a peptide linker [116]. This scFv domain is further linked to the intracellular CD3ζ domain through the transmembrane domain. CAR constructs are classified into generations, where first-generation constructs contain only the CD3ζdomain while ensuing generations have increasing numbers of additional co-stimulatory molecules (i.e., CD28, 4-1BB, OX-40) [1]. While CAR-T cell therapy has shown promising results for hematological malignancies [1,116], initial attempts at using CAR-T cell therapy to treat other cancers have not been as successful [117–119]. Specifically in metastatic melanoma, challenges include (1) selecting an optimal antigen target and (2) the influence of the immunosuppressive TME [116].

First, selecting an optimal antigen target has the dual goal of inducing an anti-tumor immune response while producing the lowest amount of off-target toxicity and immune side effects for patients. This off-target toxicity is commonly observed when the target antigen is expressed in both healthy tissue and malignant tumor tissue; consequently, multiple targets whose expression is limited to malignant tissues alone have been identified [12,120,121]. For example, CD248 is a type I transmembrane glycoprotein that is either not expressed or minimally expressed in healthy tissues [1,121]. Interestingly, CD248 has been reported to play a role in tumor vasculature and was expressed in 86% of metastatic melanoma samples analyzed by tumor microarrays [120]. Another potential target is chondroitin sulfate proteoglycan 4 (CSPG4), also known as melanoma chondroitin sulfate proteoglycan (MSCP), which is expressed in 90% of melanomas as well as in sarcomas and gliomas but rarely expressed in healthy tissues [122,123]. Whether CD248 and CSPG4 could be optimal antigen targets for metastatic melanoma in CAR-T cell therapy remains to be validated. Thus, future preclinical investigations for potential use in a clinical setting remain necessary to select the proper target antigens. Immune side effects of CAR-T cell therapies include cytokine release syndrome (CRS), encephalopathy syndrome (CRES), and immune effector cell-associated neurotoxicity (ICANS), which—with appropriate treatment and observation by clinicians—can be minimized and even reversible [124].

Second, the TME refers to the complex environment surrounding each cancer cell. Several properties of the TME (e.g., extracellular matrix, cytokines, growth factors, hypoxic conditions, common cell types such as fibroblast and immune cells) are unfavorable for CAR-T cell therapy as they can reduce the potency of the anti-tumor response and allow for continued tumor growth and invasion [1,125,126]. To combat this, significant attempts have been made to modify the CAR constructs in solid tumors like melanoma by blocking the activation of inhibitory immune checkpoint receptors on T cells, with the most common of these receptors being PD-1 and CLTA-4. Successful attempts include stable knockouts of the inhibitory receptors via CRISPR/Cas-9 and the development of CAR-T cells that are capable of constitutively secreting immune checkpoint inhibitors [127–129]. For example, Marotte et al. [130] designed PD-1 knockout TCR-engineered T cells specific for the Melan-A antigen. Their findings revealed these engineered T cells garnered higher anti-tumor efficacy and delayed PD-L1-positive melanoma tumor progression in mouse models. Given the already established role of immune checkpoint blockade as standard therapy in advanced melanoma cases, there is the potential for combination therapy that pairs anti-PD-1 and anti-CTLA-4 antibodies with ACT to produce better clinical outcomes;

some studies with lymphoma and malignant plural disease patients have already begun to move in this direction [131,132].

CAR-T cell therapy brings an innovative technique to the multifaceted space of cancer immunotherapy. Still, various barriers continue to prevent this from becoming a standard therapy in the treatment of melanoma and other solid tumors. The use of newly engineered CAR-T cells, the discovery of suitable target antigens, and combination therapy techniques to alter the TME aim to eliminate these obstacles and guide the future clinical use of CAR-T cell therapy in melanoma. Additionally, natural killer cells with chimeric antigen receptors (CAR-NK cells) are a recent development in immunotherapy [11,12]. Unlike CAR-T cell therapy's high immunologic systemic toxicity, CAR-NK cell therapy displays lower toxicity because it has a shorter in vivo duration [133]. Uniquely, NK cells are dependent on a balance between activating and inhibitory germline-encoded signals which are not susceptible to downregulation in cancerous cells [12]. Furthermore, CAR-NK therapy can be allogeneic and therefore safer and manufactured "off-the-shelf", indicating a high potential for successful future treatments [134]. For example, a phase I clinical trial using CAR-NK cell therapy against anti-PDL1/MUC1, a glycoprotein known to be overexpressed in melanoma and promote metastasis, was shown to display a stable response in a majority of patients with a range of solid tumors [135,136]. This may indicate a path forward for CAR-NK therapy's effectiveness as a personalized treatment for patients with melanoma.

3.3. *Vaccine Development*

Ideally, like the prevention of infectious diseases, administering a cancer vaccine could help the immune system detect and eliminate tumors. Unfortunately, hundreds of attempts have not made significant improvements in patients' health. However, one notable study reported that personalized vaccines for melanoma targeting mutated proteins using mRNA increased T-cell infiltration that led to antitumor activity across patients, providing optimism for the future success of this approach [137]. Vaccines can potentially create a targeted and tumor-specific immune response whose long-term memory may aid in cases of subsequent metastasis for treatment-refractory patients, especially in melanoma with high immunogenicity. The combination of vaccines with other immunotherapies also offers greater tumor control. Regardless of vaccine type and antigen or adjuvant choice, the backbone of vaccine development is the injection of tumor antigens in an immunostimulatory space to prime tumor-specific T cells or induce antibodies while breaking tolerance to self-antigens and causing tumor cell death [138]. Currently, vaccines developed for melanoma treatment have been whole-cell vaccines, peptide-based vaccines, dendritic cell (DC) vaccines, ganglioside vaccines, DNA vaccines, and RNA vaccines [139,140].

3.3.1. Whole-Cell Vaccines

Whole-cell vaccines can be split into two subtypes: autologous and allogeneic tumor cell vaccines [140]. Autologous whole-tumor cell vaccines are manufactured using either excised tumor cells or from autologous tissue culture that has undergone ex vivo irradiation to eliminate the ability to replicate [138,139]. Although this autologous subtype is patient-specific because the components are derived from the recipient, this technique lacks broad applicability. Additionally, the process is both time- and labor-intensive, requiring an adequate amount of tumor tissue from each patient, and attempts at quality vaccine preparation have been met with high degrees of failure [141].

Allogeneic vaccines derived from whole-tumor cells refer to those generated from melanoma tumor cells derived from patients who are not the intended vaccine recipient and may contain more than one tumor cell line to augment the antigen expression profile [138,139]. Like autologous whole-cell vaccines, the tissue requires prior irradiation to be rendered replication-deficient. Advantages include an expanded range of available tumor antigens, broad applicability to multiple patients, and lack of requirement for a patient's specific tumor tissue. However, there is the possibility of a lack of patient specificity. The response of allogeneic whole-cell vaccines relies on how well the tumor cells in the vaccine match the tumor cells of the treated patient. Two well-known examples of allogeneic whole-cell vaccines are Canvaxin™ (CancerVax Corporation, Carlsbad, CA, USA) and Melacine® (Corixa Corporation, Seattle, WA, USA) [138,139]. Canvaxin is composed of three melanoma cell lines, boasting over 20 melanoma-associated tumor antigens, and is administered with Bacillus Calmette–Guerin (BCG) as an immunoadjuvant; unfortunately, multiple phase III trials failed to reveal the benefit of Canvaxin over the investigated placebo [142]. Melacine comprises two melanoma cell lines that are paired with immunoadjuvant "detoxified Freund's adjuvant" (DETOX); moreover, like Canvaxin, Melacine failed to demonstrate a significant benefit in disease-free survival once reaching phase III trial stage [138,139,143].

3.3.2. DNA Vaccines

DNA vaccines comprise naked DNA expression plasmids that possess a gene encoding for the target antigen(s) from melanoma tumor cells [144]. Therefore, DNA vaccines immunize patients using plasmid-encoding antigens rather than with the antigen. The administration is commonly given through parenteral routes (i.e., intramuscular, subcutaneous, transdermal, or intradermal). However, some attention has been recently given to mucosal routes (i.e., intranasal, vaginal, and oral) due to the advantage of generating local immunity at specific sites [144,145]. DNA vaccines are traditionally low-cost, highly stable, and less laborious when compared to other vaccine therapy options. However, disadvantages include the low immunogenicity of plasmid DNA, the possibility of virus reversion, and tolerance against autoantigens if the vaccine is administered without an immunoadjuvant [138,144].

Tyrosinase, a glycoprotein that is necessary for melanin synthesis and can promote an immune response against melanogenesis-related antigens, has been a target of interest for DNA vaccines. Some studies have reported that administering tyrosinase could induce antigen-specific T-cell responses, and several DNA vaccines based on the tyrosinase antigen have been developed [144,146]. For example, the Oncept melanoma vaccine—a DNA vaccine that is used to treat melanoma in canines—uses human-DNA-encoding tyrosinase to elicit an immune response in dogs; however, while the vaccine appears to be safe, its efficacy is limited [147].

Additionally, the melanoma antigen-1 (MAGE-A1) family is known to have increased expression in human cancer types, including melanoma, and has also become a target of interest for DNA vaccines. Duperret et al. [148] found that targeting any member of the MAGE-A family, not just the commonly upregulated MAGE-A3, via DNA vaccination effectively produced a robust immune response that slowed tumor development and prolonged the median survival of mice. By targeting a wider range of proteins, the treatment is more generalized to the heterogeneity of the TME while reducing toxicity. Although some progress has been made in the treatment of melanoma with DNA vaccines at the preclinical animal model stage, more clinical studies are needed to validate DNA vaccine efficacy.

3.3.3. RNA Vaccines

Tumor-associated antigens (TAAs)—commonly cancer germline antigens or lineage-specific differentiation markers—have become the core of cancer immunotherapy and are attractive targets for RNA vaccines because they can cause cells to synthesize TAAs that are recognized by T cells and subsequently trigger a targeted immune response [140,149]. In the past however, this strategy has been clinically ineffective in many vaccine trials due to a central T-cell tolerance to TAAs [150], with this ineffectiveness especially prevalent in advanced-stage patients with lower mutational burdens [151].

Sahin et al. [149] report a novel intravenously administered nanoparticulate-liposomal RNA (RNA-LPX) vaccine known as melanoma FixVac (BNT111) that has been introduced in the first-in-human phase I trial (Lipo-MERIT, NCT02410733) using an RNA vaccine. The RNA-LPX vaccine contains optimized RNA targeting immature DC in lymphoid tissues. It is composed of four TAAs that are present on both MHC class I and class

II molecules—NY-ESO-1, MAGE-A3, tyrosinase, and TPTE—which express at restricted levels in normal tissues but have a high prevalence and immunogenicity in melanoma. Preliminary results have shown that patients experienced increased spleen metabolic activity, indicating the TLR activation of lymphoid-tissue-resident immune cells. ELISpot analyses confirmed that most patients had a strong T-cell response to at least one of the four TAAs, mostly being $CD4^+$ or a combination of $CD4^+$ and $CD8^+$ T-cell de novo responses [149,150]. These effector T cells remained stable in cohorts that received a continuing vaccine dosage, and long-term memory T cells persisted in patients who did not receive any further vaccination beyond the initial doses. Interestingly, some of the patients who had prior anti-PD1 therapy failure showed signs of tumor regression following vaccination doses and afterward responded to an ensuing round of anti-PD1 therapy [149,150]. Taken as a whole, these study results mark the beginning of what may be a promising therapeutic option for a vaccine targeting TAAs, especially when employed in combination with other immunotherapies in patients with lower mutational tumor burdens and previously treatment-refractory tumors. For example, the combination of the individualized neoantigen mRNA vaccine mRNA-4157 (V940) with pembrolizumab showed longer recurrence-free survival with a manageable safety then pembrolizumab monotherapy in resected melanomas [152].

At its current stage, vaccine therapy is not considered a standard treatment option for advanced cutaneous melanoma. Vaccines must show proven clinical efficacy against melanoma to bridge the gap from experimental therapy to standard treatment. Factors that need a more thorough investigation include optimal timing for the start of vaccine therapy and the type of adjuvant that may be considered adequate. It is largely agreed upon that the success of vaccine therapy for melanoma patients will rely on a multimodal combined approach whose actual clinical effect is yet to be elucidated.

4. Thinking Innovatively—Where to Go Next?

Although there are multiple treatment options for melanoma, significant barriers still hinder the survival rate of melanoma patients due to the nature of its various mutations and heterogeneity. Thus, it is important to consider how further research may expand on prevention, early diagnosis, disease prediction, and advancing personalized options.

4.1. *scSeq Techniques*

Single-cell sequencing (scSeq) techniques are a new and increasingly popular tool for identifying biomarkers in specific cell types. This technique involves isolating individual cells and analyzing the gene expression of each cell [153]. This information is especially helpful for analyzing melanoma samples due to their high tumor heterogeneity [154].

With scSeq, each patient cell can be analyzed to identify seemingly minute differences between tumor cells that can identify potentially more efficient molecular targets. More specific targets can be identified with this extensive and detailed analysis of cells to limit unnecessary damage and toxicity. However, as with many new technologies, greater specificity also corresponds with a high price and longer analyzing times. Additionally, as scSeq requires isolated cells, procedures to disassociate cells from each other remain challenging. However, as scSeq continues to be developed and refined, more efficient and cheaper options should become available to make this analytical method accessible to all patients beyond highly funded research institutions to minimize socioeconomic-based disparities [155]. Many also predict that the emerging Human Cell Atlas project, a common database of all cell types, will help better identify mutant and/or tumorigenic cells. Studies, such as Davidson et al. [156], have used single-cell RNA-sequencing (scRNA-seq) to further define the melanoma TME landscape and serve as a resource to identify drug candidates in a manner that other researchers can employ. Furthermore, Ho et al. [157] used scRNA-seq to analyze melanoma patient samples and identify the role of CD58 in tumor cell immune evasion. They used samples of patients before and early on in their treatment plans of nivolumab with or without ipilimumab to identify the expression of CD58 in each patient's cells. Utilizing scRNA-seq, Ho et al. discovered that the loss of CD58 confers cancer immune evasion in melanoma cells and that higher expression of CD58 is associated with anti-tumoral immunity. With this expanding database and potential applications, scSeq and its related exploratory data could be leveraged during therapeutic development. Moreover, further innovations will be needed for it to become more widely utilized [158].

4.2. AI and ML Development

More recently, artificial intelligence (AI) and machine learning (ML) are gaining attention in the field of oncology [159]. AI translates human problem-solving and comprehension skills to computers and can use ML to learn how to analyze and distill large amounts of data in less time than humans [160]. Deep learning (DL), a subset of ML, can also simulate human neural networks in order for machines to understand data automatically similarly to how humans instantaneously process sensory images to see the world.

AI/ML approaches comprise aspects that can be qualitatively as well as quantitatively superior to human analysis. In oncology, these technologies could allow clinicians to make precision-based predictions, diagnoses, and treatment decisions solely from analyzing patient data. Additionally, these technologies have the potential to improve accuracy, minimize patient sample volume collection, and detect melanoma and metastasis progression earlier [160,161]. For example, Marchetti et al. [162] demonstrated the use of an AI algorithm (ADAE) to analyze dermatoscopy images of skin lesions and subsequently predict melanoma risk. It was found that dermatologists had a significant improvement in their ability to assess melanoma risk after ADAE exposure.

With the high amounts of cellular heterogeneity in melanoma and a unique presentation in each patient, AI can be a necessary tool for clinicians to quickly analyze vast and complex information. Interestingly, the application of AI/ML/DL to existing patient data has created an improved, noninvasive method for predicting patients' intracranial $BRAF^{V600E}$ mutational status [163]. Moreover, using radiometric imaging data of patient samples, AI was able to better predict future disease progression and pembrolizumab effectiveness on early-stage melanoma samples from their baseline CT images than the standard clinician-based prediction method [164]. As a result, treatment plans can be further specified to target AI-predicted biomarkers and reduce "trial-and-error" drug therapies and resistance.

In summary, AI is a highly useful tool that can extend clinicians' knowledge and scope to give patients a higher number of accurate precision medicine treatment options. This can result in earlier diagnosis, more precise treatment plans, and better overall outcomes and quality of life for cancer patients.

4.3. AAV-Mediated Gene Delivery System for Targeting Melanoma (CRISPR-Based (AAV))

Since cancer is commonly developed from genetic mutations, gene editing is an area of medicine with high potential for it. Gene editing technology using the Clustered regularly interspersed short-palindromic repeat (CRISPR)-Cas 9 system is a recent development for treating many diseases, with the first human clinical trials conducted in 2016 [165]. The CRISPR-Cas9 system involves two main components: guide RNA sequences that bind to the target gene with high specificity and the Cas9 endonuclease that allows for genome modifications by causing a double-stranded DNA break [166]. Ideally, through the CRISPR-Cas9 system, scientists and clinicians aim to restore a patient's mutated cancerous DNA to a natural, non-tumorigenic state by altering the mutated gene, editing the mutated gene to the normal gene, or knocking out an amplificated oncogene [167].

One of the biggest hurdles to the use of CRISPR-Cas9 as a treatment is its delivery to patients. Recent studies have demonstrated that an adeno-associated virus (AAV) system could overcome this barrier [168]. AAV is a small, enveloped virus that can pack up to 5.0 kb of single-stranded DNA (ssDNA). With AAV's inverted terminal repeats (ITRs) of 0.3 kb and the commonly used Cas9 consisting of 4.2 kb DNA, less than 0.5 kb of space is left for gene regulatory elements that guide gene editing. This limited available space causes larger gene targets of CRSIPR-Cas9 to be less commonly used than smaller cancerous gene targets [169]. Because of this, variables such as tissue specificity, off-target editing, and inducible expression are more difficult to control. To account for this, dual-vector delivery methods are being investigated in which two different AAV vectors are used, but this can reduce overall efficiency [169]. Additionally, smaller-sized Cas9 proteins, such as Cas9 from *Staphylococcus aureus*, are also being investigated as an alternative [170]. Fortunately, the use of AAV in vivo for smaller-sized melanoma-associated targets, like the proteins sBTLA+HSP70 for metastatic melanoma and the GM3(Neu5Gc) ganglioside for melanoma and breast cancer, has proven successful for anti-tumor activity in mouse models, indicating potential future translational and clinical success [171,172].

The clinical application of AAV vectors for CRISPR has been approved by employing AAV-CRISPR delivery directly to the eye to target the *CEP290* gene containing the mutation for blindness [173]. Many other CRISPR treatment protocols should start to gain clinical approval, suggesting that they will be implemented as a reliable treatment option for melanoma mutations—such as $BRAF^{V600E}$—in the future.

4.4. Oncolytic Therapy Using Microorganisms (T-VEC)

4.4.1. Bacteria

The hypoxic and necrotic regions that arise within the TME have proven to be a barrier to many treatments [174]. These regions are often poorly accessible to systemically delivered therapies. Low oxygen levels can reduce the efficacy of certain treatments and can affect the function of immune cells in vivo. However, therapy involving live tumor-targeting bacteria may present a unique option in overcoming these obstacles due to their ability to thrive and colonize within these niches. Historical evidence has shown that bacterial infections could induce anti-tumor responses, but this has only recently been pursued due to the current advances in genetic engineering for creating safer, attenuated strains of bacteria [174]. Because they have a high affinity for hypoxic and necrotic cell environments, bacteria could be used to deliver cytotoxic agents, prodrug-converting enzymes, and immunomodulators directly to tumor nodes in order to decrease immunosuppression, improve tumor-targeting specificity that decreases toxicity, and disrupt the tumor vasculature [175]. Bacteria may also induce an immune response that activates specific types of host immune cells—such as T cells and inflammatory cytokines (e.g., IL-1β, GM-CSF and TNF-α)—in order to recognize cancer cells as antigens, mark them for destruction, increase inflammation, and promote antitumor activity [176]. Unfortunately, this therapy still requires further research due to complications with translating in vivo models to human studies and health concerns regarding the use of potentially infectious bacteria populations. Wang et al. [177] note that some bacteria are tumor-associated and killing these bacteria in cancer mouse models improved immune recognition of tumor cells via the release of cancer-specific microbial neoantigens. However, even with the few clinical studies, such as the bacillus BCG administration of Canvaxin mentioned previously, this method can be best utilized in combination with other therapies, such as radiation or ICIs [178]. This was recently shown in mouse models by Chen et al. [179], who demonstrated that modified *Staphylococcus epidermidis* in combination with ICIs can reduce growth in localized and metastatic melanoma tumors.

4.4.2. Viruses

Direct intralesional cancer immunotherapy is another treatment method that has been explored over the years, with a goal of inducing an effective control of disease in the injected lesions while also triggering a systemic immunological response [180]. Talimogene laherparepvec (T-VEC) marks the first oncolytic viral immunotherapy that has successfully gained FDA approval for the localized treatment of recurrent metastatic melanoma after surgery [181]. T-VEC is constituted by a genetically modified herpes simplex virus type I (HSV-1) that selectively replicates in tumor cells and transfects them with a granulocyte–macrophage colony-stimulating factor (GM-CSF) encoding plasmid, resulting in increased concentrations of GM-CSF in the TME. Locally, T-VEC causes the infected tumor cell to undergo increased antigen presentation for the recruitment of immune cells, causing lysis and a systemic polyclonal antitumor response [181,182]. T-VEC has been confirmed by pre-clinical studies to preferentially infect melanoma cells; additionally, clinical trials have demonstrated that it has promising efficacy in both monotherapy and in combination with ICIs [10,180]. When used in combination therapies, T-VEC may potentially improve the efficacy of ICIs due to its antitumor effects on the TME. This potential improvement in efficacy further supports the theory that combining immunotherapies with complementary modes of action may augment antitumor responses [183,184]. Studies remain ongoing to confirm the feasibility and efficacy of these combination strategies while producing low levels of clinical side effects [185].

5. Conclusions

Due to differences in mutational status, other genetic and non-genetic considerations that drive a patient's cancer specificity, there is not a "one-size-fits-all" solution for cancer treatment (Figure 3 and Table 1). Notably, melanoma is characterized by a higher rate of multiple gene mutations with strong intra-tumor and inter-tumor molecular heterogeneity, which makes treatment challenging. Individualized approaches are needed to determine which treatment or combination of strategies is best for each patient. Recent advances in translational treatment options, such as CAR-T cell therapy and vaccine development, are beginning to address this need for individualized therapy options. Still, more development is necessary to apply this universally to patient populations. Additionally, with emerging technologies, such as AI and CRISPR-Cas9, the coming decade of melanoma treatment research holds great promise in individualizing treatment options to improve melanoma patient outcomes and survival.

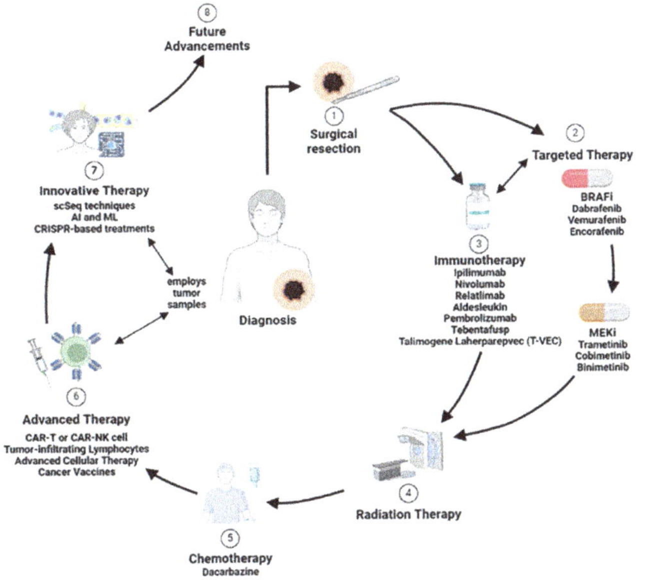

Figure 3. Optimization and personalization of treatment strategy for melanoma therapy. Due to differences in mutational status and other genetic considerations that drive a patient's cancer specificity, there is not a "one-size-fits-all" solution for cancer treatment. The treatment options for melanoma include surgical resection, targeted therapy (e.g., BRAFis and MEKis), immunotherapy (e.g., anti-CTLA-4 and anti-PD-L1), radiation therapy, chemotherapy, advanced immunotherapy (e.g., CAR-T, CAR-NK, TILs, ACT), and innovative approaches that can be personalized to the patient's disease. The ideal approach will depend on the mutational status and other genetic considerations that can drive a patient's melanoma progression.

Table 1. Current clinical and pre-clinical drugs for treatment of melanoma.

Drug Name	Target	Status	Notes	Reference
Vemurafenib	Binds to one of the ATP-binding sites of B-RAF	FDA Approved, 2011	Approved in Combination with Cobimetinib in 2015	[16]
Dabrafenib	Is an ATP-competitive inhibitor in a ATP-binding site of B-RAF	FDA Approved, 2013	Approved with Trametinib in 2022	[16,51]
Encorafenib	Binds to B-RAF and other kinases including CRAF and JNK1	FDA Approved, 2018	Approved in combination with Binimetinib in 2018	[20]
Trametinib	Targets an allosteric pocket adjacent to the ATP-binding site of MEK1 and MEK2	FDA Approved, 2013	Approved with Dabrafenib in 2022	[16,51]
Cobimetinib	Targets an allosteric pocket adjacent to the ATP-binding site of MEK1 and MEK2	FDA Approved, 2015	Approved in combination with Vemurafenib in 2015	[16]
Binimetinib	Reversibly inhibits MEK1 and MEK2	FDA Approved, 2018	Approved in combination with Encorafenib in 2018	[20]
Defactinib	Inhibits the phosphorylation of FAK	Clinical trial phase ii for uveal melanoma (with combination of RAF/MEK inhibitor VS-6766)		[47,48]
Sorafenib	Pan-RAF inhibitor targeting CRAF and BRAF	Success in pre-clinical mouse models and phase i study with selumetinib on hepatocellular carcinoma patients		[50]
AZ628	Pan-RAF inhibitor targeting CRAF, BRAF, and BRAFV600E	Success in pre-clinical mouse models		[50]
Selumetinib	Non-ATP competitive MEK1 and MEK 2 inhibitor	Success in clinical trials	Phase I trial with sorafenib on hepatocellular carcinoma patients shows promising effects	[50]
Tovorafenib	CNS-penetrant, type II pan-RAF inhibitor	Successful safety profile in phase I trial for patients with melanoma		[51]
Bemcentinib	Blocks AXL autophosphorylation and induce apoptosis	Phase 1b/2 clinical trial comparing its efficacy with pembrolizumab or dabrafenib/trametinib alone on stage III or IV unresectable melanoma	Also known as BGB324 or R428	[61,62]
Crizotinib	ATP competitive inhibitor of Met and ALK kinases	Shown to be effective with afatinib on cutaneous melanoma patient cell models	Has FDA approval for NSCLC, and combination studies with crizotinib on lung cancer and mesothelioma showed strong efficacy	[70,71]
Tivantinib	Non-ATP competitor that inhibits MET selectively	A phase I trial with sorafenib on melanoma and other solid tumors showed promising results		[70]
Quercetin	STAT3 inhibitor that inhibits MET activation through FAS inhibition	Shows promising success in pre-clinical melanoma models		[70]

Table 1. *Cont.*

Drug Name	Target	Status	Notes	Reference
Afatinib	Irreversibly inhibits ERBB family receptors including ERBB3	Shown to be effective with crizotinib on cutaneous melanoma patient cell models	Combination studies with crizotinib on lung cancer and mesothelioma showed strong efficacy	[71]
PHA665752	Blocks MET phosphorylation	Showed success with pre-clinical studies from melanoma patient tumor samples		[72]
11a-1	Specifically inhibits SHP2, blocking ERK1/2 and AKT activation	Showed success with pre-clinical tests from melanoma cell lines		[36]
SCH772984	Potent ATP-competitive compound that inhibits ERK1 and ERK2	Successfully blocked proliferation in melanoma models, including those with BRAFi/MEKi resistance		[37]
Hydroxychloroquine	Inhibitor of autophagy by impairing lysosomal function	Phase 1 trial testing hydroxycholorquine and vemurafenib in melanoma is completed		[40]
Palbociclib	Highly selective ATP-competitive inhibitor of CDK4 and CDK6	Preclinical trial combination with irradiation on donor skin cancer cells showed cell cycle arrest	FDA approved for breast cancer	[56,57]
Pembrolizumab	Monoclonal antibody that blocks programed death-ligand 1 (PD-1) on T-cell surfaces	FDA approval for metastatic melanoma in 2014 and stage iib/c melanoma in 2021		[87]
Ipilimumab	Human monoclonal antibody against CTLA-4	Approved by FDA for unresectable, metastatic melanoma in 2011 and in combination with nivolumab in 2015	Many clinical trials in combination with other drugs are in progress	[19]
Tremelimumab	Human monoclonal antibody against CTLA-4	Multiple phase I combination clinical trials showed effectiveness in advanced melanoma		[19,89]
BCD-145	Human monoclonal antibody against CTLA-4	Multiple phase i clinical trials of solo or combination BCD-145 treatments on advanced melanoma are undergoing		[19]
Nivolumab	Monoclonal antibody that blocks programed death-ligand 1 (PD-1) on T-cell surfaces	Approved solo for metastatic melanoma in 2014 and in combination with ipilimumab in 2015	Shows success with relatimab in a phase ii/iii clinical trial	[19,87]
Avelumab	Human monoclonal antibody against PD-L1	A phase I trial showed promising results in melanoma	Approved by FDA to treat Merkel cell carcinoma	[19]
Drurvalumab	Human monoclonal antibody against PD-L1	Multiple phase I combination clinical trials showed effectiveness in advanced melanoma		[19,89]
Cemiplimab	Human monoclonal antibody against PD-1	Multiple clinical trials retesting the efficacy of cemiplimab in melanoma	Approved by FDA in 2018 for cutaneous squamous cell carcinoma	[19]

Table 1. *Cont.*

Drug Name	Target	Status	Notes	Reference
Atezolizumab	Human monoclonal antibody against PD-1	Approved in combination with cobimetinib and vemurafenib for advanced melanoma in 2022		[19]
Cosibelimab	Human monoclonal antibody against PD-L1	Phase iii trials in cutaneous squamous cell carcinoma are being investigated for their efficacy		[19]
Tebentafusp	A bispecific gp100 T-cell engager	Multiple phase I combination clinical trials showed effectiveness in advanced melanoma		[89]
Relatlimab	Anti-LAG-3 antibody	A phase ii/iii trial in combination with nivolumab on advanced melanoma shows promising results		[87,93]
RO7247669	Anti-PD-1 and LAG-3 bispecific antibody	A phase I clinical trial is evaluating its efficacy in solid tumors such as melanoma		[95,96]
Lifileucel	Autologous TIL therapy product	FDA approved in 2024 to treat patients with unresectable or advanced melanoma	Also known as Amtagvi	[109]
Canvaxin	Allogenic whole-cell melanoma vaccine made of three cell lines	Multiple phase iii trials failed to show benefit over placebo		[142]
Melacine	Allogenic whole-cell melanoma vaccine made of two cell lines	Multiple phase iii trials failed to show significant benefit		[139]
Oncept	Xenogenic DNA caxxine targeting tyrosinase	USDA approved for stage ii/iii canine oral melanoma but has limited efficacy		[147]
FixVac	Encodes RNA targeting 4 TAAs: NY-ESO, MAGE-A3, tyrosinase, and TPTE	A phase I trial showed promising results in advanced melanoma patients		[149]
mRNA-4157	Encodes 34 neoantigens	A phase 2b for resected melanoma		[152]
Aldesleukin (IL-2)	Stimulates immune cells with IL-2 receptors	FDA approved for melanoma in 1998, commonly used with ACT to improve response rates		[112]
Talimogene Laherparpvec	Oncolytic viral therapy that selectively replicates in tumor cells, injecting with GM-CSF	Approved by FDA in 2015 for local treatment of unresectable stage iii/iv melanoma		[180]
Dacarbazine	Chemotherapy drug that targets cancer cell's DNA	Approved by FDA for melanoma in 1975		[22]

Author Contributions: Conceptualization, Y.Y.; Writing—Original Draft Preparation, G.R.C., A.J.I., R.G.M.B. and Y.Y.; Writing—Review and Editing, A.J.I., R.G.M.B. and Y.Y.; Writing—Reading and Revising, A.J.I., R.G.M.B., G.M. and Y.Y. All authors have read and agreed to the published version of the manuscript.

Funding: This research received no external funding.

Conflicts of Interest: The authors declare no conflicts of interest.

Abbreviations

AI: artificial intelligence; AJCC: American Joint Committee on Cancer; ACT: adoptive cellular therapy; BCG: bacillus Calmette–Guerin; BRAF: Raf proto-oncogene serine-threonine protein; CAR: chimeric antigen receptor; CLTA-4: cytotoxic T lymphocyte-associated protein 4; CSPG4: chondroitin sulphate proteoglycan 4; DC: dendritic cell; DETOX: detoxified Freund's adjuvant; GM-CSF: granulocyte–macrophage colony-stimulating factor; ICI: immune checkpoint inhibitor; LAG-3 (CD223): Lymphocyte activation gene-3; MHC: major histocompatibility complex; MAPK: mitogen-activated protein kinase; ML: machine learning; NF1: neurofibromin-1 mutant; NRAS: NRAS proto-oncogene GTPase; OS: overall survival; PD-1: programmed cell death protein; PD-L1: programmed cell death-ligand 1; PFS: progression-free survival; scFv: single-chain variable fragment; RFS: relapse-free survival; TAAs: tumor-associated antigens; T_{EX}: exhausted T cells; T_{REGS}: regulatory T cells; TCRs: T-cell receptors; TEAs: treatment-emergent adverse events; TILs: tumor-infiltrating lymphocytes; T-VEC: talimogene laherparepvec; TME: tumor microenvironment; UV: ultraviolet; V_H: antibody-variable heavy chain; V_L: antibody-variable light chain; WT: wildtype.

References

1. Soltantoyeh, T.; Akbari, B.; Karimi, A.; Mahmoodi Chalbatani, G.; Ghahri-Saremi, N.; Hadjati, J.; Hamblin, M.R.; Mirzaei, H.R. Chimeric Antigen Receptor (CAR) T Cell Therapy for Metastatic Melanoma: Challenges and Road Ahead. *Cells* **2021**, *10*, 1450. [CrossRef] [PubMed]
2. Randic, T.; Kozar, I.; Margue, C.; Utikal, J.; Kreis, S. NRAS mutant melanoma: Towards better therapies. *Cancer Treat. Rev.* **2021**, *99*, 102238. [CrossRef] [PubMed]
3. Cancer Genome Atlas Network. Genomic Classification of Cutaneous Melanoma. *Cell* **2015**, *161*, 1681–1696. [CrossRef]
4. Giugliano, F.; Crimini, E.; Tarantino, P.; Zagami, P.; Uliano, J.; Corti, C.; Trapani, D.; Curigliano, G.; Ascierto, P.A. First line treatment of BRAF mutated advanced melanoma: Does one size fit all? *Cancer Treat. Rev.* **2021**, *99*, 102253. [CrossRef] [PubMed]
5. Yu, Y. A novel combination treatment against melanoma with NRAS mutation and therapy resistance. *EMBO Mol. Med.* **2018**, *10*, e8573. [CrossRef] [PubMed]
6. Ribas, A.; Lawrence, D.; Atkinson, V.; Agarwal, S.; Miller, W.H., Jr.; Carlino, M.S.; Fisher, R.; Long, G.V.; Hodi, F.S.; Tsoi, J.; et al. Combined BRAF and MEK inhibition with PD-1 blockade immunotherapy in BRAF-mutant melanoma. *Nat. Med.* **2019**, *25*, 936–940. [CrossRef] [PubMed]
7. Sosman, J.A.; Kim, K.B.; Schuchter, L.; Gonzalez, R.; Pavlick, A.C.; Weber, J.S.; McArthur, G.A.; Hutson, T.E.; Moschos, S.J.; Flaherty, K.T.; et al. Survival in BRAF V600-mutant advanced melanoma treated with vemurafenib. *N. Engl. J. Med.* **2012**, *366*, 707–714. [CrossRef]
8. Keung, E.Z.; Gershenwald, J.E. The eighth edition American Joint Committee on Cancer (AJCC) melanoma staging system: Implications for melanoma treatment and care. *Expert Rev. Anticancer. Ther.* **2018**, *18*, 775–784. [CrossRef] [PubMed]
9. Carlino, M.S.; Larkin, J.; Long, G.V. Immune checkpoint inhibitors in melanoma. *Lancet* **2021**, *398*, 1002–1014. [CrossRef]
10. Bai, X.; Flaherty, K.T. Targeted and immunotherapies in BRAF mutant melanoma: Where we stand and what to expect. *Br. J. Dermatol.* **2021**, *185*, 253–262. [CrossRef]
11. Yu, Y. The Function of NK Cells in Tumor Metastasis and NK Cell-Based Immunotherapy. *Cancers* **2023**, *15*, 2323. [CrossRef] [PubMed]
12. Hibler, W.; Merlino, G.; Yu, Y. CAR NK Cell Therapy for the Treatment of Metastatic Melanoma: Potential & Prospects. *Cells* **2023**, *12*, 2750. [CrossRef] [PubMed]
13. Granhøj, J.S.; Witness Præst Jensen, A.; Presti, M.; Met, Ö.; Svane, I.M.; Donia, M. Tumor-infiltrating lymphocytes for adoptive cell therapy: Recent advances, challenges, and future directions. *Expert Opin. Biol. Ther.* **2022**, *22*, 627–641. [CrossRef] [PubMed]
14. Dörrie, J.; Babalija, L.; Hoyer, S.; Gerer, K.F.; Schuler, G.; Heinzerling, L.; Schaft, N. BRAF and MEK Inhibitors Influence the Function of Reprogrammed T Cells: Consequences for Adoptive T-Cell Therapy. *Int. J. Mol. Sci.* **2018**, *19*, 289. [CrossRef] [PubMed]
15. Proietti, I.; Skroza, N.; Michelini, S.; Mambrin, A.; Balduzzi, V.; Bernardini, N.; Marchesiello, A.; Tolino, E.; Volpe, S.; Maddalena, P.; et al. BRAF Inhibitors: Molecular Targeting and Immunomodulatory Actions. *Cancers* **2020**, *12*, 1823. [CrossRef] [PubMed]
16. Millet, A.; Martin, A.R.; Ronco, C.; Rocchi, S.; Benhida, R. Metastatic Melanoma: Insights Into the Evolution of the Treatments and Future Challenges. *Med. Res. Rev.* **2017**, *37*, 98–148. [CrossRef] [PubMed]
17. Chapman, P.B.; Hauschild, A.; Robert, C.; Haanen, J.B.; Ascierto, P.; Larkin, J.; Dummer, R.; Garbe, C.; Testori, A.; Maio, M.; et al. Improved survival with vemurafenib in melanoma with BRAF V600E mutation. *N. Engl. J. Med.* **2011**, *364*, 2507–2516. [CrossRef]
18. Hauschild, A.; Grob, J.J.; Demidov, L.V.; Jouary, T.; Gutzmer, R.; Millward, M.; Rutkowski, P.; Blank, C.U.; Miller, W.H., Jr.; Kaempgen, E.; et al. Dabrafenib in BRAF-mutated metastatic melanoma: A multicentre, open-label, phase 3 randomised controlled trial. *Lancet* **2012**, *380*, 358–365. [CrossRef] [PubMed]
19. Patel, H.; Yacoub, N.; Mishra, R.; White, A.; Long, Y.; Alanazi, S.; Garrett, J.T. Current Advances in the Treatment of BRAF-Mutant Melanoma. *Cancers* **2020**, *12*, 482. [CrossRef]

20. Shirley, M. Encorafenib and Binimetinib: First Global Approvals. *Drugs* **2018**, *78*, 1277–1284. [CrossRef]
21. Gonzalez-Del Pino, G.L.; Li, K.; Park, E.; Schmoker, A.M.; Ha, B.H.; Eck, M.J. Allosteric MEK inhibitors act on BRAF/MEK complexes to block MEK activation. *Proc. Natl. Acad. Sci. USA* **2021**, *118*, e2107207118. [CrossRef] [PubMed]
22. Flaherty, K.T.; Robert, C.; Hersey, P.; Nathan, P.; Garbe, C.; Milhem, M.; Demidov, L.V.; Hassel, J.C.; Rutkowski, P.; Mohr, P.; et al. Improved survival with MEK inhibition in BRAF-mutated melanoma. *N. Engl. J. Med.* **2012**, *367*, 107–114. [CrossRef] [PubMed]
23. Eroglu, Z.; Ribas, A. Combination therapy with BRAF and MEK inhibitors for melanoma: Latest evidence and place in therapy. *Ther. Adv. Med. Oncol.* **2016**, *8*, 48–56. [CrossRef] [PubMed]
24. Davis, E.J.; Johnson, D.B.; Sosman, J.A.; Chandra, S. Melanoma: What do all the mutations mean? *Cancer* **2018**, *124*, 3490–3499. [CrossRef]
25. Brodaczewska, K.; Majewska, A.; Filipiak-Duliban, A.; Kieda, C. Pten knockout affects drug resistance differently in melanoma and kidney cancer. *Pharmacol. Rep.* **2023**, *75*, 1187–1199. [CrossRef] [PubMed]
26. Bucheit, A.D.; Chen, G.; Siroy, A.; Tetzlaff, M.; Broaddus, R.; Milton, D.; Fox, P.; Bassett, R.; Hwu, P.; Gershenwald, J.E.; et al. Complete loss of PTEN protein expression correlates with shorter time to brain metastasis and survival in stage IIIB/C melanoma patients with BRAFV600 mutations. *Clin. Cancer Res.* **2014**, *20*, 5527–5536. [CrossRef]
27. Czarnecka, A.M.; Bartnik, E.; Fiedorowicz, M.; Rutkowski, P. Targeted Therapy in Melanoma and Mechanisms of Resistance. *Int. J. Mol. Sci.* **2020**, *21*, 4576. [CrossRef]
28. Tsao, H.; Goel, V.; Wu, H.; Yang, G.; Haluska, F.G. Genetic interaction between NRAS and BRAF mutations and PTEN/MMAC1 inactivation in melanoma. *J. Investig. Dermatol.* **2004**, *122*, 337–341. [CrossRef] [PubMed]
29. Zuo, Q.; Liu, J.; Huang, L.; Qin, Y.; Hawley, T.; Seo, C.; Merlino, G.; Yu, Y. AXL/AKT axis mediated-resistance to BRAF inhibitor depends on PTEN status in melanoma. *Oncogene* **2018**, *37*, 3275–3289. [CrossRef]
30. Qin, Y.; Zuo, Q.; Huang, L.; Huang, L.; Merlino, G.; Yu, Y. PERK mediates resistance to BRAF inhibition in melanoma with impaired PTEN. *NPJ Precis. Oncol.* **2021**, *5*, 68. [CrossRef]
31. Catalanotti, F.; Cheng, D.T.; Shoushtari, A.N.; Johnson, D.B.; Panageas, K.S.; Momtaz, P.; Higham, C.; Won, H.H.; Harding, J.J.; Merghoub, T.; et al. PTEN Loss-of-Function Alterations Are Associated With Intrinsic Resistance to BRAF Inhibitors in Metastatic Melanoma. *JCO Precis. Oncol.* **2017**, *1*, 1–15. [CrossRef] [PubMed]
32. Yu, Y.; Dai, M.; Huang, L.; Chen, W.; Yu, E.; Mendoza, A.; Michael, H.; Khanna, C.; Bosenberg, M.; McMahon, M.; et al. PTEN phosphatase inhibits metastasis by negatively regulating the Entpd5/IGF1R pathway through ATF6. *iScience* **2023**, *26*, 106070. [CrossRef]
33. Yu, Y.; Dai, M.; Lu, A.; Yu, E.; Merlino, G. PHLPP1 mediates melanoma metastasis suppression through repressing AKT2 activation. *Oncogene* **2018**, *37*, 2225–2236. [CrossRef]
34. Cabrita, R.; Mitra, S.; Sanna, A.; Ekedahl, H.; Lövgren, K.; Olsson, H.; Ingvar, C.; Isaksson, K.; Lauss, M.; Carneiro, A.; et al. The Role of PTEN Loss in Immune Escape, Melanoma Prognosis and Therapy Response. *Cancers* **2020**, *12*, 742. [CrossRef]
35. Pardella, E.; Pranzini, E.; Leo, A.; Taddei, M.L.; Paoli, P.; Raugei, G. Oncogenic Tyrosine Phosphatases: Novel Therapeutic Targets for Melanoma Treatment. *Cancers* **2020**, *12*, 2799. [CrossRef] [PubMed]
36. Zhang, R.Y.; Yu, Z.H.; Zeng, L.; Zhang, S.; Bai, Y.; Miao, J.; Chen, L.; Xie, J.; Zhang, Z.Y. SHP2 phosphatase as a novel therapeutic target for melanoma treatment. *Oncotarget* **2016**, *7*, 73817–73829. [CrossRef]
37. Morris, E.J.; Jha, S.; Restaino, C.R.; Dayananth, P.; Zhu, H.; Cooper, A.; Carr, D.; Deng, Y.; Jin, W.; Black, S.; et al. Discovery of a novel ERK inhibitor with activity in models of acquired resistance to BRAF and MEK inhibitors. *Cancer Discov.* **2013**, *3*, 742–750. [CrossRef]
38. Di Leo, L.; Bodemeyer, V.; De Zio, D. The Complex Role of Autophagy in Melanoma Evolution: New Perspectives From Mouse Models. *Front. Oncol.* **2019**, *9*, 1506. [CrossRef] [PubMed]
39. Karras, P.; Riveiro-Falkenbach, E.; Cañón, E.; Tejedo, C.; Calvo, T.G.; Martínez-Herranz, R.; Alonso-Curbelo, D.; Cifdaloz, M.; Perez-Guijarro, E.; Gómez-López, G.; et al. p62/SQSTM1 Fuels Melanoma Progression by Opposing mRNA Decay of a Selective Set of Pro-metastatic Factors. *Cancer Cell* **2019**, *35*, 46–63.e10. [CrossRef]
40. Ma, X.H.; Piao, S.F.; Dey, S.; McAfee, Q.; Karakousis, G.; Villanueva, J.; Hart, L.S.; Levi, S.; Hu, J.; Zhang, G.; et al. Targeting ER stress-induced autophagy overcomes BRAF inhibitor resistance in melanoma. *J. Clin. Investig.* **2014**, *124*, 1406–1417. [CrossRef]
41. Fratta, E.; Giurato, G.; Guerrieri, R.; Colizzi, F.; Dal Col, J.; Weisz, A.; Steffan, A.; Montico, B. Autophagy in BRAF-mutant cutaneous melanoma: Recent advances and therapeutic perspective. *Cell Death Discov.* **2023**, *9*, 202. [CrossRef] [PubMed]
42. LoRusso, P.M.; Schalper, K.; Sosman, J. Targeted therapy and immunotherapy: Emerging biomarkers in metastatic melanoma. *Pigment Cell Melanoma Res.* **2020**, *33*, 390–402. [CrossRef]
43. Long, G.V.; Grob, J.J.; Nathan, P.; Ribas, A.; Robert, C.; Schadendorf, D.; Lane, S.R.; Mak, C.; Legenne, P.; Flaherty, K.T.; et al. Factors predictive of response, disease progression, and overall survival after dabrafenib and trametinib combination treatment: A pooled analysis of individual patient data from randomised trials. *Lancet Oncol.* **2016**, *17*, 1743–1754. [CrossRef] [PubMed]
44. Li, S.; Balmain, A.; Counter, C.M. A model for RAS mutation patterns in cancers: Finding the sweet spot. *Nat. Rev. Cancer* **2018**, *18*, 767–777. [CrossRef] [PubMed]
45. Guida, M.; Bartolomeo, N.; Quaglino, P.; Madonna, G.; Pigozzo, J.; Di Giacomo, A.M.; Minisini, A.M.; Tucci, M.; Spagnolo, F.; Occelli, M.; et al. No Impact of NRAS Mutation on Features of Primary and Metastatic Melanoma or on Outcomes of Checkpoint Inhibitor Immunotherapy: An Italian Melanoma Intergroup (IMI) Study. *Cancers* **2021**, *13*, 475. [CrossRef] [PubMed]

46. Simanshu, D.K.; Morrison, D.K. A Structure is Worth a Thousand Words: New Insights for RAS and RAF Regulation. *Cancer Discov.* **2022**, *12*, 899–912. [CrossRef] [PubMed] [PubMed Central]
47. Del Mistro, G.; Riemann, S.; Schindler, S.; Beissert, S.; Kontermann, R.E.; Ginolhac, A.; Halder, R.; Presta, L.; Sinkkonen, L.; Sauter, T.; et al. Focal adhesion kinase plays a dual role in TRAIL resistance and metastatic outgrowth of malignant melanoma. *Cell Death Dis.* **2022**, *13*, 54. [CrossRef] [PubMed]
48. Seedor, R.S.; Orloff, M.; Gutkind, J.S.; Aplin, A.E.; Terai, M.; Sharpe-Mills, E.; Klose, H.; Mastrangelo, M.J.; Sato, T. Clinical trial in progress: Phase II trial of defactinib (VS-6063) combined with VS-6766 (CH5126766) in patients with metastatic uveal melanoma. *J. Clin. Oncol.* **2021**, *39*, TPS9588. [CrossRef]
49. Menzer, C.; Hassel, J.C. Targeted Therapy for Melanomas Without BRAF V600 Mutations. *Curr. Treat. Options Oncol.* **2022**, *23*, 831–842. [CrossRef]
50. Molnár, E.; Rittler, D.; Baranyi, M.; Grusch, M.; Berger, W.; Döme, B.; Tóvári, J.; Aigner, C.; Tímár, J.; Garay, T.; et al. Pan-RAF and MEK vertical inhibition enhances therapeutic response in non-V600 BRAF mutant cells. *BMC Cancer* **2018**, *18*, 542. [CrossRef]
51. Rasco, D.W.; Medina, T.; Corrie, P.; Pavlick, A.C.; Middleton, M.R.; Lorigan, P.; Hebert, C.; Plummer, R.; Larkin, J.; Agarwala, S.S.; et al. Phase 1 study of the pan-RAF inhibitor tovorafenib in patients with advanced solid tumors followed by dose expansion in patients with metastatic melanoma. *Cancer Chemother. Pharmacol.* **2023**, *92*, 15–28. [CrossRef]
52. Garutti, M.; Targato, G.; Buriolla, S.; Palmero, L.; Minisini, A.M.; Puglisi, F. CDK4/6 Inhibitors in Melanoma: A Comprehensive Review. *Cells* **2021**, *10*, 1334. [CrossRef]
53. Sheppard, K.E.; McArthur, G.A. The cell-cycle regulator CDK4: An emerging therapeutic target in melanoma. *Clin. Cancer Res.* **2013**, *19*, 5320–5328. [CrossRef] [PubMed]
54. Zhou, F.H.; Downton, T.; Freelander, A.; Hurwitz, J.; Caldon, C.E.; Lim, E. CDK4/6 inhibitor resistance in estrogen receptor positive breast cancer, a 2023 perspective. *Front. Cell Dev. Biol.* **2023**, *11*, 1148792. [CrossRef]
55. Dika, E.; Patrizi, A.; Lambertini, M.; Manuelpillai, N.; Fiorentino, M.; Altimari, A.; Ferracin, M.; Lauriola, M.; Fabbri, E.; Campione, E.; et al. Estrogen Receptors and Melanoma: A Review. *Cells* **2019**, *8*, 1463. [CrossRef]
56. Yoshida, A.; Lee, E.K.; Diehl, J.A. Induction of Therapeutic Senescence in Vemurafenib-Resistant Melanoma by Extended Inhibition of CDK4/6. *Cancer Res.* **2016**, *76*, 2990–3002. [CrossRef]
57. Jost, T.; Heinzerling, L.; Fietkau, R.; Hecht, M.; Distel, L.V. Palbociclib Induces Senescence in Melanoma and Breast Cancer Cells and Leads to Additive Growth Arrest in Combination With Irradiation. *Front. Oncol.* **2021**, *11*, 740002. [CrossRef] [PubMed]
58. Shao, H.; Teramae, D.; Wells, A. Axl contributes to efficient migration and invasion of melanoma cells. *PLoS ONE* **2023**, *18*, e0283749. [CrossRef] [PubMed]
59. Auyez, A.; Sayan, A.E.; Kriajevska, M.; Tulchinsky, E. AXL Receptor in Cancer Metastasis and Drug Resistance: When Normal Functions Go Askew. *Cancers* **2021**, *13*, 4864. [CrossRef]
60. Boshuizen, J.; Koopman, L.A.; Krijgsman, O.; Shahrabi, A.; van den Heuvel, E.G.; Ligtenberg, M.A.; Vredevoogd, D.W.; Kemper, K.; Kuilman, T.; Song, J.Y.; et al. Cooperative targeting of melanoma heterogeneity with an AXL antibody-drug conjugate and BRAF/MEK inhibitors. *Nat. Med.* **2018**, *24*, 203–212. [CrossRef]
61. Nyakas, M.; Fleten, K.G.; Haugen, M.H.; Engedal, N.; Sveen, C.; Farstad, I.N.; Flørenes, V.A.; Prasmickaite, L.; Mælandsmo, G.M.; Seip, K. AXL inhibition improves BRAF-targeted treatment in melanoma. *Sci. Rep.* **2022**, *12*, 5076. [CrossRef] [PubMed]
62. BGB324 in Combination with Pembrolizumab or Dabrafenib/Trametinib in Metastatic Melanoma. NCT02872259. 2023. Available online: https://clinicaltrials.gov/study/NCT02872259 (accessed on 21 September 2023).
63. Kiuru, M.; Busam, K.J. The NF1 gene in tumor syndromes and melanoma. *Lab. Investig.* **2017**, *97*, 146–157. [CrossRef] [PubMed]
64. Py, C.; Christinat, Y.; Kreutzfeldt, M.; McKee, T.A.; Dietrich, P.Y.; Tsantoulis, P. Response of NF1-Mutated Melanoma to an MEK Inhibitor. *JCO Precis. Oncol.* **2018**, *2*, 1–11. [CrossRef] [PubMed]
65. Thielmann, C.M.; Chorti, E.; Matull, J.; Murali, R.; Zaremba, A.; Lodde, G.; Jansen, P.; Richter, L.; Kretz, J.; Möller, I.; et al. NF1-mutated melanomas reveal distinct clinical characteristics depending on tumour origin and respond favourably to immune checkpoint inhibitors. *Eur. J. Cancer* **2021**, *159*, 113–124. [CrossRef] [PubMed]
66. Czyz, M. HGF/c-MET Signaling in Melanocytes and Melanoma. *Int. J. Mol. Sci.* **2018**, *19*, 3844. [CrossRef] [PubMed]
67. Huang, L.; Qin, Y.; Zuo, Q.; Bhatnagar, K.; Xiong, J.; Merlino, G.; Yu, Y. Ezrin mediates both HGF/Met autocrine and non-autocrine signaling-induced metastasis in melanoma. *Int. J. Cancer* **2018**, *142*, 1652–1663. [CrossRef]
68. Yu, Y.; Merlino, G. Constitutive c-Met signaling through a nonautocrine mechanism promotes metastasis in a transgenic transplantation model. *Cancer Res.* **2002**, *62*, 2951–2956. [PubMed]
69. Demkova, L.; Kucerova, L. Role of the HGF/c-MET tyrosine kinase inhibitors in metastasic melanoma. *Mol. Cancer* **2018**, *17*, 26. [CrossRef] [PubMed]
70. Sabbah, M.; Najem, A.; Krayem, M.; Awada, A.; Journe, F.; Ghanem, G.E. RTK Inhibitors in Melanoma: From Bench to Bedside. *Cancers* **2021**, *13*, 1685. [CrossRef]
71. Das, I.; Wilhelm, M.; Höiom, V.; Franco Marquez, R.; Costa Svedman, F.; Hansson, J.; Tuominen, R.; Egyhàzi Brage, S. Combining ERBB family and MET inhibitors is an effective therapeutic strategy in cutaneous malignant melanoma independent of BRAF/NRAS mutation status. *Cell Death Dis.* **2019**, *10*, 663. [CrossRef]
72. Chattopadhyay, C.; Ellerhorst, J.A.; Ekmekcioglu, S.; Greene, V.R.; Davies, M.A.; Grimm, E.A. Association of activated c-Met with NRAS-mutated human melanomas. *Int. J. Cancer* **2012**, *131*, E56–E65. [CrossRef] [PubMed]

73. Shakhova, O.; Sommer, L. Testing the cancer stem cell hypothesis in melanoma: The clinics will tell. *Cancer Lett.* **2013**, *338*, 74–81. [CrossRef] [PubMed]
74. Boiko, A.D.; Razorenova, O.V.; van de Rijn, M.; Swetter, S.M.; Johnson, D.L.; Ly, D.P.; Butler, P.D.; Yang, G.P.; Joshua, B.; Kaplan, M.J.; et al. Human melanoma-initiating cells express neural crest nerve growth factor receptor CD271. *Nature* **2010**, *466*, 133–137. [CrossRef] [PubMed]
75. Schatton, T.; Murphy, G.F.; Frank, N.Y.; Yamaura, K.; Waaga-Gasser, A.M.; Gasser, M.; Zhan, Q.; Jordan, S.; Duncan, L.M.; Weishaupt, C.; et al. Identification of cells initiating human melanomas. *Nature* **2008**, *451*, 345–349. [CrossRef] [PubMed]
76. Kharouf, N.; Flanagan, T.W.; Alamodi, A.A.; Al Hmada, Y.; Hassan, S.Y.; Shalaby, H.; Santourlidis, S.; Hassan, S.L.; Haikel, Y.; Megahed, M.; et al. CD133-Dependent Activation of Phosphoinositide 3-Kinase/AKT/Mammalian Target of Rapamycin Signaling in Melanoma Progression and Drug Resistance. *Cells* **2024**, *13*, 240. [CrossRef] [PubMed]
77. Simbulan-Rosenthal, C.M.; Haribabu, Y.; Vakili, S.; Kuo, L.W.; Clark, H.; Dougherty, R.; Alobaidi, R.; Carney, B.; Sykora, P.; Rosenthal, D.S. Employing CRISPR-Cas9 to Generate CD133 Synthetic Lethal Melanoma Stem Cells. *Int. J. Mol. Sci.* **2022**, *23*, 2333. [CrossRef] [PubMed]
78. Yin, Q.; Zhao, N.; Chang, Y.; Dong, M.; Xu, M.; Xu, W.; Jin, H.F.; Liu, W.; Xu, N. Melanoma stem cell vaccine induces effective tumor immunity against melanoma. *Hum. Vaccin. Immunother.* **2023**, *19*, 2158670. [CrossRef] [PubMed]
79. Hugo, W.; Shi, H.; Sun, L.; Piva, M.; Song, C.; Kong, X.; Moriceau, G.; Hong, A.; Dahlman, K.B.; Johnson, D.B.; et al. Non-genomic and Immune Evolution of Melanoma Acquiring MAPKi Resistance. *Cell* **2015**, *162*, 1271–1285. [CrossRef] [PubMed]
80. Eichhoff, O.M.; Stoffel, C.I.; Käsler, J.; Briker, L.; Turko, P.; Karsai, G.; Zila, N.; Paulitschke, V.; Cheng, P.F.; Leitner, A.; et al. ROS Induction Targets Persister Cancer Cells with Low Metabolic Activity in NRAS-Mutated Melanoma. *Cancer Res.* **2023**, *83*, 1128–1146. [CrossRef]
81. Halford, S.; Veal, G.J.; Wedge, S.R.; Payne, G.S.; Bacon, C.M.; Sloan, P.; Dragoni, I.; Heinzmann, K.; Potter, S.; Salisbury, B.M.; et al. A Phase I Dose-escalation Study of AZD3965, an Oral Monocarboxylate Transporter 1 Inhibitor, in Patients with Advanced Cancer. *Clin. Cancer Res.* **2023**, *29*, 1429–1439. [CrossRef]
82. Zhang, G.; Ji, P.; Xia, P.; Song, H.; Guo, Z.; Hu, X.; Guo, Y.; Yuan, X.; Song, Y.; Shen, R.; et al. Identification and targeting of cancer-associated fibroblast signature genes for prognosis and therapy in Cutaneous melanoma. *Comput. Biol. Med.* **2023**, *167*, 107597. [CrossRef]
83. Purcell, J.W.; Tanlimco, S.G.; Hickson, J.; Fox, M.; Sho, M.; Durkin, L.; Uziel, T.; Powers, R.; Foster, K.; McGonigal, T.; et al. LRRC15 Is a Novel Mesenchymal Protein and Stromal Target for Antibody-Drug Conjugates. *Cancer Res.* **2018**, *78*, 4059–4072. [CrossRef]
84. Jiang, Z.; He, J.; Zhang, B.; Wang, L.; Long, C.; Zhao, B.; Yang, Y.; Du, L.; Luo, W.; Hu, J.; et al. A Potential "Anti-Warburg Effect" in Circulating Tumor Cell-mediated Metastatic Progression? *Aging Dis.* **2024**. [CrossRef] [PubMed]
85. Herrscher, H.; Robert, C. Immune checkpoint inhibitors in melanoma in the metastatic, neoadjuvant, and adjuvant setting. *Curr. Opin. Oncol.* **2020**, *32*, 106–113. [CrossRef]
86. Lamba, N.; Ott, P.A.; Iorgulescu, J.B. Use of First-Line Immune Checkpoint Inhibitors and Association With Overall Survival Among Patients With Metastatic Melanoma in the Anti-PD-1 Era. *JAMA Netw. Open* **2022**, *5*, e2225459. [CrossRef] [PubMed]
87. Huang, A.C.; Zappasodi, R. A decade of checkpoint blockade immunotherapy in melanoma: Understanding the molecular basis for immune sensitivity and resistance. *Nat. Immunol.* **2022**, *23*, 660–670. [CrossRef] [PubMed]
88. Leach, D.R.; Krummel, M.F.; Allison, J.P. Enhancement of antitumor immunity by CTLA-4 blockade. *Science* **1996**, *271*, 1734–1736. [CrossRef]
89. Phase 1b/2 Study of the Combination of IMCgp100 with Durvalumab and/or Tremelimumab in Advanced Cutaneous Melanoma. NCT02535078. 2024. Available online: https://clinicaltrials.gov/study/NCT02535078 (accessed on 24 January 2024).
90. Willsmore, Z.N.; Coumbe, B.G.T.; Crescioli, S.; Reci, S.; Gupta, A.; Harris, R.J.; Chenoweth, A.; Chauhan, J.; Bax, H.J.; McCraw, A.; et al. Combined anti-PD-1 and anti-CTLA-4 checkpoint blockade: Treatment of melanoma and immune mechanisms of action. *Eur. J. Immunol.* **2021**, *51*, 544–556. [CrossRef]
91. van Zeijl, M.C.T.; van Breeschoten, J.; de Wreede, L.C.; Wouters, M.; Hilarius, D.L.; Blank, C.U.; Aarts, M.J.B.; van den Berkmortel, F.; de Groot, J.W.B.; Hospers, G.A.P.; et al. Real-world Outcomes of Ipilimumab Plus Nivolumab Combination Therapy in a Nation-wide Cohort of Advanced Melanoma Patients in the Netherlands. *J. Immunother.* **2023**, *46*, 197–204. [CrossRef]
92. Maruhashi, T.; Sugiura, D.; Okazaki, I.M.; Okazaki, T. LAG-3: From molecular functions to clinical applications. *J. Immunother. Cancer* **2020**, *8*, e001014. [CrossRef]
93. A Study of Relatlimab Plus Nivolumab Versus Nivolumab Alone in Participants with Advanced Melanoma. NCT03470922. 2018. Available online: https://clinicaltrials.gov/study/NCT03470922 (accessed on 21 September 2023).
94. Tawbi, H.A.; Schadendorf, D.; Lipson, E.J.; Ascierto, P.A.; Matamala, L.; Castillo Gutiérrez, E.; Rutkowski, P.; Gogas, H.J.; Lao, C.D.; De Menezes, J.J.; et al. Relatlimab and Nivolumab versus Nivolumab in Untreated Advanced Melanoma. *N. Engl. J. Med.* **2022**, *386*, 24–34. [CrossRef] [PubMed]
95. Kreidieh, F.Y.; Tawbi, H.A. The introduction of LAG-3 checkpoint blockade in melanoma: Immunotherapy landscape beyond PD-1 and CTLA-4 inhibition. *Ther. Adv. Med. Oncol.* **2023**, *15*, 17588359231186027. [CrossRef] [PubMed]
96. Dose Escalation Study of a PD1-LAG3 Bispecific Antibody in Patients with Advanced and/or Metastatic Solid Tumors. NCT04140500. 2024. Available online: https://clinicaltrials.gov/study/NCT04140500 (accessed on 16 April 2024).

97. Aggarwal, C.; Prawira, A.; Antonia, S.; Rahma, O.; Tolcher, A.; Cohen, R.B.; Lou, Y.; Hauke, R.; Vogelzang, N.; Dan, P.Z.; et al. Dual checkpoint targeting of B7-H3 and PD-1 with enoblituzumab and pembrolizumab in advanced solid tumors: Interim results from a multicenter phase I/II trial. *J. Immunother. Cancer* **2022**, *10*, e004424. [CrossRef]
98. Liu, C.; Zhang, G.; Xiang, K.; Kim, Y.; Lavoie, R.R.; Lucien, F.; Wen, T. Targeting the immune checkpoint B7-H3 for next-generation cancer immunotherapy. *Cancer Immunol. Immunother.* **2022**, *71*, 1549–1567. [CrossRef] [PubMed]
99. Scribner, J.A.; Brown, J.G.; Son, T.; Chiechi, M.; Li, P.; Sharma, S.; Li, H.; De Costa, A.; Li, Y.; Chen, Y.; et al. Preclinical Development of MGC018, a Duocarmycin-based Antibody-drug Conjugate Targeting B7-H3 for Solid Cancer. *Mol. Cancer Ther.* **2020**, *19*, 2235–2244. [CrossRef] [PubMed]
100. Tang, W.; Chen, J.; Ji, T.; Cong, X. TIGIT, a novel immune checkpoint therapy for melanoma. *Cell Death Dis.* **2023**, *14*, 466. [CrossRef] [PubMed]
101. Kawashima, S.; Inozume, T.; Kawazu, M.; Ueno, T.; Nagasaki, J.; Tanji, E.; Honobe, A.; Ohnuma, T.; Kawamura, T.; Umeda, Y.; et al. TIGIT/CD155 axis mediates resistance to immunotherapy in patients with melanoma with the inflamed tumor microenvironment. *J. Immunother. Cancer* **2021**, *9*, e003134. [CrossRef]
102. Mittal, D.; Lepletier, A.; Madore, J.; Aguilera, A.R.; Stannard, K.; Blake, S.J.; Whitehall, V.L.J.; Liu, C.; Bettington, M.L.; Takeda, K.; et al. CD96 Is an Immune Checkpoint That Regulates CD8(+) T-cell Antitumor Function. *Cancer Immunol. Res.* **2019**, *7*, 559–571. [CrossRef] [PubMed]
103. Blake, S.J.; Stannard, K.; Liu, J.; Allen, S.; Yong, M.C.; Mittal, D.; Aguilera, A.R.; Miles, J.J.; Lutzky, V.P.; de Andrade, L.F.; et al. Suppression of Metastases Using a New Lymphocyte Checkpoint Target for Cancer Immunotherapy. *Cancer Discov.* **2016**, *6*, 446–459. [CrossRef]
104. Prokopi, A.; Tripp, C.H.; Tummers, B.; Hornsteiner, F.; Spoeck, S.; Crawford, J.C.; Clements, D.R.; Efremova, M.; Hutter, K.; Bellmann, L.; et al. Skin dendritic cells in melanoma are key for successful checkpoint blockade therapy. *J. Immunother. Cancer* **2021**, *9*, e000832. [CrossRef]
105. Curigliano, G.; Gelderblom, H.; Mach, N.; Doi, T.; Tai, D.; Forde, P.M.; Sarantopoulos, J.; Bedard, P.L.; Lin, C.C.; Hodi, F.S.; et al. Phase I/Ib Clinical Trial of Sabatolimab, an Anti-TIM-3 Antibody, Alone and in Combination with Spartalizumab, an Anti-PD-1 Antibody, in Advanced Solid Tumors. *Clin. Cancer Res.* **2021**, *27*, 3620–3629. [CrossRef] [PubMed]
106. Bassey-Archibong, B.I.; Rajendra Chokshi, C.; Aghaei, N.; Kieliszek, A.M.; Tatari, N.; McKenna, D.; Singh, M.; Kalpana Subapanditha, M.; Parmar, A.; Mobilio, D.; et al. An HLA-G/SPAG9/STAT3 axis promotes brain metastases. *Proc. Natl. Acad. Sci. USA* **2023**, *120*, e2205247120. [CrossRef] [PubMed]
107. Seitter, S.J.; Sherry, R.M.; Yang, J.C.; Robbins, P.F.; Shindorf, M.L.; Copeland, A.R.; McGowan, C.T.; Epstein, M.; Shelton, T.E.; Langhan, M.M.; et al. Impact of Prior Treatment on the Efficacy of Adoptive Transfer of Tumor-Infiltrating Lymphocytes in Patients with Metastatic Melanoma. *Clin. Cancer Res.* **2021**, *27*, 5289–5298. [CrossRef] [PubMed]
108. Qin, S.S.; Melucci, A.D.; Chacon, A.C.; Prieto, P.A. Adoptive T Cell Therapy for Solid Tumors: Pathway to Personalized Standard of Care. *Cells* **2021**, *10*, 808. [CrossRef]
109. Sarnaik, A.A.; Hamid, O.; Khushalani, N.I.; Lewis, K.D.; Medina, T.; Kluger, H.M.; Thomas, S.S.; Domingo-Musibay, E.; Pavlick, A.C.; Whitman, E.D.; et al. Lifileucel, a Tumor-Infiltrating Lymphocyte Therapy, in Metastatic Melanoma. *J. Clin. Oncol.* **2021**, *39*, 2656–2666. [CrossRef] [PubMed]
110. Betof Warner, A.; Corrie, P.G.; Hamid, O. Tumor-Infiltrating Lymphocyte Therapy in Melanoma: Facts to the Future. *Clin. Cancer Res.* **2023**, *29*, 1835–1854. [CrossRef] [PubMed]
111. Rohaan, M.W.; van den Berg, J.H.; Kvistborg, P.; Haanen, J. Adoptive transfer of tumor-infiltrating lymphocytes in melanoma: A viable treatment option. *J. Immunother. Cancer* **2018**, *6*, 102. [CrossRef] [PubMed]
112. Goff, S.L. A Prospective Randomized and Phase 2 Trial for Metastatic Melanoma Using Adoptive Cell Therapy with Tumor Infiltrating Lymphocytes Plus IL-2 Either Alone or Following the Administration of Pembrolizumab. NCT02621021. 2023. Available online: https://clinicaltrials.gov/study/NCT02621021 (accessed on 15 March 2024).
113. Feins, S.; Kong, W.; Williams, E.F.; Milone, M.C.; Fraietta, J.A. An introduction to chimeric antigen receptor (CAR) T-cell immunotherapy for human cancer. *Am. J. Hematol.* **2019**, *94*, S3–S9. [CrossRef]
114. Gattinoni, L.; Powell, D.J., Jr.; Rosenberg, S.A.; Restifo, N.P. Adoptive immunotherapy for cancer: Building on success. *Nat. Rev. Immunol.* **2006**, *6*, 383–393. [CrossRef]
115. Kwon, M.; Iacoboni, G.; Reguera, J.L.; Corral, L.L.; Morales, R.H.; Ortiz-Maldonado, V.; Guerreiro, M.; Caballero, A.C.; Domínguez, M.L.G.; Pina, J.M.S.; et al. Axicabtagene ciloleucel compared to tisagenlecleucel for the treatment of aggressive B-cell lymphoma. *Haematologica* **2023**, *108*, 110–121. [CrossRef]
116. Simon, B.; Uslu, U. CAR-T cell therapy in melanoma: A future success story? *Exp. Dermatol.* **2018**, *27*, 1315–1321. [CrossRef] [PubMed]
117. Kershaw, M.H.; Westwood, J.A.; Parker, L.L.; Wang, G.; Eshhar, Z.; Mavroukakis, S.A.; White, D.E.; Wunderlich, J.R.; Canevari, S.; Rogers-Freezer, L.; et al. A phase I study on adoptive immunotherapy using gene-modified T cells for ovarian cancer. *Clin. Cancer Res.* **2006**, *12*, 6106–6115. [CrossRef]
118. Ahmed, N.; Brawley, V.S.; Hegde, M.; Robertson, C.; Ghazi, A.; Gerken, C.; Liu, E.; Dakhova, O.; Ashoori, A.; Corder, A.; et al. Human Epidermal Growth Factor Receptor 2 (HER2) -Specific Chimeric Antigen Receptor-Modified T Cells for the Immunotherapy of HER2-Positive Sarcoma. *J. Clin. Oncol.* **2015**, *33*, 1688–1696. [CrossRef] [PubMed]

119. Zeltsman, M.; Dozier, J.; McGee, E.; Ngai, D.; Adusumilli, P.S. CAR T-cell therapy for lung cancer and malignant pleural mesothelioma. *Transl. Res.* **2017**, *187*, 1–10. [CrossRef] [PubMed]
120. Kiyohara, E.; Donovan, N.; Takeshima, L.; Huang, S.; Wilmott, J.S.; Scolyer, R.A.; Jones, P.; Somers, E.B.; O'Shannessy, D.J.; Hoon, D.S. Endosialin Expression in Metastatic Melanoma Tumor Microenvironment Vasculature: Potential Therapeutic Implications. *Cancer Microenviron.* **2015**, *8*, 111–118. [CrossRef] [PubMed]
121. Teicher, B.A. CD248: A therapeutic target in cancer and fibrotic diseases. *Oncotarget* **2019**, *10*, 993–1009. [CrossRef] [PubMed]
122. Campoli, M.R.; Chang, C.C.; Kageshita, T.; Wang, X.; McCarthy, J.B.; Ferrone, S. Human high molecular weight-melanoma-associated antigen (HMW-MAA): A melanoma cell surface chondroitin sulfate proteoglycan (MSCP) with biological and clinical significance. *Crit. Rev. Immunol.* **2004**, *24*, 267–296. [CrossRef]
123. Teppert, K.; Winter, N.; Herbel, V.; Brandes, C.; Lennartz, S.; Engert, F.; Kaiser, A.; Schaser, T.; Lock, D. Combining CSPG4-CAR and CD20-CCR for treatment of metastatic melanoma. *Front. Immunol.* **2023**, *14*, 1178060. [CrossRef] [PubMed]
124. Adkins, S. CAR T-Cell Therapy: Adverse Events and Management. *J. Adv. Pract. Oncol.* **2019**, *10*, 21–28. [CrossRef]
125. Kosti, P.; Maher, J.; Arnold, J.N. Perspectives on Chimeric Antigen Receptor T-Cell Immunotherapy for Solid Tumors. *Front. Immunol.* **2018**, *9*, 1104. [CrossRef]
126. Kyriakou, G.; Melachrinou, M. Cancer stem cells, epigenetics, tumor microenvironment and future therapeutics in cutaneous malignant melanoma: A review. *Future Oncol.* **2020**, *16*, 1549–1567. [CrossRef]
127. Ren, J.; Zhang, X.; Liu, X.; Fang, C.; Jiang, S.; June, C.H.; Zhao, Y. A versatile system for rapid multiplex genome-edited CAR T cell generation. *Oncotarget* **2017**, *8*, 17002–17011. [CrossRef]
128. Li, S.; Siriwon, N.; Zhang, X.; Yang, S.; Jin, T.; He, F.; Kim, Y.J.; Mac, J.; Lu, Z.; Wang, S.; et al. Enhanced Cancer Immunotherapy by Chimeric Antigen Receptor-Modified T Cells Engineered to Secrete Checkpoint Inhibitors. *Clin. Cancer Res.* **2017**, *23*, 6982–6992. [CrossRef] [PubMed]
129. Rupp, L.J.; Schumann, K.; Roybal, K.T.; Gate, R.E.; Ye, C.J.; Lim, W.A.; Marson, A. CRISPR/Cas9-mediated PD-1 disruption enhances anti-tumor efficacy of human chimeric antigen receptor T cells. *Sci. Rep.* **2017**, *7*, 737. [CrossRef] [PubMed]
130. Marotte, L.; Simon, S.; Vignard, V.; Dupre, E.; Gantier, M.; Cruard, J.; Alberge, J.B.; Hussong, M.; Deleine, C.; Heslan, J.M.; et al. Increased antitumor efficacy of PD-1-deficient melanoma-specific human lymphocytes. *J. Immunother. Cancer* **2020**, *8*, e000311. [CrossRef]
131. Adusumilli, P.S.; Zauderer, M.G.; Rivière, I.; Solomon, S.B.; Rusch, V.W.; O'Cearbhaill, R.E.; Zhu, A.; Cheema, W.; Chintala, N.K.; Halton, E.; et al. A Phase I Trial of Regional Mesothelin-Targeted CAR T-cell Therapy in Patients with Malignant Pleural Disease, in Combination with the Anti-PD-1 Agent Pembrolizumab. *Cancer Discov.* **2021**, *11*, 2748–2763. [CrossRef]
132. Sang, W.; Wang, X.; Geng, H.; Li, T.; Li, D.; Zhang, B.; Zhou, Y.; Song, X.; Sun, C.; Yan, D.; et al. Anti-PD-1 Therapy Enhances the Efficacy of CD30-Directed Chimeric Antigen Receptor T Cell Therapy in Patients With Relapsed/Refractory CD30+ Lymphoma. *Front. Immunol.* **2022**, *13*, 858021. [CrossRef]
133. Li, H.; Song, W.; Li, Z.; Zhang, M. Preclinical and clinical studies of CAR-NK-cell therapies for malignancies. *Front. Immunol.* **2022**, *13*, 992232. [CrossRef] [PubMed]
134. Heipertz, E.L.; Zynda, E.R.; Stav-Noraas, T.E.; Hungler, A.D.; Boucher, S.E.; Kaur, N.; Vemuri, M.C. Current Perspectives on "Off-The-Shelf" Allogeneic NK and CAR-NK Cell Therapies. *Front. Immunol.* **2021**, *12*, 732135. [CrossRef]
135. Wang, X.; Lan, H.; Li, J.; Su, Y.; Xu, L. Muc1 promotes migration and lung metastasis of melanoma cells. *Am. J. Cancer Res.* **2015**, *5*, 2590–2604.
136. Li, Q.; Wang, Y.; Lin, M.; Xia, L.; Bao, Y.; Sun, X.; Yang, L. Abstract A014: Phase I clinical trial with PD-1/MUC1 CAR-pNK92 immunotherapy. *Cancer Immunol. Res.* **2019**, *7*, A014. [CrossRef]
137. Sahin, U.; Derhovanessian, E.; Miller, M.; Kloke, B.P.; Simon, P.; Löwer, M.; Bukur, V.; Tadmor, A.D.; Luxemburger, U.; Schrörs, B.; et al. Personalized RNA mutanome vaccines mobilize poly-specific therapeutic immunity against cancer. *Nature* **2017**, *547*, 222–226. [CrossRef] [PubMed]
138. Terando, A.M.; Faries, M.B.; Morton, D.L. Vaccine therapy for melanoma: Current status and future directions. *Vaccine* **2007**, *25* (Suppl. S2), B4–B16. [CrossRef] [PubMed]
139. Lens, M. The role of vaccine therapy in the treatment of melanoma. *Expert Opin. Biol. Ther.* **2008**, *8*, 315–323. [CrossRef]
140. Kwak, M.; Leick, K.M.; Melssen, M.M.; Slingluff, C.L., Jr. Vaccine Strategy in Melanoma. *Surg. Oncol. Clin. N. Am.* **2019**, *28*, 337–351. [CrossRef]
141. Terando, A.; Sabel, M.S.; Sondak, V.K. Melanoma: Adjuvant therapy and other treatment options. *Curr. Treat. Options Oncol.* **2003**, *4*, 187–199. [CrossRef]
142. Faries, M.B.; Mozzillo, N.; Kashani-Sabet, M.; Thompson, J.F.; Kelley, M.C.; DeConti, R.C.; Lee, J.E.; Huth, J.F.; Wagner, J.; Dalgleish, A.; et al. Long-Term Survival after Complete Surgical Resection and Adjuvant Immunotherapy for Distant Melanoma Metastases. *Ann. Surg. Oncol.* **2017**, *24*, 3991–4000. [CrossRef] [PubMed]
143. Sondak, V.K.; Liu, P.Y.; Tuthill, R.J.; Kempf, R.A.; Unger, J.M.; Sosman, J.A.; Thompson, J.A.; Weiss, G.R.; Redman, B.G.; Jakowatz, J.G.; et al. Adjuvant immunotherapy of resected, intermediate-thickness, node-negative melanoma with an allogeneic tumor vaccine: Overall results of a randomized trial of the Southwest Oncology Group. *J. Clin. Oncol.* **2002**, *20*, 2058–2066. [CrossRef] [PubMed]
144. Rezaei, T.; Davoudian, E.; Khalili, S.; Amini, M.; Hejazi, M.; de la Guardia, M.; Mokhtarzadeh, A. Strategies in DNA vaccine for melanoma cancer. *Pigment Cell Melanoma Res.* **2021**, *34*, 869–891. [CrossRef]

145. Farris, E.; Brown, D.M.; Ramer-Tait, A.E.; Pannier, A.K. Micro- and nanoparticulates for DNA vaccine delivery. *Exp. Biol. Med.* **2016**, *241*, 919–929. [CrossRef]
146. Colluru, V.T.; Johnson, L.E.; Olson, B.M.; McNeel, D.G. Preclinical and clinical development of DNA vaccines for prostate cancer. *Urol. Oncol.* **2016**, *34*, 193–204. [CrossRef] [PubMed]
147. Pellin, M.A. The Use of Oncept Melanoma Vaccine in Veterinary Patients: A Review of the Literature. *Vet. Sci.* **2022**, *9*, 597. [CrossRef]
148. Duperret, E.K.; Liu, S.; Paik, M.; Trautz, A.; Stoltz, R.; Liu, X.; Ze, K.; Perales-Puchalt, A.; Reed, C.; Yan, J.; et al. A Designer Cross-reactive DNA Immunotherapeutic Vaccine that Targets Multiple MAGE-A Family Members Simultaneously for Cancer Therapy. *Clin. Cancer Res.* **2018**, *24*, 6015–6027. [CrossRef]
149. Sahin, U.; Oehm, P.; Derhovanessian, E.; Jabulowsky, R.A.; Vormehr, M.; Gold, M.; Maurus, D.; Schwarck-Kokarakis, D.; Kuhn, A.N.; Omokoko, T.; et al. An RNA vaccine drives immunity in checkpoint-inhibitor-treated melanoma. *Nature* **2020**, *585*, 107–112. [CrossRef] [PubMed]
150. Bordon, Y. An RNA vaccine for advanced melanoma. *Nat. Rev. Drug. Discov.* **2020**, *19*, 671. [CrossRef] [PubMed]
151. Romero, P.; Banchereau, J.; Bhardwaj, N.; Cockett, M.; Disis, M.L.; Dranoff, G.; Gilboa, E.; Hammond, S.A.; Hershberg, R.; Korman, A.J.; et al. The Human Vaccines Project: A roadmap for cancer vaccine development. *Sci. Transl. Med.* **2016**, *8*, 334ps339. [CrossRef] [PubMed]
152. Weber, J.S.; Carlino, M.S.; Khattak, A.; Meniawy, T.; Ansstas, G.; Taylor, M.H.; Kim, K.B.; McKean, M.; Long, G.V.; Sullivan, R.J.; et al. Individualised neoantigen therapy mRNA-4157 (V940) plus pembrolizumab versus pembrolizumab monotherapy in resected melanoma (KEYNOTE-942): A randomised, phase 2b study. *Lancet* **2024**, *403*, 632–644. [CrossRef] [PubMed]
153. Tang, X.; Huang, Y.; Lei, J.; Luo, H.; Zhu, X. The single-cell sequencing: New developments and medical applications. *Cell Biosci.* **2019**, *9*, 53. [CrossRef] [PubMed]
154. He, L.F.; Mou, P.; Yang, C.H.; Huang, C.; Shen, Y.; Zhang, J.D.; Wei, R.L. Single-cell sequencing in primary intraocular tumors: Understanding heterogeneity, the microenvironment, and drug resistance. *Front. Immunol.* **2023**, *14*, 1194590. [CrossRef]
155. Haque, A.; Engel, J.; Teichmann, S.A.; Lönnberg, T. A practical guide to single-cell RNA-sequencing for biomedical research and clinical applications. *Genome Med.* **2017**, *9*, 75. [CrossRef]
156. Davidson, S.; Efremova, M.; Riedel, A.; Mahata, B.; Pramanik, J.; Huuhtanen, J.; Kar, G.; Vento-Tormo, R.; Hagai, T.; Chen, X.; et al. Single-Cell RNA Sequencing Reveals a Dynamic Stromal Niche That Supports Tumor Growth. *Cell Rep.* **2020**, *31*, 107628. [CrossRef] [PubMed]
157. Ho, P.; Melms, J.C.; Rogava, M.; Frangieh, C.J.; Poźniak, J.; Shah, S.B.; Walsh, Z.; Kyrysyuk, O.; Amin, A.D.; Caprio, L.; et al. The CD58-CD2 axis is co-regulated with PD-L1 via CMTM6 and shapes anti-tumor immunity. *Cancer Cell* **2023**, *41*, 1207–1221. [CrossRef] [PubMed]
158. Kim, N.; Eum, H.H.; Lee, H.O. Clinical Perspectives of Single-Cell RNA Sequencing. *Biomolecules* **2021**, *11*, 1161. [CrossRef]
159. Yoon, J.; Lee, E.; Koo, J.S.; Yoon, J.H.; Nam, K.H.; Lee, J.; Jo, Y.S.; Moon, H.J.; Park, V.Y.; Kwak, J.Y. Artificial intelligence to predict the BRAFV600E mutation in patients with thyroid cancer. *PLoS ONE* **2020**, *15*, e0242806. [CrossRef] [PubMed]
160. Das, K.; Cockerell, C.J.; Patil, A.; Pietkiewicz, P.; Giulini, M.; Grabbe, S.; Goldust, M. Machine Learning and Its Application in Skin Cancer. *Int. J. Environ. Res. Public Health* **2021**, *18*, 13409. [CrossRef]
161. Guerrisi, A.; Falcone, I.; Valenti, F.; Rao, M.; Gallo, E.; Ungania, S.; Maccallini, M.T.; Fanciulli, M.; Frascione, P.; Morrone, A.; et al. Artificial Intelligence and Advanced Melanoma: Treatment Management Implications. *Cells* **2022**, *11*, 3965. [CrossRef]
162. Marchetti, M.A.; Cowen, E.A.; Kurtansky, N.R.; Weber, J.; Dauscher, M.; DeFazio, J.; Deng, L.; Dusza, S.W.; Haliasos, H.; Halpern, A.C.; et al. Prospective validation of dermoscopy-based open-source artificial intelligence for melanoma diagnosis (PROVE-AI study). *NPJ Digit. Med.* **2023**, *6*, 127. [CrossRef] [PubMed]
163. Meißner, A.K.; Gutsche, R.; Galldiks, N.; Kocher, M.; Jünger, S.T.; Eich, M.L.; Montesinos-Rongen, M.; Brunn, A.; Deckert, M.; Wendl, C.; et al. Radiomics for the noninvasive prediction of the BRAF mutation status in patients with melanoma brain metastases. *Neuro Oncol.* **2022**, *24*, 1331–1340. [CrossRef] [PubMed]
164. Dercle, L.; Zhao, B.; Gönen, M.; Moskowitz, C.S.; Firas, A.; Beylergil, V.; Connors, D.E.; Yang, H.; Lu, L.; Fojo, T.; et al. Early Readout on Overall Survival of Patients With Melanoma Treated With Immunotherapy Using a Novel Imaging Analysis. *JAMA Oncol.* **2022**, *8*, 385–392. [CrossRef]
165. Gostimskaya, I. CRISPR-Cas9: A History of Its Discovery and Ethical Considerations of Its Use in Genome Editing. *Biochemistry* **2022**, *87*, 777–788. [CrossRef]
166. Redman, M.; King, A.; Watson, C.; King, D. What is CRISPR/Cas9? *Arch. Dis. Child Educ. Pract. Ed.* **2016**, *101*, 213–215. [CrossRef]
167. Wang, D.; Zhang, F.; Gao, G. CRISPR-Based Therapeutic Genome Editing: Strategies and In Vivo Delivery by AAV Vectors. *Cell* **2020**, *181*, 136–150. [CrossRef] [PubMed]
168. Hacker, U.T.; Bentler, M.; Kaniowska, D.; Morgan, M.; Büning, H. Towards Clinical Implementation of Adeno-Associated Virus (AAV) Vectors for Cancer Gene Therapy: Current Status and Future Perspectives. *Cancers* **2020**, *12*, 1889. [CrossRef] [PubMed]
169. Xu, C.L.; Ruan, M.Z.C.; Mahajan, V.B.; Tsang, S.H. Viral Delivery Systems for CRISPR. *Viruses* **2019**, *11*, 28. [CrossRef]
170. Friedland, A.E.; Baral, R.; Singhal, P.; Loveluck, K.; Shen, S.; Sanchez, M.; Marco, E.; Gotta, G.M.; Maeder, M.L.; Kennedy, E.M.; et al. Characterization of Staphylococcus aureus Cas9: A smaller Cas9 for all-in-one adeno-associated virus delivery and paired nickase applications. *Genome Biol.* **2015**, *16*, 257. [CrossRef]

171. Han, L.; Wang, W.; Lu, J.; Kong, F.; Ma, G.; Zhu, Y.; Zhao, D.; Zhu, J.; Shuai, W.; Zhou, Q.; et al. AAV-sBTLA facilitates HSP70 vaccine-triggered prophylactic antitumor immunity against a murine melanoma pulmonary metastasis model in vivo. *Cancer Lett.* **2014**, *354*, 398–406. [CrossRef]
172. Piperno, G.M.; López-Requena, A.; Predonzani, A.; Dorvignit, D.; Labrada, M.; Zentilin, L.; Burrone, O.R.; Cesco-Gaspere, M. Recombinant AAV-mediated in vivo long-term expression and antitumour activity of an anti-ganglioside GM3(Neu5Gc) antibody. *Gene Ther.* **2015**, *22*, 960–967. [CrossRef]
173. Uddin, F.; Rudin, C.M.; Sen, T. CRISPR Gene Therapy: Applications, Limitations, and Implications for the Future. *Front. Oncol.* **2020**, *10*, 1387. [CrossRef] [PubMed]
174. Zhou, S.; Gravekamp, C.; Bermudes, D.; Liu, K. Tumour-targeting bacteria engineered to fight cancer. *Nat. Rev. Cancer* **2018**, *18*, 727–743. [CrossRef]
175. Duong, M.T.; Qin, Y.; You, S.H.; Min, J.J. Bacteria-cancer interactions: Bacteria-based cancer therapy. *Exp. Mol. Med.* **2019**, *51*, 1–15. [CrossRef]
176. Huang, X.; Pan, J.; Xu, F.; Shao, B.; Wang, Y.; Guo, X.; Zhou, S. Bacteria-Based Cancer Immunotherapy. *Adv. Sci.* **2021**, *8*, 2003572. [CrossRef] [PubMed]
177. Wang, M.; Rousseau, B.; Qiu, K.; Huang, G.; Zhang, Y.; Su, H.; Le Bihan-Benjamin, C.; Khati, I.; Artz, O.; Foote, M.B.; et al. Killing tumor-associated bacteria with a liposomal antibiotic generates neoantigens that induce anti-tumor immune responses. *Nat. Biotechnol.* 2023; *online ahead of print*. [CrossRef] [PubMed]
178. Cardillo, F.; Bonfim, M.; da Silva Vasconcelos Sousa, P.; Mengel, J.; Ribeiro Castello-Branco, L.R.; Pinho, R.T. Bacillus Calmette-Guérin Immunotherapy for Cancer. *Vaccines* **2021**, *9*, 439. [CrossRef] [PubMed]
179. Chen, Y.E.; Bousbaine, D.; Veinbachs, A.; Atabakhsh, K.; Dimas, A.; Yu, V.K.; Zhao, A.; Enright, N.J.; Nagashima, K.; Belkaid, Y.; et al. Engineered skin bacteria induce antitumor T cell responses against melanoma. *Science* **2023**, *380*, 203–210. [CrossRef] [PubMed]
180. Ferrucci, P.F.; Pala, L.; Conforti, F.; Cocorocchio, E. Talimogene Laherparepvec (T-VEC): An Intralesional Cancer Immunotherapy for Advanced Melanoma. *Cancers* **2021**, *13*, 1383. [CrossRef] [PubMed]
181. Fukuhara, H.; Ino, Y.; Todo, T. Oncolytic virus therapy: A new era of cancer treatment at dawn. *Cancer Sci.* **2016**, *107*, 1373–1379. [CrossRef]
182. Marabelle, A.; Tselikas, L.; de Baere, T.; Houot, R. Intratumoral immunotherapy: Using the tumor as the remedy. *Ann. Oncol.* **2017**, *28*, xii33–xii43. [CrossRef] [PubMed]
183. Rohaan, M.W.; Stahlie, E.H.A.; Franke, V.; Zijlker, L.P.; Wilgenhof, S.; van der Noort, V.; van Akkooi, A.C.J.; Haanen, J. Neoadjuvant nivolumab + T-VEC combination therapy for resectable early stage or metastatic (IIIB-IVM1a) melanoma with injectable disease: Study protocol of the NIVEC trial. *BMC Cancer* **2022**, *22*, 851. [CrossRef] [PubMed]
184. Chesney, J.A.; Puzanov, I.; Collichio, F.A.; Singh, P.; Milhem, M.M.; Glaspy, J.; Hamid, O.; Ross, M.; Friedlander, P.; Garbe, C.; et al. Talimogene laherparepvec in combination with ipilimumab versus ipilimumab alone for advanced melanoma: 5-year final analysis of a multicenter, randomized, open-label, phase II trial. *J. Immunother. Cancer* **2023**, *11*, e006270. [CrossRef]
185. Chesney, J.A.; Ribas, A.; Long, G.V.; Kirkwood, J.M.; Dummer, R.; Puzanov, I.; Hoeller, C.; Gajewski, T.F.; Gutzmer, R.; Rutkowski, P.; et al. Randomized, Double-Blind, Placebo-Controlled, Global Phase III Trial of Talimogene Laherparepvec Combined With Pembrolizumab for Advanced Melanoma. *J. Clin. Oncol.* **2023**, *41*, 528–540. [CrossRef]

MDPI AG
Grosspeteranlage 5
4052 Basel
Switzerland
Tel.: +41 61 683 77 34

International Journal of Molecular Sciences Editorial Office
E-mail: ijms@mdpi.com
www.mdpi.com/journal/ijms

www.ingramcontent.com/pod-product-compliance
Lightning Source LLC
Chambersburg PA
CBHW061631210926
51850CB00009B/2507